Nursing School and Allied Health Entrance Exams

16th Edition

Nursing School and Allied Health Entrance Exams

16th Edition

Marion F. Gooding, RN, Ph.D.

Professor of Nursing
North Carolina Central University
Durham, North Carolina

CONTRIBUTING EDITORS

Mattie Moss, Ed.D.
Mathematics

Duana A. Dreyer, Ph.D.
Anatomy and Physiology

Charles R. George, Ph.D.
Biology

Doris E. Wilson, B.A.
Language Arts

James M. Schooler, Ph.D.
Chemistry

Australia • Canada • Mexico • Singapore • Spain • United Kingdom • United States

An ARCO Book

ARCO is a registered trademark of Thomson Learning, Inc., and is used herein under license by Peterson's.

About The Thomson Corporation and Peterson's

With revenues of US$7.8 billion, The Thomson Corporation (www.thomson.com) is a leading global provider of integrated information solutions for business, education, and professional customers. Its Learning businesses and brands (www.thomsonlearning.com) serve the needs of individuals, learning institutions, and corporations with products and services for both traditional and distributed learning.

Peterson's, part of The Thomson Corporation, is one of the nation's most respected providers of lifelong learning online resources, software, reference guides, and books. The Education Supersite[SM] at www.petersons.com—the Internet's most heavily traveled education resource—has searchable databases and interactive tools for contacting U.S.-accredited institutions and programs. In addition, Peterson's serves more than 105 million education consumers annually.

For more information, contact Peterson's, 2000 Lenox Drive, Lawrenceville, NJ 08648; 800-338-3282; or find us on the World Wide Web at www.petersons.com/about.

Sixteenth Edition

ISBN 0-7689-1195-8

Printed in the United States of America

10 9 8 7 6 5 4 3   05 04

Contents

PART III: PRACTICE FOR ALLIED HEALTH SCHOOL ENTRANCE EXAMINATIONS **293**

PART IV: PRACTICE FOR PRACTICAL/VOCATIONAL NURSING SCHOOL ENTRANCE EXAMINATIONS... **381**

PART I

INFORMATION ABOUT NURSING AND ALLIED HEALTH PROGRAMS AND ENTRANCE EXAMINATIONS

About the Nursing Profession

SELECTING A NURSING CAREER

Regardless of which kind of nursing program you choose to enter, you will have opportunities to provide an important service to humanity. You may enter nursing at one level and expand your skills through practice and additional education. Advancement within the nursing profession comes about in several ways. A practical nurse may decide to become a registered nurse, an upward move. A registered nurse may decide to move from the hospital setting into community-based care, a lateral move that expands the types of services a nurse can provide. A registered nurse who does not have a baccalaureate degree may decide to earn one in order to step up to a management position.

There are four kinds of programs that provide preparation for entrance into nursing:

The practical-nurse programs are usually offered in vocational schools, hospitals, and community colleges. The program varies from nine to eighteen months. The courses include the basic sciences and medical-surgical, pediatric, and obstetrical nursing. Some mental health concepts are included. The major focus is on technical skills. A practical nurse works under the supervision of a registered nurse (RN).

The associate-degree nurse is a graduate of a two-year college program that is designed with a balance between clinical nursing courses (medical, surgical, psychiatric, obstetrical, and pediatric nursing) and general education courses (biological and physical sciences, behavioral sciences, humanities, and electives) to provide a background for making important judgments about patient care. The graduate is prepared for technical expertise in the assessment, planning, and delivery of direct patient care in the hospital setting.

The graduate of the hospital-based diploma program functions on the nursing team in the same manner as the associate-degree nurse. Most diploma programs are twenty-four to thirty months in length, and the non-nursing courses may be offered through a college.

The baccalaureate nursing program is four years in length and is offered in senior colleges and universities. The required courses in the biological, physical, and behavioral sciences are both basic and advanced. These general education requirements, along with courses that provide a broad liberal arts background, are taken during the first two years. The major clinical courses are offered in the third and fourth years and include the five clinical areas identified above, with an emphasis on community health nursing and the role of the professional nurse as manager. Most nursing programs offering the professional baccalaureate degree admit graduates from the diploma and associate-degree programs with varying degrees of advanced standing.

The graduates of all four programs take a licensing examination. At the present time, there are two kinds of licenses: the practical-nurse license and the registered-nurse license for graduates of the diploma, associate-degree, and baccalaureate-degree programs.

A nurse may continue studies to receive a master's degree and a doctorate with a major in clinical specialties, teaching, administration, or research, depending on his or her career choice. There is a great demand for nurses in hospitals, schools, clinics, public health agencies, and many other settings throughout the world. Nurses may become anesthetists, enter the military, or become writers, consultants, or private practitioners. Nursing provides a foundation for many career opportunities and, more importantly, a personally and financially satisfying vocation.

SELECTING A NURSING PROGRAM

The first consideration you should make when selecting a nursing program is your career goal. Do you plan to work in a hospital or as a member of the health team? Is your ultimate goal to function as a manager or an administrator? Are you primarily interested in teaching? Do you want to specialize in a specific clinical area? Are you planning to work in a community setting, providing services to families? Is your ultimate goal to become an entrepreneur?

The rapidly moving trend in nursing today is to license two levels of nursing for entry into the professional services. The assistant level will be represented by graduates of the associate-degree nursing programs; the professional level, by graduates of the baccalaureate nursing programs. Baccalaureate education in nursing forms the foundation for graduate education in nursing, where specialization as a clinical practitioner, administrator, and teacher occurs. Other types of graduates (practical nurse and diploma) will achieve these credentials through career mobility programs.

A second factor to consider is cost. The demands of full-time study and the length of the program may necessitate resigning from your job.

A third factor is your qualification for admission. As the levels of performance increase, so do the academic requirements. In some cases, a student may enter at the associate degree level and, upon graduating and receiving a license (RN), enter the baccalaureate program because the requirements are different for RNs.

Once you have matched your career goals with a program, you should use the guidelines listed below to make your final choice.

1. Is the program approved by the state regulating body (Board of Nursing)?

2. Is the program accredited by a voluntary agency (National League for Nursing)?

3. What is the program's reputation in terms of graduate performance?

4. How does the social and academic environment meet your needs?

SELECTING AN ALLIED HEALTH PROGRAM

Occupations related to allied health are rapidly expanding. The criteria for selecting a program are similar to those for nursing:

1. If a license is required to practice, be certain that the program is approved by the regulating body.

2. Check to see if the program is accredited by the appropriate voluntary agency.

3. Find out how well the graduates are performing on the licensing examination.

4. How well does the program meet your short- and long-term career goals?

The most popular allied health careers are described below.

Occupation	Work Description	Education Needed
Clinical and Medical Lab Technician	Perform tests in labs to get information for doctors to use. Use chemicals, microscopes, and other technical equipment.	OJT, Two-Year CC, Bachelor's, Master's
Emergency Medical Technician	Administer first aid treatment to sick or injured persons and transport them to medical facilities. Work as a member of an emergency medical team.	OJT, One-Year CC, Two-Year CC
Medical Lab Technician	Perform routine tests in medical laboratories for use in the treatment and diagnosis of diseases.	OJT, Two-Year CC, Bachelor's, Master's
Medical Record Technician	Compile and maintain medical records of hospital clinic patients.	OJT, Two-Year CC
Occupational Therapist	Plan, organize, and conduct programs to facilitate rehabilitation of mentally, physically, or emotionally handicapped people.	Bachelor's, Master's
Physical Therapist	Plan, organize, and administer treatment in order to restore mobility and prevent and relieve pain for those suffering from a disabling injury or disease.	Bachelor's, Master's
Radiologic Technologist	Take X rays to help doctors diagnose illness. Also use radioactive materials to treat patients.	Two-Year CC
Respiratory Therapist	Specialize in the evaluation, treatment, and care of patients with breathing disorders.	Two-Year CC, Bachelor's

Key: OJT—On-the-Job Training, CC—Community College, HS—High School.

FINANCIAL AID SOURCES

With education costs on the rise and the decline in federal sources for financial aid, competition for funds is increasing. Therefore, it is important to be familiar with the sources of funding, the eligibility requirements, and the application procedures. It is also important to apply as early as possible to a variety of programs.

To initiate the application process, get a financial aid form from your local high school counseling office, or directly from the school to which you are seeking admission. This form must be completed and mailed to the *College Scholarship Service* (address is on the form). In approximately six weeks, a report is sent back that identifies whether you are eligible for financial aid. This report must be sent to the school of your selection so that the amount you are eligible for and amount you will have to pay can be determined.

The amount of money a recipient can receive is dependent upon the need analysis derived from the financial aid form and the financial aid program in which the nursing school, college, or university is participating. The school usually prepares a financial aid package that includes a combination of financial sources to make up the difference between the amount the student can contribute and the total costs of the nursing program.

Some financial aid programs are loans, which must be paid back at a low interest rate over a prolonged period of time. Other sources are grants and scholarships, which do not have to be paid back. The obligation for debt payment requires serious thought on the part of the student, since a default on a loan can affect credit ranking.

When shopping for financial aid, check the accreditation status of the nursing program and the institution's eligibility for aid. All accredited nursing programs are eligible for federal funding, but some institutions have limited federal sources due to high default rates.

FEDERAL SOURCES OF FINANCIAL AID

Pell Grants are awarded to undergraduate students who have not previously earned a degree. The grant does not have to be repaid and may be supplemented by other funds. Eligibility is based on need, which is calculated by a formula. The amounts of the awards vary yearly and depend on program funding. The maximum award for 2002–2003 was $4,000 per year. The maximum grant for the 2000–2001 award year was $3,750 per year. You do not have to be a full-time student.

Direct and FFEL Stafford Loans

These federal loans are of two kinds; subsidized, which are awarded on the basis of need and accrue no interest before repayment, and unsubsidized, which are not based on need and accrue interest from the time of disbursement. Dependent students may borrow $2,625 the first year, $3,500 the second year, and $5,500 the third and the fourth years. Independent students may receive $6,625 the first year, $7,500 the second year, and $10,500 a year for the remaining two years.

Plus Loans

Plus loans enable parents with stable credit histories to borrow for the education expenses of each dependent child who is an undergraduate student enrolled at least half-time. The yearly time is equal to your cost of attendance minus any additional financial aid received.

Consolidation Loans

These loans are designed to help students and parents simplify loan repayment by consolidating several types of federal loans into one loan with one repayment schedule.

Campus-Based Programs (Administered by Financial Aid Office)

- **Federal Supplemental Educational Opportunity Grants (SEOG)** are for undergraduates with exceptional financial need and give priority to students who received Federal Pell Grants. You can receive between $100 to $4,000 per year depending on need, the financial level of the school, and the financial aid policies.

- **Federal Work Study** provides a work-study program for undergraduate and graduate students in financial need. Students are allowed to earn money through community service and work related to their course of study.

- **Federal Perkins Loan** is a low-interest (5 percent) loan for both undergraduate and graduate students with exceptional financial need. Your school is the lender and the loan must be repaid to the school. Loans may be granted in the amount of $4,000 up to $20,000 for each year of undergraduate study and $6,000 up to $40,000 for each year of graduate/professional study.

For additional information on federal loans, call 1-800-4-FED-AID or pick up the U.S. Department of Education's guide, *The Student Guide: Financial Aid*, from your local campus financial aid office.

OTHER SOURCES OF FINANCIAL AID

Your public library is a helpful source for information on foundations, religious organizations, fraternities and sororities, and civic groups that provide scholarships and/or loans for educational purposes. In addition, the military offers scholarships through the ROTC Program. You should also seek sources from the organizations related to your field of interest. Once you identify your program of choice, you can obtain specific information and assistance.

SPECIAL FEATURES OF THIS BOOK

SIMULATED TESTS

Studying the more than 1,300 test questions in this book, which are similar to the items included in the entrance examinations, will allow you to review material you already know, gain new knowledge, and become familiar with the format of timed tests. The sections for the registered-nurse and practical-nurse examinations are separated; however, the entire book may be used to prepare for all examinations.

TEST-TAKING SKILLS

By following the guidelines presented on test-taking skills, you will be able to increase your chances for success using the "educated guess" technique.

PRESENTATION OF BASIC CONCEPTS

The verbal ability, mathematics, and science sections include a summary of basic facts, principles, and concepts related to the content area. These summaries function as a study guide designed to help you select correct answers.

EXPLANATORY ANSWERS

For the practice test, explanations of the correct answers are given. This section provides another opportunity to reinforce principles that apply to test items.

SPECIAL FEATURES OF THE SIXTEENTH EDITION

- Expanded sections for Nursing and Allied Health exams
- Updated test material
- Expanded contributions from distinguished item writers
- Hundreds of new test question items
- New critical thinking items

ABOUT THE EXAMINATIONS

Registered nursing programs, practical/vocational nursing programs, and allied health programs require different entrance examinations.

For registered nursing programs, you may be required to take either the Entrance Examination for Schools of Nursing (RNEE), the Pre-Admission Examination-RN, the PSB-Nursing School Aptitude Examination (RN), the Nurse Entrance Test (NET), or the Test of Essential Academic Skills (TEAS). All exams evaluate the academic ability of applicants in key areas of the basic nursing curriculum.

For information about the Entrance Examination for Schools of Nursing (RNEE), write to:
The Psychological Corporation
555 Academic Court
San Antonio, Texas 78204-2498

For information about the Pre-Admission Examination-RN, write to:
National League for Nursing
350 Hudson Street
New York, New York 10014

For information about the PSB-Nursing School Aptitude Examination (RN), write to:
Psychological Services Bureau
P.O. Box 327
St. Thomas, Pennsylvania 17252

For information about the Nurse Entrance Test (NET), write to:
Educational Resources, Inc.
10200 W. 75th Street
Shawnee Mission, Kansas 66204

For more information about the Test of Essential Academic Skills (TEAS), write to:
Assessment Technologies, Inc. (ATI)
P.O. Box 26050
Overland Park, Kansas 66225

The entrance examinations for practical/vocational nursing programs assess your knowledge of areas essential to the basic practical/vocational nursing curriculum. You may be required to take either the Entrance Examination for Schools of Practical/Vocational Nursing (PNEE), the Pre-Admission Examination-PN, or the PSB-Aptitude for Practical Nursing Examination. For information about the PNEE, write to the Psychological Corporation. For information about the Pre-Admission Examination-PN, write to the National League for Nursing. For information about the PSB-Aptitude for Practical Nursing Examination, write to the Psychological Services Bureau.

Allied health programs entrance examinations measure academic ability and scientific knowledge in order to identify qualified applicants. The Allied Health Professions Admissions Test (AHPAT) is administered by the Psychological Corporation; the Psychological Services Bureau offers the PSB-Health Occupations Aptitude Examination.

CONTENT AND FORMAT OF THE EXAMINATIONS

Registered Nursing Entrance Exams

The Psychological Corporation's Entrance Examination for Schools of Nursing (RNEE) contains approximately 230 multiple-choice questions, and takes about three and one-half hours to complete. There is a break midway through the test. The test format is as follows:

Test Section	Content	No. of Questions
Verbal Ability	Uses synonym and antonym identification to measure vocabulary and verbal reasoning.	Approximately 50 questions
Numerical Ability	Emphasizes arithmetic operations, including word problems, percentages and fractions, and fundamental algebra and geometry.	Approximately 40 questions
Life Sciences	Focuses on principles and concepts of the biological sciences specifically related to body structure and functions, heredity and development, microorganisms and health.	Approximately 40 questions
Physical Sciences	Measures understanding of principles and concepts of chemistry and physics, which include the nature of matter, changes, and energy.	Approximately 40 questions
Reading Skill	Determines ability to draw inferences, interpret, and evaluate reading passages from natural and social sciences.	Approximately 45 questions

NOTE: Occasionally, there is an extra experimental section included on the exam. It will be based on one of the five content areas. This section has no effect on your score; however, you will not be told which section is the experimental one.

The National League for Nursing's Pre-Admission Examination-RN contains three multiple-choice tests and takes approximately three and one-half hours to complete. The test format is as follows:

Test Section	Content	Time
Verbal Ability (2 subtests)	1. Word knowledge: uses word identification to test vocabulary.	Approximately one hour
	2. Reading comprehension: presents five reading passages of a scientific or general nature; tests ability to identify main idea and supporting details, and to analyze and interpret material.	
Mathematics	Includes computation and word problems; emphasizes proportions, decimals, percentages, basic algebra and geometry.	Approximately one hour
Science	Measures understanding of general principles of biology, chemistry, physics, general science.	Approximately one hour

NOTE: Experimental items are included that do not affect your test score.

The Psychological Services Bureau's Nursing School Aptitude Examination (RN) contains five tests and three subtests, and takes about one hour and forty-five minutes to complete. The test format is as follows:

Test Section	Content	No. of Questions
Academic Aptitude (3 subtests)	1. Verbal: emphasizes vocabulary-related questions.	Subtest 1: 30 questions
	2. Arithmetic: focuses on skill and computational speed with arithmetic.	Subtest 2: 30 questions
	3. Non-Verbal: deals with recognizing relationships and differences between objects; measures mental manipulation and reasoning.	Subtest 3: 30 questions
Spelling	Measures written expression or communication skills.	50 questions
Reading Comprehension	Determines ability to interpret passages, understand direct statements, infer ideas and purposes, and derive author's intent.	40 questions
Information in the Natural Sciences	Tests understanding of biology, chemistry, health, safety, etc., at an elementary level.	90 questions
Vocational Adjustment Index	Ascertains an individual's characteristic lifestyle by examining his or her educational and occupational adjustment.	90 questions

The Test of Essential Academic Skills (TEAS) contains the areas listed below in the sample student report.

Name:　　　　　J DOE
Test Date:　　　03/30/01　5:00:23 P.M.
Institution:　　Sample University
Program Type:　BSN
Booklet #:　　　33,357

Raw Score:
Percentage Correct: 81.8%

Your Percentile Rank By:
Test:　　94

Score Explanation

Percentage Correct: Number of items answered correctly divided by the total number possible.

Percentile Rank: A value (1–99) used for ranking a student against a sample of similar students taking the exam.

Summary Overview

Content Area	Percentage Correct	Percentile Rank
Reading	92.5%	89
Paragraph Comprehension	83.3%	76
Passage Comprehension	92.9%	82
Inferences/Conclusions	100.0%	99
Math	80.0%	96
Whole Numbers	86.7%	97
Fractions & Decimals	100.0%	99
Percentages	50.0%	70
Ratio & Proportion	80.0%	94
Metric Conversions	100.0%	99
Algebraic Equations	50.0%	73
Diagrams/Graphs	83.3%	96
Science	73.3%	89
Science Reasoning	60.0%	83
Science Knowledge	76.0%	90
Biology	80.0%	81
Chemistry	66.7%	89
Anatomy & Physiology	66.7%	78
Physics	75.0%	69
General Science	85.07%	98
English	80.0%	87
Punctuation	100.0%	99
Grammar	64.0%	66
Sentence Structure	100.0%	99
Contextual Words	100.0%	89
Spelling	100.0%	99

The Nurse Entrance Test (NET) given by Educational Resources is the newest type of entrance examination for registered nursing programs. It takes approximately two and one-half hours to complete and is divided into seven subtests. Of these, three cover subjects considered to be *cognitive* (related to knowledge and achievement), and four cover subjects considered to be *noncognitive* (related to psychological-social factors). You do not have to study for the noncognitive tests. The test format is as follows:

Type	Subtest	Content
COGNITIVE	Essential Math Skills	Tests basic arithmetic operations, including whole numbers, fractions, decimals, percentages, ratios, and basic algebra.
	Reading Comprehension Skills	Evaluates inferential reading level for science-related material; reading passages have a tenth-grade level of vocabulary and sentence syntax.
	Reading Rate	Estimates the number of words per minute that the student is able to read in a test or study situation.
NONCOGNITIVE	Test-Taking Skills	Measures student's writing ability on objective, essay, and standardized examinations.
	Stress Level Profile	Judges student's ability to cope with five personal stressors: family life, social life, the work place, academics, and time/money.
	Social Interaction Profile	Assesses passive and aggressive social interaction attitudes of the student within a group.
	Learning Style Inventory	Determines auditory, visual, group, solitary, oral and writing-dependent learner styles.

Practical Nursing Entrance Exams

The Entrance Examination for Schools of Practical/Vocational Nursing (PNEE) given by the Psychological Corporation contains approximately 300 multiple-choice questions, and takes about three and one-half hours to complete, including a break period. The test format is as follows:

Test Section	Content	No. of Questions
Verbal Ability	Uses synonym and antonym identification to measure vocabulary and verbal reasoning.	Approximately 75 questions
Numerical Ability	Emphasizes arithmetic operations, including word problems, percentages and ratios, and fundamental algebra. Focuses on understanding and applying quantitative concepts and relationships.	Approximately 60 questions
Science	Measures understanding of principles and concepts of biology, chemistry, health, and the physical sciences.	Approximately 75 questions
Reading Skill	Determines ability to read and understand passages from natural and social sciences.	Approximately 45 questions

NOTE: Occasionally, there is an extra experimental section included on the exam. It will be based on one of the five content areas. This section has no effect on your score; however, you will not be told which section is the experimental one.

The National League for Nursing's Pre-Admission Examination-PN has the same test format as their registered nursing exam; however, its contents are at a level appropriate for applicants to practical/vocational programs. The test format is as follows:

Test Section	Content	Time
Verbal Ability (2 subtests)	1. Word knowledge: uses word identification to test vocabulary. 2. Reading comprehension: presents five reading passages of a scientific or general nature: tests ability to identify main idea and supporting details, and to analyze and interpret material.	Approximately one hour
Mathematics	Includes computation and word problems; emphasizes proportions, decimals, percentages, basic algebra and geometry.	Approximately one hour
Science	Measures understanding of general principles of biology, chemistry, physics, general science.	Approximately one hour

NOTE: Experimental items are included that do not affect your test score.

The Psychological Services Bureau's Aptitude for Practical Nursing Examination contains five tests and three subtests, and takes about two hours and fifteen minutes to complete. The test format is as follows:

Test Section	Content	No. of Questions
Academic Aptitude (3 subtests)	1. Verbal: emphasizes vocabulary-related questions. 2. Arithmetic: focuses on skill and computational speed with arithmetic. 3. Non-Verbal: deals with recognizing relationships and differences between objects; measures mental manipulation and reasoning.	Subtest 1: 30 questions Subtest 2: 30 questions Subtest 3: 30 questions
Spelling	Measures written expression or communication skills.	50 questions
Information in the Natural Sciences	Determines understanding of biology, chemistry, health, safety, hygiene, etc., at an elementary level.	90 questions
Judgment and Comprehension in Practical Nursing Situations	Evaluates how a nurse—both as a student and as a practitioner—exercises judgment in his/her working relationships.	50 questions
Vocational Adjustment Index	Ascertains an individual's characteristic lifestyle by examining his or her educational and occupational adjustment.	90 questions

Allied Health Programs Entrance Exams

The Psychological Corporation's Allied Health Professions Admissions Test (AHPAT) contains about 300 multiple-choice questions and lasts approximately three and one-half hours, including a short break period. The test format is as follows:

Test Section	Content	No. of Questions
Verbal Ability	Uses synonym and antonym identification to measure vocabulary and verbal reasoning.	Approximately 75 questions
Quantitative Ability	Emphasizes nonverbal arithmetic exercises, problem solving, and applications in algebra, geometry, and basic trigonometry to interpret ability to reason through and understand quantitative concepts.	Approximately 50 questions
Biology	Focuses on the principles and concepts of basic biology, especially human biology, including cell biology, heredity, human structure and function, bacteria and viruses, evolution, and plants.	Approximately 50 questions
Chemistry	Focuses on the principles and concepts of basic chemistry, including atoms and molecules, formulas, equations, bonding, element and periodic relationships, states of matter, solutions, chemical equilibrium, acids, bases, electrochemistry, kinetics, and nuclear and organic chemistry.	Approximately 50 questions
Reading Comprehension	Determines ability to comprehend, analyze, and interpret reading passages on science-oriented topics.	Approximately 45 questions

The Psychological Services Bureau's Health Occupations Aptitude Examination contains five tests and three subtests, and takes about two hours and fifteen minutes to complete. The test format is as follows:

Test Section	Content	No. of Questions
Academic Aptitude (3 subtests)	1. Verbal: emphasizes vocabulary-related questions. 2. Arithmetic: focuses on skill and computational speed with arithmetic. 3. Non-Verbal: deals with recognizing relationships and differences between objects; measures mental manipulation and reasoning.	Subtest 1: 30 questions Subtest 2: 30 questions Subtest 3: 30 questions
Spelling	Measures written expression or communication skills.	60 questions
Reading Comprehension	Determines ability to interpret passages, understand direct statements, infer ideas and purposes, and derive author's intent.	50 questions
Information in the Natural Sciences	Tests understanding of biology, chemistry, health, safety, hygiene, etc., at an elementary level.	90 questions
Vocational Adjustment Index	Ascertains an individual's characteristic lifestyle by examining his or her educational and occupational adjustment.	90 questions

How to Apply for an Entrance Examination

The procedures for applying for an entrance examination for nursing school or for an allied health program will be provided by the specific school that you have selected. The school will notify you which examination it requires, where the local testing centers are located, and the specific time you are scheduled to take the examination. An application card must be completed and submitted with a test fee. You must follow all instructions given by the specific program to which you are applying. All applications and test results are handled through the specific schools.

Administration of the Examinations

The examinations are administered by qualified persons, usually in a testing center. You will be scheduled to take the tests along with other candidates. Specific directions for taking the examinations will be given by the person proctoring the examination. All tests are timed. The proctor will tell you when to begin and when to stop.

All answers are placed on a separate answer sheet so that your results can be analyzed by computer. The computerized answer sheets are similar to the answer sheets in this book.

Answer sheets are sent to the respective testing centers for analysis. A computerized report is sent to the program from which the application was obtained, and the person taking the examination can also receive a report. The average time for receiving the test results is three weeks.

The tests are developed from a blueprint that identifies the number and type of items. There are several forms for each examination. If the blueprint calls for ten items related to understanding electrolytes, each form will have ten such items, but the specific test items may differ. That is why this book provides a variety of test items along with basic guidelines for answering similar questions.

PREPARING FOR THE EXAMINATIONS

Reducing Test Anxiety

Anxiety results from a threat to our well-being that might be real or perceived. This threat makes us uncomfortable and affects our feelings of self-esteem. We then change our behavior in an attempt to seek relief.

Many people become anxious or "uptight" about taking a test because they anticipate that someone is going to make a judgment about them based on their test performance. Is your self-esteem strong enough for you to think, "I can pass this test!" Or, do you lack confidence in yourself, and assume, "I am going to fail." What can you do to prevent this kind of negative thinking?

First, you must realize that anxiety can be both productive and destructive. Anxiety can be energizing if you direct the energy toward your goals and away from the imagined threats. For example, you may have the idea that the admission test will determine your entire future. If you don't pass the test, you imagine that you won't be admitted to the program of your choice. The fact is that admission tests are used along with many other kinds of information to determine your eligibility for entering a program. Therefore, this is not a real threat. On the other hand, if you have made no effort to prepare for this test, then your chances for admission might be threatened.

■ **The secret to success is confidence.** You can gain that confidence by completing the practice tests in this book with a score of 80 percent or above in all areas. This would assure you that you can perform well on the admission test.

- **There are several things that you can do to relieve anxiety.** First, you can set up a time-frame for studying this book. Schedule a few pages per day to avoid a last minute rush.

- **Sharing your anxiety helps to reduce it.** Talk to a friend. Explore the "what if" situations and the related options for achieving your career goals.

- **Provide an outlet for yourself**—perhaps exercise or some other physical activity that you enjoy.

- **Think back to how you have handled stress and anxiety in your past experiences.** Draw on those experiences.

- **Positive thinking is a must.** Imagine yourself receiving the results of your test enclosed in a letter of congratulations that you share with your family and friends. Make plans for the next step toward achieving your career goals. Imagine the pleasurable feeling and comfort that comes from a job well done. You'll do just fine!

ANSWERING TEST ITEMS

After completing the overview of a section, answer the sample test questions. Many questions are multiple choice, requiring an educated guess if you do not know the answer. (You are not penalized for guessing incorrectly on these examinations.) Therefore, you should go through the entire test, answering the questions you know, and then making educated guesses on the questions you don't know. Here is how to make an educated guess:

1. *Carefully* read the question (the *stem*). Look for the clues or the main ideas in the stem that will lead you to the correct answer.

2. Go through the entire examination, answering all the questions that you feel sure about. This will give you an overall idea of what the test is about and lessen the time pressure, and you may run across related information that will help you to answer the questions you don't know.

3. Now go back to those items you didn't answer and use the test-taking techniques. First, look for the key word(s) or clue(s) in the stem. Keeping that in mind, try to eliminate the choices that do not relate to the clue. Look at the remaining choices to identify similarities and differences to the stem or clue. Compare the differences with the clue to see if you can eliminate another choice. Select the remaining choice.

Example:

Which of the following observations may be an indication of high blood pressure?

- **(A)** Flushed skin
- **(B)** Pale skin
- **(C)** Cold skin
- **(D)** Weak pulse

What is the *clue*?

Answer: high pressure

Can I eliminate any choices?

Answer: Yes. There is a direct relationship between pressure and force; therefore, choice (D) cannot be the correct answer.

What are the similarities and differences among choices (A), (B), and (C)?

Answer: They all relate to changes in skin characteristics. However, choices (B) and (C) are similar. As a matter of fact, if choice (B) were correct, choice (C) would also be correct.

The corrected answer, then, is choice (A).

Now, let's assume that the following question is also on the test.

Why do some people with high blood pressure have flushed skin?

(A) The pulse weakens, and blood pools in the skin.
(B) The skin temperature lowers, and the skin blood vessels dilate.
(C) The increased pressure increases the volume of blood to the arteries.
(D) The increased pressure forces the arteries to dilate.

Based on your experience with the previous item, you would immediately eliminate choices (A) and (B). Looking at choices (C) and (D), you might think that both would cause reddened skin. However, you would either eliminate choice (D) because it contradicts the relationship between pressure and volume, or you would select choice (C) because it supports the relationship between pressure and volume.

PLEASE PRACTICE THIS TECHNIQUE WITH THE SAMPLE ITEMS!

A summary of the steps for preparing to take a nursing school entrance examination is presented below:

1. Study the concepts and principles presented in each section so that you will have a good base of knowledge.

2. Study one section at a time over a period of time—whatever is reasonable for your learning style. Do not cram!

3. Take the tests related to each section immediately after studying the explanatory materials.

4. Follow all directions for each test carefully.

5. Utilize the guidelines for test-taking as presented in this section.

6. Check your answers in order to diagnose your strengths and weaknesses.

7. Seek additional information from reliable resources in the areas in which you are weak.

PART II

PRACTICE FOR REGISTERED NURSING SCHOOL ENTRANCE EXAMINATIONS

VERBAL ABILITY

WHAT VERBAL ABILITY IS AND HOW IT IS MEASURED

Verbal ability may be defined as skill with word usage and comprehension. It is often evaluated in the form of written vocabulary tests. These vocabulary tests measure the test taker's ability to recall and produce *lexical units*. A lexical unit is a word or group of words possessing a specific meaning. A single word can have a variety of meanings in different contexts (that is, phrases or sentences). For this reason, a single word may represent several lexical units. Consider the following example:

Her answer to the question was *right*.

She handed the paper to the person on her *right*.

She has a *right* to know the results of the test.

She felt compelled to help *right* the wrong that was done.

The vocabulary test usually includes words from your *active* vocabulary—words that you see, hear, and use frequently—and words from your *passive* vocabulary—words that you have heard and seen, and might comprehend, but that you rarely, if ever, use. It also includes words that may be common in written language but are not often used in spoken expression, and vice versa.

Measurement of verbal skill encompasses many elements. Although vocabulary test items may or may not appear on your test, it is advisable to study and practice with the kind of material presented in this verbal ability section. Words and their meanings are vital for good scores on tests of reading comprehension, effective writing, and current usage. Expanding your vocabulary will result in a marked improvement in your scores in these and similar subjects.

EXTENDING YOUR VOCABULARY

A good command of words is essential to most aspects of your life. Words can broaden your horizons and reveal new interests in your daily environment and activities. Such discoveries may never be accessible to you if your vocabulary remains restricted or too specialized.

Effective expression is essential to making and maintaining meaningful social relationships. An extensive vocabulary will help you to convey ideas, desires, and information. If you are enrolled in school, regardless of the level, you will learn faster and enjoy the process more if you are "fortified" with a large, effective vocabulary. Your comprehension of a broad range of words will help you to determine what you do *not* understand and will help you remedy the situation by posing intelligent questions.

Your word power directly affects your work. If you are seeking to improve your occupational status through a job change or a promotion from your present position, a better command of words will undoubtedly help you to succeed. This fact has been proven time and again through scientific studies conducted by educators, psychologists, sociologists, and personnel specialists. Many employers require a battery of tests, the results of which are used in determining which applicants are best suited to an available position. Frequently these tests incorporate a number of items designed to measure verbal ability.

Attaining a leadership role depends on, among other things, the extent of your vocabulary. Leadership tasks demand that you get your ideas across, that you speak and are heard. You will need to use all your expressive powers to voice your opinion with conviction. Articulation can furnish you with an astonishing amount of persuasive power.

A larger vocabulary will help you feel secure and competent in every undertaking. Let's explore the means by which this vocabulary may be acquired.

The following strategies are designed to increase your vocabulary and help you achieve word mastery. Word mastery implies reaching a level of verbal ability at which you can both recognize and comprehend words—and use them frequently and appropriately.

1. Read as much as you can, taking care not to confine yourself to one kind of reading material. Seek variety in what you read—periodicals, newspapers, nonfiction, novels and other fiction, poetry, prose, essays, etc. Reading from a broad range of material will accelerate your vocabulary growth. You will learn the meaning of words by context. This means that at times you will not know the definition of an isolated word, but the words or phrase within which this word appears will be familiar and therefore provide a clue to its meaning.

2. Take vocabulary tests. There are many practice books containing word tests; we recommend *Webster's New World*™ *Power Vocabulary*. These tests are challenging and make an enjoyable leisure-time activity. More importantly, they are fast vocabulary builders.

3. Listen to lectures, discussion, and talks given by people who speak well. TV and radio are excellent means of learning new terminology coming into common usage in the English language. A word of caution: You cannot always rely on a speaker's pronunciation. Always check your dictionary for proper pronunciation.

4. Use a dictionary when you are not certain of a word's meaning. If you do not have access to a dictionary when you encounter the word, make a note of it (and its context) and research it at your earliest convenience. Find out how it is pronounced, what words are related to it, its finer shades of meaning, and its correct usage. A good dictionary is a must! Any one of the following is highly recommended:

    Funk and Wagnall's Standard College Dictionary
    Webster's New World™ *Dictionary*
    Random House College Dictionary
    Merriam Webster Dictionary of Synonyms and Antonyms
    Webster's Synonyms and Antonyms
    Bell's Pocket Guide to Synonyms

5. Word games, such as Scrabble and Boggle, are an effective and pleasurable means of encountering new words. Crossword puzzles, anagrams, and similar word games provide a relaxing method of acquiring new vocabulary. Most of these puzzles are published in varying degrees of difficulty. Start with the easy level and progress to the expert level. You will find it a challenging learning experience.

6. Review the etymological charts and diagrams in this book, which explain word derivations. A knowledge of roots, or stems, of words will enable you to infer the meaning of new words having roots similar to words you already know.

7. Study words by central ideas. It is difficult to study and retain isolated words. Even context clues sometimes are not enough to help you remember a word, its meaning, or its appropriate use. Studying vocabulary by central idea encourages you to consider groups of related words. As you learn each term, you associate it with some other word. For example: The words *ingest, devour, consume, voracious, edible, delectable*, and *palatable* are all tied to the principle idea of eating. The central idea strategy of studying words will not only provide you with a basis for remembering the word but will also motivate you to use the word in your everyday oral and written expression. Frequent use of the word will in turn ensure your ability to recall its meaning in a testing situation. This word study method also fosters comprehension of jargon or word usage peculiar to specific fields. A number of workbooks and study materials present words according to a central idea and feature exercises formatted to this method. Such books may be found in the "study aids" section of most bookstores.

Be sure to record all new words in a notebook dedicated to that purpose. Make notes alongside each entry that include a simple definition or synonym, finer shades of meaning, related forms, and sample sentences of the word in context. Finally, make these words your own. Use them in your writing and speaking. Remember—verbal ability is a skill you can improve at any age.

The purpose of this section is to provide you with practice exercises representative of the three most common kinds of verbal-ability test items: synonyms, antonyms, and verbal analogies. This section covers these question types in three separate subsections.

An explanation of each kind of test item, helpful study hints, and test-taking strategies precede each subsection. Subsections also include a 75-question, multiple-choice test. An answer key follows each sample test to help you immediately evaluate your performance and determine areas of weakness. You may wish to use these answer keys to compile a word study list.

ETYMOLOGY—KEY TO WORD RECOGNITION

Etymology is the study of the history and origin of words. It explains how a word came into being, the place of its beginning, and how it has been used through the ages. The etymology of a word also outlines alterations in its meaning, usage, and spelling through the years.

Although the term "etymology" sounds somewhat complex and weighty, the science itself is not difficult to understand. Etymologies may be simple and concise or lengthy and intricate. To find them, you should use your dictionary. Etymologies are usually found at the beginning of a definition of a principal entry (the word you are looking up, usually printed in heavy type), enclosed in brackets and placed directly before the definition.

arris ar ə s\n, pl **arris** or **arrises** [probably modif. of MF *areste*, lit., fishbone, fr LL *arista*, ear of grain]: the sharp edge or salient angle formed by the meeting of two surfaces, esp. in moldings.

You probably should familiarize yourself with the abbreviations used to denote the origin of words. Consult the front pages of your dictionary where you will find a guide to the use of that particular publication. Look for a heading that refers to etymologies or abbreviations and symbols used in etymologies. These keys will help you interpret a word's entry. For instance, the entry on the previous page uses the abbreviations MF and LL indicating that the entry *arris* is derived from Middle French or Late Latin.

Many English words have their origin in Greek and Roman myths and legends. If you are well-read, you may already have an edge in using the etymological method of determining word meaning. For instance, if you have read the story of the mythical king Tantalus, you would understand the derivation of the verb *tantalize*. King Tantalus, after his death, was punished for his wickedness by being placed in water up to his chin. When he stooped to drink, the water would recede. Above his head, branches laden with fruit bobbed out of his reach. So from the name Tantalus came the word *tantalize*, meaning "to tease."

A great many of the words we use daily came into our language from the Latin and Greek. Approximately half the words in the dictionary are derived from Latin. Many Latin words and phrases have been borrowed and adopted by other languages. European languages such as French and Spanish came directly from Latin and are known as Romance languages. Consequently, if you are or have been a student of Latin, you will find it easier to build your vocabulary.

Many foreign terms were absorbed into English as parts of several different words related in meaning to each other. These parts of words fall into three groups.

Roots (or stems)—These carry the basic meaning and are combined with each other and with prefixes and suffixes to create other words with related meanings.

Prefixes—Letter combinations with their own particular meaning that appear at the beginning of a word.

Suffixes—Letter combinations with their own particular meaning that appear at the end of a word.

The lists of roots, prefixes, and suffixes in this section are accompanied by words in which the letter combinations appear. Use the dictionary to look up any words that are not clear in your mind.

Remember that this section is not meant for easy reading. It is a guide to a program of study that will prove invaluable if you do your part. Do not try to absorb too much at one time. If you can put in a half-hour every day, your study will yield better results.

After you have done your preliminary work and have a better idea of how words are formed in English, attempt the various vocabulary tests we have provided. They cover a wide variety of the vocabulary questions commonly encountered on examinations. These lengthy tests are not meant to be taken all at once. Space them out. Adhere closely to the directions, which differ depending on the test. Keep an honest record of your scores. Study your corrected mistakes and look them up in your dictionary. Concentrate closely on each sample test, and watch your scores improve.

KNOW YOUR ROOTS

ROOTS OR STEMS

The root or stem is that part of the word that conveys the basic meaning of the word. For example, in the word *introduction*, *duct* is the root. It means "lead." *Intro-* means *within, into,* and *-tion* is a noun ending. Hence, the meaning of introduction—a "leading into."

Below is a chart of common stems. See how well you "know your roots."

COMMON STEMS

Stem	Meaning	Example
ag, ac	do	agenda, action
agri	farm	agriculture
aqua	water	aquatic
auto	self	automatic
biblio	book	bibliography
bio	life	biography
cad, cas	fall	cadence, casual
cap, cep, cept	take	captive, accept
capit	head	capital, decapitate
ced, cede, ceed, cess	go	intercede
celer	speed	accelerate
chrom	color	monochromatic
chron	time	chronological
cide, cis	cut	incision
clude, clud, clus	close, close in	include, cluster
cog, cogn	knowledge of	recognize
cur, curs	run	recur, cursive
ded	give	dedicate
dent, dont	tooth	dental
duce, duct	lead	induce, deduct
fact, fect, fict	make, do	perfect, fiction, factory
fer, late	carry	refer, dilate, transfer, translate
flect, flex	bend, turn	reflect
fring, fract	break	infringe, refract
graph, gram	picture, writing	graphic, telegram
greg	group, gather	gregarious, congregation

COMMON STEMS—*continued*

Stem	Meaning	Example
gress, grad	step, walk	progress, degrade
hydr	water	hydrate
ject	throw	inject
jud	right	judicial
junct	join	conjunction
juris	law, justice	jurist
lect, leg	read, choose	collect, legible
logue	speech, speaking	dialogue
logy	study of	psychology
loq, loc	speak	elocution
lude, lus	play, perform	elude, ludicrous
manu	by hand	manuscript
mand	order	remand
mar	sea	maritime
med	middle	intermediate
ment, mem	mind, memory	mention
meter	measure	thermometer
micro	small	microscope
min	lessen	miniature
mis, miss, mit	send	remit, dismiss
mot, mov	move	remote, remove
mute	change	commute, mutation
naut	sailor, sail	nautical
nounce, nunci	declare, state	announce, enunciate
ped, pod	foot	pedal
pel, pulse	drive, push	dispel, impulse
pend, pense	hang	depend, dispenser
plac	please	placate
plic	fold	implicate
port	carry	portable
pose, pone	put, place	depose, component
reg, rect	rule	regulate, direct
rupt	break	disruption
sec, sect	cut	bisect
sed	remain	sedentary
sert	weave, bind	insert
serve	keep, save	preserve
scend, scent	climb	ascent
scribe, script	write	describe, transcript
sist	stand, set	insist
spect	look	inspect
spire, spirat	breath, breathe	perspire
strict	tighten	restrict
tain	hold	detain
term	end	terminate
tract	draw, drag	detract
tort	twist	distort
vene, vent	come	intervene, invent
vict	overcome, conquer	evict
volve, volu	roll, turn	evolve, evolution

PREFIXES AND SUFFIXES

Prefixes and suffixes are the "beginning and end." We will begin by reviewing the term *prefix*. A prefix is a letter-combination attached to the beginning of a word; it usually carries a meaning independent of the word to which it is attached. For example, the prefix *semi* means "half." It can be added to many words—*semicircle, semilunar, semiprofessional, semiformal*. Attaching a prefix sometimes requires the placement of a hyphen between the prefix and the root word. A hyphen is used when the prefix is attached to a proper noun: *all-American, pro-British, anti-Fascist, un-Christian*.

A suffix is a combination of letters attached to the end of a word and usually possesses a meaning separate from the word to which it is affixed, for example, *-less* (without)—*careless, hopeless, meaningless*. Usually, affixing a suffix to a word changes its part of speech, for example, *assert* (verb)—*assertion* (noun), *beautiful* (adjective)—*beautifully* (adverb).)

Study the following prefix and suffix charts to increase your understanding of related words and inflected (changed) forms.

PREFIXES

Prefix	Meaning	Example
a	not	amoral
ab, a	away from	absent
ad, ac, ag, at	to	advent, accrue, attract, aggressive
an	without	anarchy
ante	before	antedate
anti	against	antipathy
aud, audit	hear	auditor
bene	well	beneficent
bi	two	bicameral
cap, capt, cept	take, seize, hold	capture
ced, cess	go, yield	rescind, recess
circum	around	circumspect
com, con, col	together	commit, confound, collate
contra	against	contraband
cred, credit	believe	credible
de	from, down	descend
dic, dict	say	dictionary
dis, di	apart	distract, divert
dom	home, rule	domicile, dominate
duc, duct	lead	induce
ex, e	out	exit, emit
extra	beyond	extracurricular
fac, fact	make	facsimile
in, im, ir, il, un	not	inept, irregular, illegal
in, im	in, into	interest, imbibe
inter	between	interscholastic
intra, intro	within	intramural
mal	bad	malcontent
mis	wrong	misnomer

PREFIXES—*continued*

Prefix	Meaning	Example
non	not	nonentity
ob	against	obstacle
omni	all	omnivorous
per	through	permeate
peri	around	periscope
poly	many	polytheism
post	after	postmortem
pre	before	premonition
pro	forward	propose
re	again	review
se	apart	seduce
semi	half	semicircle
sub	under	subvert
sui	self	suicide
super	above	superimpose
sur	on, upon	surcharge
trans	across	transpose
un	not	unwelcome
vice	instead of	vice-president

SUFFIXES

Suffix	Meaning	Example
able, ible	capable of being	capable, reversible
age	state of	storage
al	pertaining to	instructional
ance	relating to	reliance
ary	relating to	dictionary
ate	act	confiscate
ation	action	radiation
cy	quality	democracy
ed	past action	subsided
ence	relating to	confidence
er, or	one who	adviser, actor
ic	pertaining to	democratic
ing	present action	surmising
ious	full of	rebellious
ish	like, as	childish
ive	having the quality of	creative
ize	to make like	harmonize
less	without	hopeless
ly	the quality of	carefully
ment	result	amusement
ness	the quality of being	selfishness
ty	condition	sanity

INCREASED WORD POWER FROM BEGINNING TO END

Using the etymological approach can simplify the process by which you attack the monumental feat of learning medical terminology. By knowing that the suffix *itis* implies inflammation and *ectomy* means "the cutting out or removal of," you can easily deduce that the term *appendicitis* means "inflammation of the appendix" and *appendectomy* means "the cutting out or removal of the appendix."

Now that you have studied the various letter combinations or word components, see if you can make an educated guess at the meanings of the terms listed below. Start with the root or stem. Next, add the suffix and/or prefix to the interpretation in the order that provides a clear definition. The result will be increased word power from "beginning to end." It's as challenging as a jigsaw puzzle! Be sure to compare your definitions with those in the dictionary.

decapitate	colloquy
emissary	aggregation
incursion	retractable
involuted	implacable
convocation	celerity

SYNONYMS

THE NAME'S THE SAME

Synonyms are words that share meanings. The English language abounds in synonyms. In your effort to acquire word mastery, you must learn to express your ideas without redundancy and constant use of overworked words. Effective writing and speaking may be achieved through the precise use of synonyms.

Words such as *brave* and *courageous*, which may allude to an identical quality, can be used interchangeably. Some synonyms, however, differ in definition or usage. For example, *fewer* refers to number, while *less* refers to quantity: John has *fewer* books and *less* money than his brother. These words are indeed similar in meaning, but one cannot be substituted for the other.

The adjectives *beautiful* and *handsome* both describe someone or something attractive or pleasing to the eye. Nevertheless, you would not usually speak of a "beautiful man" or a "handsome young lady." In our society, common usage would cause one to reverse these expressions to "beautiful young lady" and a "handsome man."

A study of the finer shades of meaning of synonyms will help you be more precise when you convey your feelings or mental picture of an object or scene. For instance, if you were to say, "The *bottom* of the lamp is made of Indian brass and features intricate carvings," one might simply envision the underside of the lamp. However, if you were to substitute *base* for the word *bottom*, one would instead get a visual image of something highly decorative that supports the upper structure of the lamp. So even though the "name" appears to be the same, an investigation into various shades of definition will assist you in distinguishing variations in usage.

If you wish to expand your vocabulary of synonyms and familiarize yourself with their correct usage, you will find the following reference books helpful:

Webster's Dictionary of Synonyms
Roget's International Thesaurus
Merriam-Webster's Concise Dictionary of English Usage

FAMILIAR SURROUNDINGS?

The most common way of testing vocabulary on a standardized test is in context, that is, to present the items in a sentence or phrase so that you can see how a word is used. You can then determine whether the word is used as a noun, a verb, an adjective, etc. The test, therefore, is designed to encourage the extraction of word meaning from context; however, the context will not be so explicit that you can easily infer the meaning of a word.

More specifically, the synonym test item is usually a multiple-choice item that appears in one of three formats:

Type A

Given an underlined or italicized word in a complete sentence, the test-taker is required to identify which of the four other words is a synonym for the underlined or italicized word.

Example

The disinterested witness was able to give a *candid* account of the incident.

- **(A)** complete
- **(B)** impartial
- **(C)** biased
- **(D)** candescent

Type B

Given an underlined or italicized word in a phrase, the test-taker is required to identify which of the four other words is a synonym for the underlined or italicized word.

Example

The *emaciated* patient

- **(A)** discharged
- **(B)** emancipated
- **(C)** emotional
- **(D)** shriveled

Type C

Given a sentence with a missing word, the test-taker is required to identify which of the four other words best completes the sentence.

Example

An *apology* is appropriate when a person feels

- **(A)** sorry.
- **(B)** apathetic.
- **(C)** rejected.
- **(D)** elated.

OR

Example

He is a *staunch* supporter of the presidential candidate. Staunch means

- **(A)** stubborn.
- **(B)** faithful.
- **(C)** inflexible.
- **(D)** hopeful.

Nursing School and Allied Health Entrance Exams

Context Clues

Examining the various types of context clues is another means of understanding how to extract the meaning of a word from the words surrounding it. The sample sentences below illustrate the different kinds of context clues.

1. Since the *litigation* would be costly, the lawyers advised that such a suit should be settled out of court. (**DEFINITION**)

2. The crumbling *edifice*, a building located on the north side of town, is targeted for implosion early in June. (**DEFINITION**)

3. He exhibits his *sloth* by resting on the couch while his wife and elderly father shovel snow. (**DESCRIPTION**)

4. She had indeed turned into a *shrew* with her screaming, nagging, and quarrelsome manner. (**DESCRIPTION**)

5. Tyler was anything but *amenable* to the proposal of another coed dorm on campus; on the contrary, he vehemently protested the board's recommendation for such action. (**CONTRAST**)

6. Crestville was a *quaint*, little town until the relocation of several large corporations turned it into a bustling metropolis. (**CONTRAST**)

7. Charles, like his brave and dauntless father, was fearless in the face of trouble. (**COMPARISON**)

8. She was stricken with the disease at an early age; her daughter likewise was *infirm* while very young. (**COMPARISON**)

9. The sentence of five years in prison hardly seemed adequate *retribution* for this dreadful crime. (**EXAMPLES**)

10. Peas and beans are two kinds of *legumes*. (**EXAMPLES**)

11. The disease is considered *infectious*, or contagious. (**SYNONYMS**)

12. The *cardiologist*, or heart specialist, ordered several tests for his patient. (**SYNONYMS**)

13. Karin was *elated* at the news of her job transfer; however, her mother appeared sad. (**ANTONYMS**)

14. The *arid* climate was a welcomed change from the dampness I experienced in London. (**ANTONYMS**)

Especially Special: Scientific Terms

When preparing for an entrance exam for programs leading to science-related careers, it is beneficial to familiarize yourself with the specialized vocabulary of this discipline. Remember, even though the general public considers scientific jargon confusing, technical terms are imperative for scientific communication. If you plan to study science, your ability to comprehend the terminology of the field could indicate how well you will do in the related course work. Your entrance exam may measure your scientific vocabulary skills.

Mastery of specialized vocabulary—or any vocabulary for that matter—can best be achieved by learning words as you encounter them in your reading. However, when preparing for an entrance exam, you may want to employ the following strategies:

1. Review "Know Your Roots" and "Prefixes and Suffixes" on pages 25–28 of this publication.

2. Read a variety of scientific articles, science textbook chapters, etc.

3. Try to understand the unfamiliar words that you encounter in these readings as they are used in context.

4. If you cannot grasp the meaning from context, then put your knowledge of roots and affixes to work. Take the word apart and see if you can determine a meaning that fits the context (or if you are in the testing situation, a meaning that comes close to one of the multiple-choice items).

5. If Step 4 does not yield a reasonable definition, then check the footnotes, glossary, or index of the text you are reading. If you find the word in the index, skim the pages listed for that word, checking for either its definition or its contextual usage.

6. If you cannot find a definition of the word in the material that you are reading, look it up in a dictionary. It would be best to use a scientific dictionary or encyclopedia. There are dictionaries that are for specific areas of study, such as geography, modern history, politics, and biology.

7. Once you have come up with a definition for the word, you may want to write it on an index card (word on one side, definition on the other). After accumulating a number of these vocabulary cards, carry them in your pocket or book bag. Flip through them when you have a spare moment (commuting by train or bus, sitting in the waiting room of the dentist or doctor, etc.).

8. Become accustomed to recognizing words that stand for concepts rather than facts. To a scientist, a concept is a generalization or an idea based on information or knowledge that explains a phenomenon. Read the following paragraph and underline those words which you feel represent scientific concepts.

   Karotyping is a process that enables scientists to study the chromosomes of human beings. Sometimes the study can be made even before birth. Chromosomes can best be observed during metaphase in mitosis. At this point they are coiled. Skin cells are good to use in making a Karyotype because they divide frequently. Some genetic disorders can be identified just by looking at the Karyotype of a person.

   If you underlined Karyotype process, metaphase, mitosis, and genetic disorders, you would be correct. These words represent ideas. They cannot be touched and they have no exact physical form or boundaries, yet they are real because they represent scientific facts.

9. Finally, learn to connect symbols to words. A scientific symbol is an abbreviation that stands for a word or concept.

   Example

   $C_6H_{12}O_6$ represents glucose, a chemical compound.

You will have the opportunity to practice your use of these vocabulary expansion strategies as you encounter scientific terms on the verbal ability practice test and final verbal ability examination in this book. The answers to several of the questions in the reading comprehension test involve scientific terms. These questions are indicated by asterisks.

In completing a synonym test item, remember to look for a word which means the same, or almost the same, as the target word in the item (the underlined or italicized word). Do not be distracted by a word that is a look-alike, that is, one that looks similar or begins with the same three or four letters but is unrelated in meaning. When possible, apply the etymological approach of interpreting roots, prefixes, and suffixes. Now try completing the sample synonym test. There is a total of 75 items. An answer key appears on page 41.

ANSWER SHEET

1. Ⓐ Ⓑ Ⓒ Ⓓ   16. Ⓐ Ⓑ Ⓒ Ⓓ   31. Ⓐ Ⓑ Ⓒ Ⓓ   46. Ⓐ Ⓑ Ⓒ Ⓓ   61. Ⓐ Ⓑ Ⓒ Ⓓ

2. Ⓐ Ⓑ Ⓒ Ⓓ   17. Ⓐ Ⓑ Ⓒ Ⓓ   32. Ⓐ Ⓑ Ⓒ Ⓓ   47. Ⓐ Ⓑ Ⓒ Ⓓ   62. Ⓐ Ⓑ Ⓒ Ⓓ

3. Ⓐ Ⓑ Ⓒ Ⓓ   18. Ⓐ Ⓑ Ⓒ Ⓓ   33. Ⓐ Ⓑ Ⓒ Ⓓ   48. Ⓐ Ⓑ Ⓒ Ⓓ   63. Ⓐ Ⓑ Ⓒ Ⓓ

4. Ⓐ Ⓑ Ⓒ Ⓓ   19. Ⓐ Ⓑ Ⓒ Ⓓ   34. Ⓐ Ⓑ Ⓒ Ⓓ   49. Ⓐ Ⓑ Ⓒ Ⓓ   64. Ⓐ Ⓑ Ⓒ Ⓓ

5. Ⓐ Ⓑ Ⓒ Ⓓ   20. Ⓐ Ⓑ Ⓒ Ⓓ   35. Ⓐ Ⓑ Ⓒ Ⓓ   50. Ⓐ Ⓑ Ⓒ Ⓓ   65. Ⓐ Ⓑ Ⓒ Ⓓ

6. Ⓐ Ⓑ Ⓒ Ⓓ   21. Ⓐ Ⓑ Ⓒ Ⓓ   36. Ⓐ Ⓑ Ⓒ Ⓓ   51. Ⓐ Ⓑ Ⓒ Ⓓ   66. Ⓐ Ⓑ Ⓒ Ⓓ

7. Ⓐ Ⓑ Ⓒ Ⓓ   22. Ⓐ Ⓑ Ⓒ Ⓓ   37. Ⓐ Ⓑ Ⓒ Ⓓ   52. Ⓐ Ⓑ Ⓒ Ⓓ   67. Ⓐ Ⓑ Ⓒ Ⓓ

8. Ⓐ Ⓑ Ⓒ Ⓓ   23. Ⓐ Ⓑ Ⓒ Ⓓ   38. Ⓐ Ⓑ Ⓒ Ⓓ   53. Ⓐ Ⓑ Ⓒ Ⓓ   68. Ⓐ Ⓑ Ⓒ Ⓓ

9. Ⓐ Ⓑ Ⓒ Ⓓ   24. Ⓐ Ⓑ Ⓒ Ⓓ   39. Ⓐ Ⓑ Ⓒ Ⓓ   54. Ⓐ Ⓑ Ⓒ Ⓓ   69. Ⓐ Ⓑ Ⓒ Ⓓ

10. Ⓐ Ⓑ Ⓒ Ⓓ   25. Ⓐ Ⓑ Ⓒ Ⓓ   40. Ⓐ Ⓑ Ⓒ Ⓓ   55. Ⓐ Ⓑ Ⓒ Ⓓ   70. Ⓐ Ⓑ Ⓒ Ⓓ

11. Ⓐ Ⓑ Ⓒ Ⓓ   26. Ⓐ Ⓑ Ⓒ Ⓓ   41. Ⓐ Ⓑ Ⓒ Ⓓ   56. Ⓐ Ⓑ Ⓒ Ⓓ   71. Ⓐ Ⓑ Ⓒ Ⓓ

12. Ⓐ Ⓑ Ⓒ Ⓓ   27. Ⓐ Ⓑ Ⓒ Ⓓ   42. Ⓐ Ⓑ Ⓒ Ⓓ   57. Ⓐ Ⓑ Ⓒ Ⓓ   72. Ⓐ Ⓑ Ⓒ Ⓓ

13. Ⓐ Ⓑ Ⓒ Ⓓ   28. Ⓐ Ⓑ Ⓒ Ⓓ   43. Ⓐ Ⓑ Ⓒ Ⓓ   58. Ⓐ Ⓑ Ⓒ Ⓓ   73. Ⓐ Ⓑ Ⓒ Ⓓ

14. Ⓐ Ⓑ Ⓒ Ⓓ   29. Ⓐ Ⓑ Ⓒ Ⓓ   44. Ⓐ Ⓑ Ⓒ Ⓓ   59. Ⓐ Ⓑ Ⓒ Ⓓ   74. Ⓐ Ⓑ Ⓒ Ⓓ

15. Ⓐ Ⓑ Ⓒ Ⓓ   30. Ⓐ Ⓑ Ⓒ Ⓓ   45. Ⓐ Ⓑ Ⓒ Ⓓ   60. Ⓐ Ⓑ Ⓒ Ⓓ   75. Ⓐ Ⓑ Ⓒ Ⓓ

SYNONYMS TEST

75 QUESTIONS ■□ TIME—35 MINUTES

Directions: In each of the sentences below, one word is italicized. Following each sentence are four words or phrases. For each sentence, choose the word or phrase that most nearly corresponds in meaning with the italicized word.

1. The *diction* acceptable in speech is usually more informal than that required in writing.

   (A) conviction
   (B) language
   (C) discourse
   (D) decrement

2. It is apparent that Mr. Smith is the most *sedulous* and active member of the group.

   (A) hideous
   (B) generous
   (C) infirm
   (D) industrious

3. During the hockey game several *altercations* took place.

   (A) fracases
   (B) substitutions
   (C) alterations
   (D) plays

4. The carrot is a perfect illustration of a *biennial*.

   (A) occurring quarterly
   (B) occurring once in two years
   (C) perennial
   (D) bisection

5. She has run the *gamut* of clerical jobs in this office.

   (A) periphery
   (B) margin
   (C) range
   (D) imperception

6. His deeds amounted to nothing more than those of a *sanctimonious* hypocrite.

   (A) parsimonious
   (B) perpetual
   (C) intrinsic
   (D) affectedly pious

7. He displayed the manners of an *urbane* gentleman.

   (A) suave
   (B) poignant
   (C) spasmodic
   (D) pensive

8. The *slogan* is appropriate for both the product and its service.

   (A) catchword
   (B) sample
   (C) design
   (D) passage

9. The *chloroplasts* in plant cells is where photosynthesis takes place.

   (A) organelles
   (B) mitochondria
   (C) ribosomes
   (D) vacuoles

10. He was determined to *foil* the scheme of his opponent.

    (A) heighten
    (B) secure
    (C) disencumber
    (D) thwart

GO ON TO THE NEXT PAGE

11. The examiner *purported* to be an official representative.
    - (A) addressed
    - (B) claimed
    - (C) propitiated
    - (D) conciliated

12. The ship carried refugees of every *persuasion*.
    - (A) mediocrity
    - (B) sort
    - (C) prospectus
    - (D) compendium

13. The child could not *recollect* the incident.
    - (A) remember
    - (B) dubitate
    - (C) interrogate
    - (D) illumine

14. The Supreme Court *rescinded* the law.
    - (A) complicated
    - (B) inveigled
    - (C) revoked
    - (D) accepted

15. The implementation of the plan was given *scant* consideration.
    - (A) audacious
    - (B) fervid
    - (C) little
    - (D) clothed

16. The key speaker, in his lengthy presentation, *scoffed* at religion.
    - (A) exonerated
    - (B) amplified
    - (C) confuted
    - (D) mocked

17. She completed the *sprint* with a sudden surge of energy.
    - (A) relaxation
    - (B) adventure
    - (C) run
    - (D) convergence

18. The content of the message was *urgent*.
    - (A) privileged
    - (B) amendable
    - (C) pressing
    - (D) absolved

19. A *simulated* rescue mission was conducted by the forest rangers.
    - (A) pretended
    - (B) superficial
    - (C) stimulated
    - (D) simultaneous

20. A *histamine* is released from the tissues when the cells are injured.
    - (A) a histone
    - (B) an amine
    - (C) a stimulant
    - (D) an isoenzyme

21. Her quickening gait seemed regulated by the *pulse* of the big city.
    - (A) utility
    - (B) pace
    - (C) reverence
    - (D) solace

22. The language of the publication is *unsophisticated* but informative.
    - (A) ponderous
    - (B) elaborate
    - (C) simple
    - (D) superficial

23. All the evidence presented pointed to *willful* execution of a crime.
    - (A) deliberate
    - (B) eminent
    - (C) amicable
    - (D) remorseful

24. There is no *provision* for deadlines in the contract.
    - (A) improvement
    - (B) convenience
    - (C) aggregation
    - (D) stipulation

25. The furnishings *impart* an air of elegance to the room.

(A) communicate
(B) indemnify
(C) reinforce
(D) disguise

26. She exhibited great *valor* in handling the emergency.

(A) ingeniousness
(B) courage
(C) discretion
(D) optimism

27. Various courses were *fused* in the revision of the curriculum.

(A) required
(B) implicated
(C) combined
(D) involved

28. Production of complex molecules is accomplished by *replication*.

(A) duplication
(B) synthesis
(C) fixation
(D) reproduction

29. The task of choosing one from so many qualified applicants *bewildered* the employer.

(A) perplexed
(B) aggravated
(C) subdued
(D) infuriated

30. The revision of the city plan incorporated adjustments in the projected *modes* of transportation.

(A) increments
(B) expenditures
(C) means
(D) modifications

31. The politician sought to *aggrandize* himself at the expense of the people.

(A) exhaust
(B) subjugate
(C) sacrifice
(D) exalt

32. The newcomer made an effort to *mingle* with the crowd.

(A) argue
(B) mix
(C) disrupt
(D) flout

33. If an organization's programs were described as *philanthropic*, the programs would be

(A) primitive.
(B) deleterious.
(C) extraneous.
(D) benevolent.

34. If the traits of a nation's leader were *covetous*, they were

(A) greedy.
(B) exemplary.
(C) disparate.
(D) adventitious.

35. Rabbits *breed* offspring rapidly.

(A) raise
(B) gather
(C) propagate
(D) destroy

36. It was necessary to *iterate* one procedure of the experiment.

(A) adjust
(B) defend
(C) ferment
(D) repeat

37. A shadow of a man *loomed* ominously in the dimly lit corridor.

(A) asserted
(B) yielded
(C) appeared
(D) rebuffed

38. Alcohol consumption often exerts a *malign* influence on an individual.

(A) ecstatic
(B) injurious
(C) luminous
(D) gloomy

GO ON TO THE NEXT PAGE

39. The girl is reported to have left of her own *volition*.

    (A) flight
    (B) will
    (C) repudiation
    (D) recognizance

40. The most important *mutation* is one occurring in the gametes.

    (A) fertilization
    (B) meiosis
    (C) deamination
    (D) change

41. The *similitude* between the original painting and the reproduction is remarkable.

    (A) incongruity
    (B) connection
    (C) resemblance
    (D) relationship

42. A *prudent* individual will save some portion of his or her wage.

    (A) judicious
    (B) terse
    (C) audacious
    (D) laconic

43. His decision to return home was *instinctive*.

    (A) spontaneous
    (B) turbid
    (C) premeditated
    (D) irrelevant

44. The mountain *torrent* flowed over the rocks.

    (A) slide
    (B) avalanche
    (C) deluge
    (D) air

45. The book was written to embody all aspects of life science.

    (A) combat
    (B) eliminate
    (C) abjure
    (D) incorporate

46. Her sudden decision is typical of her *impetuous* behavior.

    (A) contemptible
    (B) sophisticated
    (C) impulsive
    (D) fallacious

47. It is fitting that we *eulogize* one who has contributed so greatly to our society.

    (A) promulgate
    (B) praise
    (C) denigrate
    (D) append

48. The convention hall swelled with the *vociferation* of various campaign groups.

    (A) clamor
    (B) taciturnity
    (C) oblivion
    (D) discernment

49. The blackmailer has placed her in a *precarious* position.

    (A) mellifluous
    (B) intrusive
    (C) unusual
    (D) unstable

50. Her display of so much fine china was too *ostentatious*.

    (A) pretentious
    (B) inconspicuous
    (C) ascribable
    (D) candid

51. To *manifest* interest

    (A) conceal
    (B) diminish
    (C) augment
    (D) display

52. *Banter* and laughter

    (A) discourse
    (B) singing
    (C) toasting
    (D) raillery

53. *Aesthetic* value

(A) practical
(B) artistic
(C) monetary
(D) intrinsic

54. Confirmed his *apostasy*

(A) defiance
(B) defection
(C) belief
(D) inference

55. The *cryptic* message

(A) cynical
(B) mysterious
(C) critical
(D) censorious

56. New witnesses *emerged*

(A) deviated
(B) divested
(C) declined
(D) appeared

57. The *contumacious* youngster

(A) exuberant
(B) rebellious
(C) awkward
(D) mischievous

58. *Cognizant* of the ill will

(A) ignorant
(B) aware
(C) insensitive
(D) remorseful

59. *Glacial* region

(A) glass-like
(B) illiberal
(C) frigid
(D) reticent

60. *Instigated* the rebellion

(A) quelled
(B) incited
(C) assisted
(D) depressed

61. A fight *ensued*

(A) followed
(B) terminated
(C) was avoided
(D) culminated

62. *Retrospect* of events

(A) review
(B) concept
(C) knowledge
(D) awareness

63. *Malice* toward my friend

(A) adoration
(B) sympathy
(C) ill will
(D) apathy

64. *Saturated* with moisture

(A) void of
(B) mixed with
(C) full of
(D) replaced with

65. *Debilitating* to people

(A) invigorating
(B) stimulating
(C) tolerable
(D) weakening

66. Ten years' *servitude*

(A) freedom
(B) lethargy
(C) vicissitude
(D) bondage

67. *Relish* the thought

(A) enjoy
(B) dread
(C) spread
(D) implant

68. A *lackadaisical* attitude

(A) enthusiastic
(B) complacent
(C) profound
(D) indifferent

GO ON TO THE NEXT PAGE

69. To *hoist* the sails

    (A) cast
    (B) raise
    (C) prepare
    (D) repair

70. *Asperse* the family's good name

    (A) slander
    (B) fathom
    (C) extol
    (D) palliate

71. *Sordid* details

    (A) bizarre
    (B) wretched
    (C) primordial
    (D) exaggerated

72. Sudden *alienation*

    (A) agitation
    (B) inception
    (C) subsidence
    (D) isolation

73. *Biotin* is widely distributed in organisms.

    (A) vitamin H
    (B) vitamin D
    (C) chyme
    (D) plasmodia

74. *Accede* to the request

    (A) attend
    (B) refer
    (C) adjust
    (D) agree

75. The *proximity* of the lake

    (A) worthlessness
    (B) nearness
    (C) level
    (D) ebullition

STOP   If you finish before time is called, you may check your work on this section only. Do not turn to any other section in the test.

ANSWER KEY

1. **B**	16. **D**	31. **D**	46. **C**	61. **A**
2. **D**	17. **C**	32. **B**	47. **B**	62. **A**
3. **A**	18. **C**	33. **D**	48. **A**	63. **C**
4. **B**	19. **A**	34. **A**	49. **D**	64. **C**
5. **C**	20. **B**	35. **C**	50. **A**	65. **D**
6. **D**	21. **B**	36. **D**	51. **D**	66. **D**
7. **A**	22. **C**	37. **C**	52. **D**	67. **A**
8. **A**	23. **A**	38. **B**	53. **B**	68. **D**
9. **A**	24. **D**	39. **B**	54. **B**	69. **B**
10. **D**	25. **A**	40. **D**	55. **B**	70. **A**
11. **B**	26. **B**	41. **C**	56. **D**	71. **B**
12. **B**	27. **C**	42. **A**	57. **B**	72. **D**
13. **A**	28. **A**	43. **A**	58. **B**	73. **A**
14. **C**	29. **A**	44. **C**	59. **C**	74. **D**
15. **C**	30. **C**	45. **D**	60. **B**	75. **B**

ANTONYMS

THE TURNABOUTS

In the preceding part of this section, emphasis was placed on synonyms, or words with similar or identical meanings. You are now ready to increase your word power from a contrasting point of view. Antonyms are words that are opposite in meaning. Some simple examples are: *hot/cold*, *strong/weak*, *sit/stand*, *night/day*, and *lazy/industrious*.

Antonyms are extremely useful to express contrast. The use of certain antonyms can result in the verbal creation of a universal portrait or concept. For instance, everyone associates the name "Scrooge" with *penny-pinching* or *miserly* traits. The Dickens character was anything but philanthropic, a term that characterizes people or agencies who devote themselves to helping and giving to humanity. Therefore, if you read that "a former Scrooge has transformed himself into a philanthropist" you would surmise that the person being described has had a complete change of heart. The term *philanthropist* has been contrasted with a symbol of *miserly* and *penny-pinching* traits.

When taking a test measuring your comprehension of verbal contrasts, be certain to select a response that is the same part of speech as the term in question. Although *discourtesy* and *insolent* share the same shade of meaning, one could not be substituted for the other—the former is a noun and the latter an adjective. Therefore, they could not play identical roles in a sentence.

If you are stumped by any one test item, move on quickly to the next. When you have completed the test, and if time permits, return to any test item(s) you have skipped. Mentally put the various word choices, including the test item, in a sentence. Then remove the test item again.

Example
Polite

- **(A)** desperate
- **(B)** discourtesy
- **(C)** insolent
- **(D)** discriminate

For the above example, make up a sentence using the word *polite* and then substitute the choices, such as "The boy is *discourtesy*" and "The boy is *insolent*." Obviously, *insolent* is the correct response, as it is the word opposite in meaning to *polite* and best fits the sentence pattern "The boy is . . ."

USING PREFIXES

Another helpful technique in taking antonym tests is the close examination of prefixes. Review the etymological information before attempting the sample antonym test, and pay special attention to prefixes. Prefixes can often be the key to contrast in meaning. For example, the prefixes *un*, *im*, and *in* frequently denote the opposite meaning of the word to which they are affixed: *happy/unhappy*; *adequate/inadequate*; *polite/impolite*. These examples make it apparent that the actual meaning of the prefixes is "not." The prefixes *in* and *ex* are opposite in meaning. *In* means, "in," "into," "inside"; and *ex* means "out," "outside of."

If the target word is *internal*, which of the following words would you select as its antonym?

- **(A)** interior
- **(B)** ephemeral
- **(C)** illegal
- **(D)** external

Of course, *external* is the correct response. Study the list of contrasting prefixes below. Then try your hand at making the "turnabout."

CONTRASTING PREFIXES

ad, ac, ag, at (to)   *ab, a* (away from)
ante (before)   *post* (after)
anti, contra (against)   *pro* (for)
bene (well, good)   *mal* (bad)
corn, con, col (together)   *dis, di* (apart)
con, com (with)   *an* (without)
eu (good)   *dys* (bad)
in, im (in)   *e, ex* (out)
hypo (under)   *hyper* (over)
pro (forward)   *retro* (backward)
sub (under)   *super, sur* (above)

Another strategy for the study of antonyms would be to review the antonym notations of a current edition of *Roget's Thesaurus* or *Bolander's Instant Synonyms and Antonyms*. Browsing through these two sources will help you think in terms of contrasting meanings.

ANSWER SHEET

1. Ⓐ Ⓑ Ⓒ Ⓓ   16. Ⓐ Ⓑ Ⓒ Ⓓ   31. Ⓐ Ⓑ Ⓒ Ⓓ   46. Ⓐ Ⓑ Ⓒ Ⓓ   61. Ⓐ Ⓑ Ⓒ Ⓓ

2. Ⓐ Ⓑ Ⓒ Ⓓ   17. Ⓐ Ⓑ Ⓒ Ⓓ   32. Ⓐ Ⓑ Ⓒ Ⓓ   47. Ⓐ Ⓑ Ⓒ Ⓓ   62. Ⓐ Ⓑ Ⓒ Ⓓ

3. Ⓐ Ⓑ Ⓒ Ⓓ   18. Ⓐ Ⓑ Ⓒ Ⓓ   33. Ⓐ Ⓑ Ⓒ Ⓓ   48. Ⓐ Ⓑ Ⓒ Ⓓ   63. Ⓐ Ⓑ Ⓒ Ⓓ

4. Ⓐ Ⓑ Ⓒ Ⓓ   19. Ⓐ Ⓑ Ⓒ Ⓓ   34. Ⓐ Ⓑ Ⓒ Ⓓ   49. Ⓐ Ⓑ Ⓒ Ⓓ   64. Ⓐ Ⓑ Ⓒ Ⓓ

5. Ⓐ Ⓑ Ⓒ Ⓓ   20. Ⓐ Ⓑ Ⓒ Ⓓ   35. Ⓐ Ⓑ Ⓒ Ⓓ   50. Ⓐ Ⓑ Ⓒ Ⓓ   65. Ⓐ Ⓑ Ⓒ Ⓓ

6. Ⓐ Ⓑ Ⓒ Ⓓ   21. Ⓐ Ⓑ Ⓒ Ⓓ   36. Ⓐ Ⓑ Ⓒ Ⓓ   51. Ⓐ Ⓑ Ⓒ Ⓓ   66. Ⓐ Ⓑ Ⓒ Ⓓ

7. Ⓐ Ⓑ Ⓒ Ⓓ   22. Ⓐ Ⓑ Ⓒ Ⓓ   37. Ⓐ Ⓑ Ⓒ Ⓓ   52. Ⓐ Ⓑ Ⓒ Ⓓ   67. Ⓐ Ⓑ Ⓒ Ⓓ

8. Ⓐ Ⓑ Ⓒ Ⓓ   23. Ⓐ Ⓑ Ⓒ Ⓓ   38. Ⓐ Ⓑ Ⓒ Ⓓ   53. Ⓐ Ⓑ Ⓒ Ⓓ   68. Ⓐ Ⓑ Ⓒ Ⓓ

9. Ⓐ Ⓑ Ⓒ Ⓓ   24. Ⓐ Ⓑ Ⓒ Ⓓ   39. Ⓐ Ⓑ Ⓒ Ⓓ   54. Ⓐ Ⓑ Ⓒ Ⓓ   69. Ⓐ Ⓑ Ⓒ Ⓓ

10. Ⓐ Ⓑ Ⓒ Ⓓ   25. Ⓐ Ⓑ Ⓒ Ⓓ   40. Ⓐ Ⓑ Ⓒ Ⓓ   55. Ⓐ Ⓑ Ⓒ Ⓓ   70. Ⓐ Ⓑ Ⓒ Ⓓ

11. Ⓐ Ⓑ Ⓒ Ⓓ   26. Ⓐ Ⓑ Ⓒ Ⓓ   41. Ⓐ Ⓑ Ⓒ Ⓓ   56. Ⓐ Ⓑ Ⓒ Ⓓ   71. Ⓐ Ⓑ Ⓒ Ⓓ

12. Ⓐ Ⓑ Ⓒ Ⓓ   27. Ⓐ Ⓑ Ⓒ Ⓓ   42. Ⓐ Ⓑ Ⓒ Ⓓ   57. Ⓐ Ⓑ Ⓒ Ⓓ   72. Ⓐ Ⓑ Ⓒ Ⓓ

13. Ⓐ Ⓑ Ⓒ Ⓓ   28. Ⓐ Ⓑ Ⓒ Ⓓ   43. Ⓐ Ⓑ Ⓒ Ⓓ   58. Ⓐ Ⓑ Ⓒ Ⓓ   73. Ⓐ Ⓑ Ⓒ Ⓓ

14. Ⓐ Ⓑ Ⓒ Ⓓ   29. Ⓐ Ⓑ Ⓒ Ⓓ   44. Ⓐ Ⓑ Ⓒ Ⓓ   59. Ⓐ Ⓑ Ⓒ Ⓓ   74. Ⓐ Ⓑ Ⓒ Ⓓ

15. Ⓐ Ⓑ Ⓒ Ⓓ   30. Ⓐ Ⓑ Ⓒ Ⓓ   45. Ⓐ Ⓑ Ⓒ Ⓓ   60. Ⓐ Ⓑ Ⓒ Ⓓ   75. Ⓐ Ⓑ Ⓒ Ⓓ

ANTONYMS TEST

75 QUESTIONS ▪▢ TIME—35 MINUTES

Directions: For each of the following questions, select the word opposite in meaning to the word printed in capital letters.

1. DEFACE

   (A) defame
   (B) embellish
   (C) vilify
   (D) disfigure

2. SUPERFLUOUS

   (A) coarse
   (B) transient
   (C) insufficient
   (D) abundant

3. ASSUAGE

   (A) presume
   (B) agitate
   (C) alleviate
   (D) absorb

4. AUGURY

   (A) gentility
   (B) relentlessness
   (C) supremacy
   (D) science

5. TERMINATE

   (A) withhold
   (B) construe
   (C) repel
   (D) initiate

6. VITIATE

   (A) liquidate
   (B) revive
   (C) validate
   (D) slander

7. JUBILANT

   (A) lugubrious
   (B) irrepressible
   (C) discernible
   (D) jocular

8. HOSTILE

   (A) affable
   (B) awkward
   (C) judicious
   (D) coxcombical

9. TACITURN

   (A) tactful
   (B) talkative
   (C) crucial
   (D) impetuous

10. LAGGARDLY

    (A) laboriously
    (B) languidly
    (C) briskly
    (D) cowardly

11. PHLEGMATIC

    (A) vital
    (B) apparent
    (C) conversant
    (D) apprehensive

12. LOATHSOME

    (A) alluring
    (B) mournful
    (C) indifferent
    (D) preposterous

GO ON TO THE NEXT PAGE

13. EXALT
    (A) degrade
    (B) gratify
    (C) expose
    (D) desiderate

14. PACIFY
    (A) conciliate
    (B) palliate
    (C) quell
    (D) exasperate

15. SUBSEQUENT
    (A) worthless
    (B) inactive
    (C) preceding
    (D) demeaning

16. ULTIMATE
    (A) initial
    (B) equitable
    (C) irrefutable
    (D) turbid

17. LEEWAY
    (A) relevance
    (B) restriction
    (C) protection
    (D) satisfaction

18. PRETENTIOUS
    (A) flagrant
    (B) diabolical
    (C) officious
    (D) modest

19. QUANDARY
    (A) certainty
    (B) mediocrity
    (C) ruthlessness
    (D) criterion

20. SAGACIOUS
    (A) obtuse
    (B) scurrilous
    (C) indulgent
    (D) impertinent

21. SAVANT
    (A) savage
    (B) master
    (C) neophyte
    (D) constituent

22. SQUALID
    (A) staunch
    (B) stately
    (C) avaricious
    (D) equivocal

23. EXQUISITE
    (A) exorbitant
    (B) inobscure
    (C) extraneous
    (D) ordinary

24. FACILITATE
    (A) falsify
    (B) delude
    (C) hinder
    (D) assimilate

25. FLAWLESS
    (A) pertinent
    (B) conventional
    (C) defective
    (D) complacent

26. RECOMPENSE
    (A) renovate
    (B) misrequite
    (C) miscompute
    (D) sanction

27. FERVENT
    (A) nonchalant
    (B) lenient
    (C) meager
    (D) liable

28. AVERT
    (A) pursue
    (B) forestall
    (C) reject
    (D) relinquish

29. ARID

   (A) fragrant
   (B) moist
   (C) parched
   (D) odoriferous

30. IMPERATIVE

   (A) conceptive
   (B) illustrative
   (C) speculative
   (D) optional

31. SUCCINCT

   (A) corporeal
   (B) graphic
   (C) princely
   (D) loquacious

32. JEOPARDY

   (A) security
   (B) discernment
   (C) curiosity
   (D) tedium

33. SOMBER

   (A) insipid
   (B) congruous
   (C) festive
   (D) voluminous

34. EXOTIC

   (A) diachronic
   (B) erotic
   (C) common
   (D) harmonious

35. AFFILIATE

   (A) annihilate
   (B) disassociate
   (C) proffer
   (D) disparage

36. SINISTER

   (A) auspicious
   (B) immaculate
   (C) fanatical
   (D) transitory

37. INEXTRICABLE

   (A) intricate
   (B) judicious
   (C) disentangled
   (D) desperate

38. PROFLIGATE

   (A) insolvent
   (B) virtuous
   (C) redundant
   (D) incessant

39. TURBULENT

   (A) diaphanous
   (B) tranquil
   (C) formidable
   (D) diffident

40. UNWARRANTED

   (A) justifiable
   (B) baneful
   (C) depleted
   (D) contemplated

41. PLAINTIVE

   (A) embellished
   (B) peccant
   (C) rational
   (D) gleeful

42. ORNATE

   (A) unadorned
   (B) deft
   (C) subtle
   (D) conspicuous

43. ABROGATE

   (A) ratify
   (B) reconcile
   (C) abridge
   (D) alleviate

44. ABASE

   (A) cede
   (B) dignify
   (C) repudiate
   (D) engulf

GO ON TO THE NEXT PAGE

45. RENOUNCE

    (A) claim
    (B) deride
    (C) conceive
    (D) alienate

46. SABOTAGE

    (A) compensate
    (B) reinforce
    (C) restrain
    (D) release

47. OBLIVIOUS

    (A) latent
    (B) integrant
    (C) repugnant
    (D) cognizant

48. SUBMISSIVE

    (A) offensive
    (B) tactless
    (C) incompliant
    (D) manifest

49. NURTURE

    (A) distinguish
    (B) impart
    (C) neglect
    (D) disclose

50. PRUDENCE

    (A) compunction
    (B) dilemma
    (C) anticipation
    (D) recklessness

51. LAMENT

    (A) rejoice
    (B) acclaim
    (C) surmise
    (D) deceive

52. GRUELING

    (A) relaxing
    (B) satisfying
    (C) taming
    (D) suppressing

53. TRIVIAL

    (A) nugatory
    (B) ungainly
    (C) critical
    (D) solicitous

54. ZENITH

    (A) vitality
    (B) rage
    (C) reverence
    (D) nadir

55. UNOBTRUSIVE

    (A) resonant
    (B) interfering
    (C) controlled
    (D) subjective

56. REFRACTIVE

    (A) cryptic
    (B) interruptive
    (C) applicable
    (D) direct

57. REBUFF

    (A) exclusion
    (B) disturbance
    (C) recall
    (D) encouragement

58. ADVERSARY

    (A) opponent
    (B) administrator
    (C) accomplice
    (D) enemy

59. ANTAGONIST

    (A) rival
    (B) protagonist
    (C) analyst
    (D) pessimist

60. ALIEN

    (A) native
    (B) anonymous
    (C) verified
    (D) copious

61. ERUDITE

    (A) contagious
    (B) inadvertent
    (C) benevolent
    (D) ignorant

62. PARAMOUNT

    (A) admissible
    (B) inconsequential
    (C) tolerable
    (D) supreme

63. SURREPTITIOUS

    (A) authoritative
    (B) candid
    (C) vulnerable
    (D) subjugated

64. MENDACIOUS

    (A) meddlesome
    (B) incomparable
    (C) malicious
    (D) creditable

65. UNCTUOUS

    (A) awkward
    (B) dubious
    (C) furtive
    (D) disputable

66. IMPETUOUS

    (A) subdued
    (B) unmitigated
    (C) substantial
    (D) egregious

67. PENURIOUS

    (A) frugal
    (B) extravagant
    (C) plausible
    (D) absurd

68. ODIOUS

    (A) attentive
    (B) considerate
    (C) acceptable
    (D) unascertained

69. OSTENSIBLE

    (A) hidden
    (B) preliminary
    (C) authentic
    (D) unsuitable

70. DELETERIOUS

    (A) distressing
    (B) beneficial
    (C) grievous
    (D) delirious

71. IGNOMINY

    (A) honor
    (B) aversion
    (C) perplexity
    (D) remoteness

72. COMPATIBLE

    (A) dexterous
    (B) repugnant
    (C) incongruous
    (D) captivating

73. PREMEDITATED

    (A) devoted
    (B) condescending
    (C) improvised
    (D) supposed

74. PERNICIOUS

    (A) restorative
    (B) conclusive
    (C) tractable
    (D) capricious

75. UMBRAGE

    (A) pique
    (B) monstrous
    (C) reliance
    (D) amity

STOP If you finish before time is called, you may check your work on this section only. Do not turn to any other section in the test.

ANSWER KEY

1. **B**	16. **A**	31. **D**	46. **B**	61. **D**
2. **C**	17. **B**	32. **A**	47. **D**	62. **B**
3. **B**	18. **D**	33. **C**	48. **C**	63. **B**
4. **D**	19. **A**	34. **C**	49. **C**	64. **D**
5. **D**	20. **A**	35. **B**	50. **D**	65. **A**
6. **C**	21. **C**	36. **A**	51. **A**	66. **A**
7. **A**	22. **B**	37. **C**	52. **A**	67. **B**
8. **A**	23. **D**	38. **B**	53. **C**	68. **C**
9. **B**	24. **C**	39. **B**	54. **D**	69. **A**
10. **C**	25. **C**	40. **A**	55. **B**	70. **B**
11. **A**	26. **B**	41. **D**	56. **D**	71. **A**
12. **A**	27. **A**	42. **A**	57. **D**	72. **C**
13. **A**	28. **A**	43. **A**	58. **C**	73. **C**
14. **D**	29. **B**	44. **B**	59. **B**	74. **A**
15. **C**	30. **D**	45. **A**	60. **A**	75. **D**

SKILL WITH VERBAL ANALOGIES

The verbal analogy is one variation of the vocabulary question often encountered on nursing school tests. It tests your understanding of word meanings and your ability to grasp relationships between words and ideas. This practice in mental agility will help you do better with all the other questions on the test.

In addition to their simple meanings, words carry subtle shades of implication that depend in some degree upon the relationship they bear to other words. There are various classifications of relationship, such as similarity (synonyms) and opposition (antonyms). Careful students will try to examine each shade of meaning they encounter.

The ability to detect the exact nature of the relationship between words is a function of your intelligence. In a sense, the verbal analogy test is a vocabulary test. But it is also a test of your ability to analyze meanings, think things out, and see the relationships between ideas and words. In mathematics, this kind of situation is expressed as a proportion problem: 3:5::6:X. Sometimes, verbal analogies are written in this mathematical form:

CLOCK : TIME :: THERMOMETER :

- **(A)** hour
- **(B)** degrees
- **(C)** climate
- **(D)** temperature

Or the question may be put:

CLOCK is to TIME as THERMOMETER is to

- **(A)** hour
- **(B)** degrees
- **(C)** climate
- **(D)** temperature

The challenge is to determine which one of the lettered words has the same relationship to *thermometer* as *time* has to *clock*. The best way to determine the correct answer is to provide a word or phrase that shows the relationship between these words. In the above example, "measures" is a word expressing the relationship. However, this may not be enough. The analogy must be exact. *Climate* or *weather* would not be exact enough. *Temperature*, of course, is the correct answer.

You will find that many of the choices have some relationship to the third word. Select the one with a relationship that *best* approximates the relationship between the first two words.

THREE FORMATS FOR VERBAL ANALOGY QUESTIONS

Some standardized tests provide four answer choices (A,B,C,D) and some five (A,B,C,D,E).

Type 1

From the four pairs of words that follow, select the pair related in the same way as are the words of the first pair.

SPELLING: PUNCTUATION ::

(A) pajamas : fatigue
(B) powder : shaving
(C) bandage : cut
(D) biology : physics

Spelling and *punctuation* are elements of the mechanics of English; *biology* and *physics* are two of the subjects that make up the field of science. The other choices do not possess this part : part relationship. Therefore, (D) is the correct answer.

Type 2

Another popular format gives two words followed by a third word. The latter is related to one word in a group of choices in the same way that the first two words are related.

WINTER : SUMMER :: COLD :

(A) wet
(B) future
(C) hot
(D) freezing

Winter and *summer* bear an opposite relationship. *Cold* and *hot* have the same kind of opposite relationship. Therefore, (C) is the correct answer.

Type 3

Still another analogy format has a variable construction. Any four relationship elements may not be specified. From choices offered—regardless of position—you are to select the one choice that completes the relationship with the other three items. In this example the third element is not specified.

SUBMARINE: FISH :: ____ : BIRD

(A) kite
(B) limousine
(C) feather
(D) chirp

Both a *submarine* and a *fish* are usually found in the water; both a *kite* and a *bird* are customarily seen in the air. Consequently, (A) is the correct answer.

This third type is used in the Miller Analogy Test, considered one of the most reliable and valid tests for selection of graduate students for universities and high-level personnel for government, industry, and business.

CATEGORIZING THE KINDS OF ANALOGY RELATIONSHIPS

1. Purpose Relationship

   GLOVE : BALL ::

   (A) hook : fish
   (B) winter : weather
   (C) game : pennant
   (D) stadium : seats

   The correct answer is (A).

2. Cause-and-Effect Relationship

   RACE : FATIGUE ::

   (A) track : athlete
   (B) ant : bug
   (C) fast : hunger
   (D) walking : running

   The correct answer is (C).

3. Part : Whole Relationship

   SNAKE : REPTILE ::

   (A) patch : thread
   (B) removal : snow
   (C) struggle : wrestle
   (D) hand : clock

   The correct answer is (D).

4. Part : Part Relationship

   GILL : FIN ::

   (A) tube : antenna
   (B) instrument : violin
   (C) sea : fish
   (D) salad : supper

   The correct answer is (A).

5. Action : Object Relationship

   KICK : FOOTBALL ::

   (A) kill : bomb
   (B) break : pieces
   (C) question : team
   (D) smoke : pipe

   The correct answer is (D).

6. Object : Action Relationship

   STEAK : BROIL ::

   (A) bread : bake
   (B) food : eat
   (C) wine : pour
   (D) sugar : spill

   The correct answer is (A).

7. Synonym Relationship

   ENORMOUS : HUGE ::

   (A) rogue : rock
   (B) muddy : unclear
   (C) purse : kitchen
   (D) black : white

   The correct answer is (B).

8. Antonym Relationship

   PURITY : EVIL ::

   (A) suavity : bluntness
   (B) north : climate
   (C) angel : horns
   (D) boldness : victory

   The correct answer is (A).

9. Place Relationship

   MIAMI : FLORIDA ::

   (A) Chicago : United States
   (B) New York : Albany
   (C) United States : Chicago
   (D) Albany : New York

   The correct answer is (D).

10. Degree Relationship

    WARM : HOT ::

    (A) glue : paste
    (B) climate : weather
    (C) fried egg : boiled egg
    (D) bright : genius

    The correct answer is (D).

11. Characteristic Relationship

    IGNORANCE : POVERTY ::

    (A) blood : wound
    (B) money : dollar
    (C) schools : elevators
    (D) education : stupidity

    The correct answer is (A).

12. Sequence Relationship

    SPRING : SUMMER ::

    (A) Thursday : Wednesday
    (B) Wednesday : Monday
    (C) Monday : Sunday
    (D) Wednesday : Thursday

    The correct answer is (D).

13. Grammatical Relationship

    RESTORE : CLIMB ::

    (A) segregation : seem
    (B) into : nymph
    (C) tearoom : although
    (D) overpower : seethe

    The correct answer is (D).

14. Association Relationship

    DEVIL : WRONG ::

    (A) color : sidewalk
    (B) slipper : state
    (C) ink : writing
    (D) picture : bed

    The correct answer is (C).

15. Numerical Relationship

    4 : 12 ::

    (A) 10 : 16
    (B) 9 : 27
    (C) 3 : 4
    (D) 12 : 6

    The correct answer is (B).

POINTS TO REMEMBER

In many analogy questions, the incorrect choices may be related in some way to the first two words. Don't let this association mislead you. For example, in number four (part : part relationship), (A), *tube : antenna* is the correct answer. Choice (C), *sea : fish*, is incorrect, although these two latter words are associated in a general sense with the first two words (*gill : fin*).

Often, the relationship of the first two words may apply to *more than one* of the choices given. In such a case, you must narrow down the initial relationship in order to get the correct choice. For example, in number six (object: action relationship), a *steak* is something that you *broil*. Now let us consider the choices: *bread* is something that you *bake*; food is something that you *eat*; wine is something that you *pour;* and *sugar* is something that you (can) *spill*. Thus far, each choice seems correct. Let us now narrow down the relationship: a *steak* is something that you *broil* with *heat*. The only choice that fulfills this *complete* relationship is (A), *bread*—something that you bake with *heat*. It follows that (A) is the correct answer.

Remember that the keys to analogy success are:

Step One: Determine the relationship between the first two words.

Step Two: Find the same relationship among the choices that follow the first two words.

ANSWER SHEET

PART A

1. Ⓐ Ⓑ Ⓒ Ⓓ	6. Ⓐ Ⓑ Ⓒ Ⓓ	11. Ⓐ Ⓑ Ⓒ Ⓓ	16. Ⓐ Ⓑ Ⓒ Ⓓ	21. Ⓐ Ⓑ Ⓒ Ⓓ
2. Ⓐ Ⓑ Ⓒ Ⓓ	7. Ⓐ Ⓑ Ⓒ Ⓓ	12. Ⓐ Ⓑ Ⓒ Ⓓ	17. Ⓐ Ⓑ Ⓒ Ⓓ	22. Ⓐ Ⓑ Ⓒ Ⓓ
3. Ⓐ Ⓑ Ⓒ Ⓓ	8. Ⓐ Ⓑ Ⓒ Ⓓ	13. Ⓐ Ⓑ Ⓒ Ⓓ	18. Ⓐ Ⓑ Ⓒ Ⓓ	23. Ⓐ Ⓑ Ⓒ Ⓓ
4. Ⓐ Ⓑ Ⓒ Ⓓ	9. Ⓐ Ⓑ Ⓒ Ⓓ	14. Ⓐ Ⓑ Ⓒ Ⓓ	19. Ⓐ Ⓑ Ⓒ Ⓓ	24. Ⓐ Ⓑ Ⓒ Ⓓ
5. Ⓐ Ⓑ Ⓒ Ⓓ	10. Ⓐ Ⓑ Ⓒ Ⓓ	15. Ⓐ Ⓑ Ⓒ Ⓓ	20. Ⓐ Ⓑ Ⓒ Ⓓ	25. Ⓐ Ⓑ Ⓒ Ⓓ

PART B

1. Ⓐ Ⓑ Ⓒ Ⓓ	6. Ⓐ Ⓑ Ⓒ Ⓓ	11. Ⓐ Ⓑ Ⓒ Ⓓ	16. Ⓐ Ⓑ Ⓒ Ⓓ	21. Ⓐ Ⓑ Ⓒ Ⓓ
2. Ⓐ Ⓑ Ⓒ Ⓓ	7. Ⓐ Ⓑ Ⓒ Ⓓ	12. Ⓐ Ⓑ Ⓒ Ⓓ	17. Ⓐ Ⓑ Ⓒ Ⓓ	22. Ⓐ Ⓑ Ⓒ Ⓓ
3. Ⓐ Ⓑ Ⓒ Ⓓ	8. Ⓐ Ⓑ Ⓒ Ⓓ	13. Ⓐ Ⓑ Ⓒ Ⓓ	18. Ⓐ Ⓑ Ⓒ Ⓓ	23. Ⓐ Ⓑ Ⓒ Ⓓ
4. Ⓐ Ⓑ Ⓒ Ⓓ	9. Ⓐ Ⓑ Ⓒ Ⓓ	14. Ⓐ Ⓑ Ⓒ Ⓓ	19. Ⓐ Ⓑ Ⓒ Ⓓ	24. Ⓐ Ⓑ Ⓒ Ⓓ
5. Ⓐ Ⓑ Ⓒ Ⓓ	10. Ⓐ Ⓑ Ⓒ Ⓓ	15. Ⓐ Ⓑ Ⓒ Ⓓ	20. Ⓐ Ⓑ Ⓒ Ⓓ	25. Ⓐ Ⓑ Ⓒ Ⓓ

PART C

1. Ⓐ Ⓑ Ⓒ Ⓓ	6. Ⓐ Ⓑ Ⓒ Ⓓ	11. Ⓐ Ⓑ Ⓒ Ⓓ	16. Ⓐ Ⓑ Ⓒ Ⓓ	21. Ⓐ Ⓑ Ⓒ Ⓓ
2. Ⓐ Ⓑ Ⓒ Ⓓ	7. Ⓐ Ⓑ Ⓒ Ⓓ	12. Ⓐ Ⓑ Ⓒ Ⓓ	17. Ⓐ Ⓑ Ⓒ Ⓓ	22. Ⓐ Ⓑ Ⓒ Ⓓ
3. Ⓐ Ⓑ Ⓒ Ⓓ	8. Ⓐ Ⓑ Ⓒ Ⓓ	13. Ⓐ Ⓑ Ⓒ Ⓓ	18. Ⓐ Ⓑ Ⓒ Ⓓ	23. Ⓐ Ⓑ Ⓒ Ⓓ
4. Ⓐ Ⓑ Ⓒ Ⓓ	9. Ⓐ Ⓑ Ⓒ Ⓓ	14. Ⓐ Ⓑ Ⓒ Ⓓ	19. Ⓐ Ⓑ Ⓒ Ⓓ	24. Ⓐ Ⓑ Ⓒ Ⓓ
5. Ⓐ Ⓑ Ⓒ Ⓓ	10. Ⓐ Ⓑ Ⓒ Ⓓ	15. Ⓐ Ⓑ Ⓒ Ⓓ	20. Ⓐ Ⓑ Ⓒ Ⓓ	25. Ⓐ Ⓑ Ⓒ Ⓓ

VERBAL ANALOGIES TEST

75 Questions ▪▫ Time— 30 Minutes

Directions: In the following questions, determine the relationship between the first pair of capitalized words and then decide which of the answer choices shares a similar relationship with the third capitalized word. Parts A and B of this test are written in mathematical form (expressed as proportion problems). Part A's questions have four answer choices, Part B's questions have five. Part C is written so that relationships are expressed with "is to" and "as."

Part A

25 Questions ▪▫ Time—10 Minutes

1. GUN : SHOTS :: KNIFE :
   - (A) run
   - (B) cuts
   - (C) hat
   - (D) bird

2. EAR : HEAR :: EYE :
   - (A) table
   - (B) hand
   - (C) see
   - (D) foot

3. FUR : MAMMAL :: FEATHERS :
   - (A) bird
   - (B) neck
   - (C) feet
   - (D) bill

4. HANDLE : HAMMER :: KNOB :
   - (A) key
   - (B) room
   - (C) shut
   - (D) door

5. SHOE : FOOT :: HAT :
   - (A) coat
   - (B) nose
   - (C) head
   - (D) collar

6. WATER : DRINK :: BREAD :
   - (A) cake
   - (B) coffee
   - (C) eat
   - (D) pie

7. FOOD : MAN :: GASOLINE :
   - (A) gas
   - (B) oil
   - (C) automobile
   - (D) spark

8. EAT : FAT :: STARVE :
   - (A) thin
   - (B) food
   - (C) bread
   - (D) thirsty

9. MAN : HOUSE :: BIRD :
   - (A) fly
   - (B) insect
   - (C) worm
   - (D) nest

10. GO : COME :: SELL :
    - (A) leave
    - (B) buy
    - (C) money
    - (D) papers

11. PENINSULA : LAND :: BAY :
    - (A) boats
    - (B) pay
    - (C) ocean
    - (D) colony

12. HOUR : MINUTE :: MINUTE :
   (A) hour
   (B) week
   (C) second
   (D) short

13. ABIDE : DEPART :: STAY :
   (A) over
   (B) home
   (C) play
   (D) leave

14. JANUARY : FEBRUARY :: JUNE :
   (A) July
   (B) May
   (C) month
   (D) year

15. BOLD : TIMID :: ADVANCE :
   (A) proceed
   (B) retreat
   (C) campaign
   (D) soldiers

16. ABOVE : BELOW :: TOP :
   (A) spin
   (B) bottom
   (C) surface
   (D) side

17. LION : ANIMAL :: ROSE :
   (A) smell
   (B) leaf
   (C) plant
   (D) thorn

18. TIGER : CARNIVOROUS :: HORSE :
   (A) cow
   (B) nervous
   (C) omnivorous
   (D) herbivorous

19. SAILOR : NAVY :: SOLDIER :
   (A) gun
   (B) cap
   (C) hill
   (D) army

20. PICTURE : SEE :: SOUND :
   (A) noise
   (B) music
   (C) hear
   (D) bark

21. SUCCESS : JOY :: FAILURE :
   (A) sadness
   (B) success
   (C) fail
   (D) work

22. HOPE : DESPAIR :: HAPPINESS :
   (A) frolic
   (B) fun
   (C) joy
   (D) sadness

23. PRETTY : UGLY :: ATTRACT :
   (A) fine
   (B) repel
   (C) nice
   (D) draw

24. PUPIL : TEACHER :: CHILD :
   (A) parent
   (B) dolly
   (C) youngster
   (D) obey

25. CITY : MAYOR :: ARMY :
   (A) navy
   (B) soldier
   (C) general
   (D) private

GO ON TO THE NEXT PAGE

PART B

25 QUESTIONS ▄▭ TIME—10 MINUTES

1. REMUNERATIVE : PROFITABLE ::
   FRAUDULENT:

   (A) lying
   (B) slander
   (C) fallacious
   (D) plausible
   (E) reward

2. AX : WOODSMAN :: AWL :

   (A) cut
   (B) hew
   (C) plumber
   (D) pierce
   (E) cobbler

3. SURGEON : SCALPEL :: BUTCHER :

   (A) mallet
   (B) cleaver
   (C) chisel
   (D) wrench
   (E) medicine

4. CAT : FELINE :: HORSE :

   (A) equine
   (B) tiger
   (C) quadruped
   (D) carnivore
   (E) vulpine

5. ADVERSITY : HAPPINESS ::
   VEHEMENCE :

   (A) misfortune
   (B) gaiety
   (C) troublesome
   (D) petulance
   (E) serenity

6. NECKLACE : ADORNMENT :: MEDAL :

   (A) jewel
   (B) metal
   (C) bravery
   (D) bronze
   (E) decoration

7. GUN : HOLSTER :: SWORD :

   (A) pistol
   (B) scabbard
   (C) warrior
   (D) slay
   (E) plunder

8. ARCHEOLOGIST : ANTIQUITY ::
   ICHTHYOLOGIST :

   (A) theology
   (B) ruins
   (C) horticulture
   (D) marine life
   (E) mystic

9. SHOE : LEATHER :: HIGHWAY :

   (A) passage
   (B) road
   (C) asphalt
   (D) trail
   (E) journey

10. SERFDOM : FEUDALISM ::
    ENTREPRENEUR :

    (A) laissez faire
    (B) captain
    (C) radical
    (D) agriculture
    (E) capitalism

11. FIN : FISH :: PROPELLER :

    (A) automobile
    (B) airplane
    (C) grain elevator
    (D) water
    (E) canoe

12. PULP : PAPER :: HEMP :

    (A) rope
    (B) baskets
    (C) yarn
    (D) cotton
    (E) wood

13. SKIN : MAN :: HIDE :
   (A) scales
   (B) fur
   (C) animal
   (D) hair
   (E) fish

14. RAIN : DROP :: SNOW :
   (A) ice
   (B) cold
   (C) zero
   (D) flake
   (E) sleet

15. WING : BIRD :: HOOF :
   (A) dog
   (B) foot
   (C) horse
   (D) girl
   (E) horseshoe

16. CONSTELLATION : STAR ::
    ARCHIPELAGO :
   (A) continent
   (B) peninsula
   (C) country
   (D) island
   (E) river

17. ACCOUNTANCY : BOOKKEEPING ::
    COURT REPORTING :
   (A) law
   (B) judgment
   (C) stenography
   (D) lawyer
   (E) judge

18. ABSENCE : PRESENCE :: STABLE :
   (A) steady
   (B) secure
   (C) safe
   (D) changeable
   (E) influential

19. RUBBER : FLEXIBILITY :: PIPE :
   (A) iron
   (B) copper
   (C) pliability
   (D) elasticity
   (E) rigidity

20. SAFETY VALVE : BOILER :: FUSE :
   (A) motor
   (B) house
   (C) wire
   (D) city
   (E) factory

21. SCHOLARLY : UNSCHOLARLY ::
    LEARNED :
   (A) ignorant
   (B) wise
   (C) skilled
   (D) scholarly
   (E) literary

22. IMMIGRANT : ARRIVAL :: EMIGRATION :
   (A) leaving
   (B) alienation
   (C) native
   (D) welcoming
   (E) emigrant

23. GOVERNOR : STATE :: GENERAL :
   (A) lieutenant
   (B) navy
   (C) army
   (D) captain
   (E) admiral

24. LETTER CARRIER : MAIL ::
    MESSENGER :
   (A) value
   (B) dispatches
   (C) easy
   (D) complicated
   (E) fast

GO ON TO THE NEXT PAGE

25. CLOTH : COAT :: GINGHAM :

- (A) doll
- (B) cover
- (C) washable
- (D) dress
- (E) dressmaker

PART C

25 QUESTIONS ■□ TIME—10 MINUTES

1. BOAT is to DOCK as AIRPLANE is to

- (A) wing
- (B) strut
- (C) engine
- (D) wind
- (E) hangar

2. OAT is to BUSHEL as DIAMOND is to

- (A) gram
- (B) hardness
- (C) usefulness
- (D) carat
- (E) ornament

3. MEDICINE is to EXAMINATION as LAW is to

- (A) jurist
- (B) court
- (C) interrogation
- (D) contract
- (E) suit

4. PARENT is to COMMAND as CHILD is to

- (A) obey
- (B) will
- (C) women
- (D) love
- (E) achieve

5. CAPTAIN is to VESSEL as DIRECTOR is to

- (A) touring party
- (B) board
- (C) travel
- (D) orchestra
- (E) musician

6. FATHER is to DAUGHTER as UNCLE is to

- (A) son
- (B) daughter
- (C) son-in-law
- (D) niece
- (E) aunt

7. PISTOL is to TRIGGER as MOTOR is to

- (A) wire
- (B) dynamo
- (C) amperes
- (D) barrel
- (E) switch

8. CUBE is to PYRAMID as SQUARE is to

- (A) box
- (B) solid
- (C) pentagon
- (D) triangle
- (E) cylinder

9. PROFIT is to SELLING as FAME is to

- (A) buying
- (B) cheating
- (C) bravery
- (D) praying
- (E) loving

10. BINDING is to BOOK as WELDING is to

- (A) box
- (B) tank
- (C) chair
- (D) wire
- (E) pencil

11. GYMNASIUM is to HEALTH as SCHOOL is to

- (A) sick
- (B) study
- (C) books
- (D) knowledge
- (E) library

12. RIGHT is to WRONG as SUCCEED is to
    (A) aid
    (B) profit
    (C) fail
    (D) error
    (E) gain

13. INDIAN is to AMERICA as ABORIGINE is to
    (A) Hindustan
    (B) Mexico
    (C) soil
    (D) magic
    (E) Australia

14. WEALTH is to MERCENARY as GOLD is to
    (A) lucre
    (B) miner
    (C) fame
    (D) eleemosynary
    (E) South Africa

15. BOTTLE is to BRITTLE as TIRE is to
    (A) elastic
    (B) scarce
    (C) rubber
    (D) spheroid
    (E) automobile

16. SOPRANO is to HIGH as BASS is to
    (A) violin
    (B) good
    (C) low
    (D) fish
    (E) soft

17. OLFACTORY is to NOSE as TACTILE is to
    (A) tacit
    (B) bloody
    (C) finger
    (D) handkerchief
    (E) stomach

18. STREET is to HORIZONTAL as BUILDING is to
    (A) tall
    (B) brick
    (C) broad
    (D) vertical
    (E) large

19. ALLEGIANCE is to LOYALTY as TREASON is to
    (A) obedience
    (B) rebellion
    (C) murder
    (D) felony
    (E) homage

20. CANVAS is to PAINT as MOLD is to
    (A) clay
    (B) cloth
    (C) statue
    (D) art
    (E) aesthetic

21. FISH is to FIN as BIRD is to
    (A) wing
    (B) five
    (C) feet
    (D) beak
    (E) feathers

22. CONQUEST is to ASCENDANCY as DEFEAT is to
    (A) omission
    (B) frustration
    (C) censure
    (D) subjugation
    (E) mastery

23. SOLUTION is to MYSTERY as COMPLETION is to
    (A) puzzle
    (B) books
    (C) college
    (D) school
    (E) detective

GO ON TO THE NEXT PAGE

24. ALUMNUS is to ALUMNA as PRINCE is to

(A) castle
(B) king
(C) knight
(D) country
(E) princess

25. OCCULT is to OVERT as SECRET is to

(A) abstract
(B) outward
(C) science
(D) tarry
(E) concealed

STOP If you finish before time is called, you may check your work on this section only. Do not turn to any other section in the test.

ANSWER KEY

PART A	PART B	PART C
1. B	1. C	1. E
2. C	2. E	2. D
3. A	3. B	3. C
4. D	4. A	4. A
5. C	5. E	5. B
6. C	6. E	6. D
7. C	7. B	7. E
8. A	8. D	8. D
9. D	9. C	9. C
10. B	10. E	10. B
11. C	11. B	11. D
12. C	12. A	12. C
13. D	13. C	13. E
14. A	14. D	14. A
15. B	15. C	15. A
16. B	16. D	16. C
17. C	17. C	17. C
18. D	18. D	18. D
19. D	19. E	19. B
20. C	20. A	20. A
21. A	21. A	21. A
22. D	22. A	22. D
23. B	23. C	23. A
24. A	24. B	24. E
25. C	25. D	25. B

LET'S PUT YOU TO THE TEST

Now that you have thoroughly reviewed the various kinds of verbal-ability items and are familiar with the test-taking strategies associated with them, let's put you to the test.

Pay strict attention to the time allotted for each section of the test and do your best to adhere to the time limits. Read the directions for each part of the test before attempting to answer any of the questions.

This test has three parts: A—Synonyms; B—Antonyms; C—Verbal Analogies. The total time allotted for this test is 50 minutes. Have extra pencils available in case of point breakage, so as not to lose testing time.

An answer key is provided at the end of the test so that you can evaluate your performance. Remember, this is a simulation of the "real thing," so be honest with yourself and look at the answer key only after you have completed the test.

ANSWER SHEET

Part A: Synonyms

1. Ⓐ Ⓑ Ⓒ Ⓓ	8. Ⓐ Ⓑ Ⓒ Ⓓ	15. Ⓐ Ⓑ Ⓒ Ⓓ	22. Ⓐ Ⓑ Ⓒ Ⓓ	29. Ⓐ Ⓑ Ⓒ Ⓓ
2. Ⓐ Ⓑ Ⓒ Ⓓ	9. Ⓐ Ⓑ Ⓒ Ⓓ	16. Ⓐ Ⓑ Ⓒ Ⓓ	23. Ⓐ Ⓑ Ⓒ Ⓓ	30. Ⓐ Ⓑ Ⓒ Ⓓ
3. Ⓐ Ⓑ Ⓒ Ⓓ	10. Ⓐ Ⓑ Ⓒ Ⓓ	17. Ⓐ Ⓑ Ⓒ Ⓓ	24. Ⓐ Ⓑ Ⓒ Ⓓ	31. Ⓐ Ⓑ Ⓒ Ⓓ
4. Ⓐ Ⓑ Ⓒ Ⓓ	11. Ⓐ Ⓑ Ⓒ Ⓓ	18. Ⓐ Ⓑ Ⓒ Ⓓ	25. Ⓐ Ⓑ Ⓒ Ⓓ	32. Ⓐ Ⓑ Ⓒ Ⓓ
5. Ⓐ Ⓑ Ⓒ Ⓓ	12. Ⓐ Ⓑ Ⓒ Ⓓ	19. Ⓐ Ⓑ Ⓒ Ⓓ	26. Ⓐ Ⓑ Ⓒ Ⓓ	33. Ⓐ Ⓑ Ⓒ Ⓓ
6. Ⓐ Ⓑ Ⓒ Ⓓ	13. Ⓐ Ⓑ Ⓒ Ⓓ	20. Ⓐ Ⓑ Ⓒ Ⓓ	27. Ⓐ Ⓑ Ⓒ Ⓓ	34. Ⓐ Ⓑ Ⓒ Ⓓ
7. Ⓐ Ⓑ Ⓒ Ⓓ	14. Ⓐ Ⓑ Ⓒ Ⓓ	21. Ⓐ Ⓑ Ⓒ Ⓓ	28. Ⓐ Ⓑ Ⓒ Ⓓ	35. Ⓐ Ⓑ Ⓒ Ⓓ

Part B: Antonyms

1. Ⓐ Ⓑ Ⓒ Ⓓ	9. Ⓐ Ⓑ Ⓒ Ⓓ	17. Ⓐ Ⓑ Ⓒ Ⓓ	25. Ⓐ Ⓑ Ⓒ Ⓓ	33. Ⓐ Ⓑ Ⓒ Ⓓ
2. Ⓐ Ⓑ Ⓒ Ⓓ	10. Ⓐ Ⓑ Ⓒ Ⓓ	18. Ⓐ Ⓑ Ⓒ Ⓓ	26. Ⓐ Ⓑ Ⓒ Ⓓ	34. Ⓐ Ⓑ Ⓒ Ⓓ
3. Ⓐ Ⓑ Ⓒ Ⓓ	11. Ⓐ Ⓑ Ⓒ Ⓓ	19. Ⓐ Ⓑ Ⓒ Ⓓ	27. Ⓐ Ⓑ Ⓒ Ⓓ	35. Ⓐ Ⓑ Ⓒ Ⓓ
4. Ⓐ Ⓑ Ⓒ Ⓓ	12. Ⓐ Ⓑ Ⓒ Ⓓ	20. Ⓐ Ⓑ Ⓒ Ⓓ	28. Ⓐ Ⓑ Ⓒ Ⓓ	36. Ⓐ Ⓑ Ⓒ Ⓓ
5. Ⓐ Ⓑ Ⓒ Ⓓ	13. Ⓐ Ⓑ Ⓒ Ⓓ	21. Ⓐ Ⓑ Ⓒ Ⓓ	29. Ⓐ Ⓑ Ⓒ Ⓓ	37. Ⓐ Ⓑ Ⓒ Ⓓ
6. Ⓐ Ⓑ Ⓒ Ⓓ	14. Ⓐ Ⓑ Ⓒ Ⓓ	22. Ⓐ Ⓑ Ⓒ Ⓓ	30. Ⓐ Ⓑ Ⓒ Ⓓ	38. Ⓐ Ⓑ Ⓒ Ⓓ
7. Ⓐ Ⓑ Ⓒ Ⓓ	15. Ⓐ Ⓑ Ⓒ Ⓓ	23. Ⓐ Ⓑ Ⓒ Ⓓ	31. Ⓐ Ⓑ Ⓒ Ⓓ	39. Ⓐ Ⓑ Ⓒ Ⓓ
8. Ⓐ Ⓑ Ⓒ Ⓓ	16. Ⓐ Ⓑ Ⓒ Ⓓ	24. Ⓐ Ⓑ Ⓒ Ⓓ	32. Ⓐ Ⓑ Ⓒ Ⓓ	40. Ⓐ Ⓑ Ⓒ Ⓓ

Part C: Verbal Analogies

1. Ⓐ Ⓑ Ⓒ Ⓓ	6. Ⓐ Ⓑ Ⓒ Ⓓ	11. Ⓐ Ⓑ Ⓒ Ⓓ	16. Ⓐ Ⓑ Ⓒ Ⓓ	21. Ⓐ Ⓑ Ⓒ Ⓓ
2. Ⓐ Ⓑ Ⓒ Ⓓ	7. Ⓐ Ⓑ Ⓒ Ⓓ	12. Ⓐ Ⓑ Ⓒ Ⓓ	17. Ⓐ Ⓑ Ⓒ Ⓓ	22. Ⓐ Ⓑ Ⓒ Ⓓ
3. Ⓐ Ⓑ Ⓒ Ⓓ	8. Ⓐ Ⓑ Ⓒ Ⓓ	13. Ⓐ Ⓑ Ⓒ Ⓓ	18. Ⓐ Ⓑ Ⓒ Ⓓ	23. Ⓐ Ⓑ Ⓒ Ⓓ
4. Ⓐ Ⓑ Ⓒ Ⓓ	9. Ⓐ Ⓑ Ⓒ Ⓓ	14. Ⓐ Ⓑ Ⓒ Ⓓ	19. Ⓐ Ⓑ Ⓒ Ⓓ	24. Ⓐ Ⓑ Ⓒ Ⓓ
5. Ⓐ Ⓑ Ⓒ Ⓓ	10. Ⓐ Ⓑ Ⓒ Ⓓ	15. Ⓐ Ⓑ Ⓒ Ⓓ	20. Ⓐ Ⓑ Ⓒ Ⓓ	25. Ⓐ Ⓑ Ⓒ Ⓓ

FINAL VERBAL ABILITY EXAMINATION

100 QUESTIONS ■ TIME—50 MINUTES

PART A: SYNONYMS

35 QUESTIONS ■ TIME— 20 MINUTES

Directions: In each of the sentences below, one word is in italics. Following each sentence are four words or phrases. For each sentence, select the word or phrase that best corresponds in meaning to the italicized word.

1. The chart *classifies* these organisms.

   (A) fuses
   (B) categorizes
   (C) controls
   (D) camouflages

2. On many teams, a player may face a *penalty* for irresponsible or unruly behavior.

   (A) arrangement
   (B) gratification
   (C) punishment
   (D) precaution

3. He used the *allotted* study time to complete his assignments.

   (A) authorized
   (B) designated
   (C) agreed
   (D) alerted

4. When examining the *notochord*, you will find it to be a flexible, rodlike structure.

   (A) backbone
   (B) muscle
   (C) tissue
   (D) pharynx

5. It was apparent that he had attempted to *concoct* an alibi.

   (A) inculcate
   (B) conceal
   (C) reveal
   (D) fabricate

6. The City Council could have avoided this *sanction* by passing the ordinance.

   (A) preliminary plan
   (B) obliteration
   (C) veneration
   (D) penalty

7. *Lipids* are organic compounds that store and release large amounts of energy.

   (A) enzymes
   (B) diatoms
   (C) proteins
   (D) fats

8. The soldiers retreated to a position of *comparative* safety.

   (A) objective
   (B) relative
   (C) subjective
   (D) scientific

9. Geologists *assure* us that our earth is a few billion years old.

   (A) guarantee
   (B) instruct
   (C) deny
   (D) assail

10. It has been said that he is a *connoisseur* of fine wines.

    (A) expert on
    (B) taster of
    (C) procurer of
    (D) vendor of

11. He *spurned* the name that had won him this dishonor.

    (A) lauded
    (B) extolled
    (C) acclaimed
    (D) repudiated

12. The well-dressed gentleman bowed *ceremoniously*.

    (A) without ritual
    (B) disrespectfully
    (C) serenely
    (D) formally

13. Food is moved through the digestive system by *peristalsis*.

    (A) periosteum
    (B) contractions
    (C) metabolism
    (D) protists

14. The annual parade *traversed* this magnificent city from the east to the west side.

    (A) was patronized
    (B) extended
    (C) crossed
    (D) augmented

15. *Enraptured* by the beauty of the mountains, they had not spoken for twenty minutes.

    (A) summoned
    (B) impeded
    (C) exonerated
    (D) entranced

16. The results of the experiment upheld the *contention* of those who supported the hypothesis.

    (A) realization
    (B) contiguity
    (C) argument
    (D) exhilaration

17. The *consensus* of the group

    (A) stipulation
    (B) regulation
    (C) conviction
    (D) collective opinion

18. Arthritis is a *chronic* disease that results from a faulty immune system.

    (A) long-lasting
    (B) serious
    (C) contagious
    (D) infectious

19. Mayan magnificence *abounds* in the small resort village of Kailuum.

    (A) is remote
    (B) is abundant
    (C) is significant
    (D) is inadequate

20. If enthusiasm for the project *waxed* under the direction of a newly appointed administrator, the level of excitement

    (A) stirred.
    (B) waned.
    (C) vanished.
    (D) increased.

21. *Void* of intellectual stimuli

    (A) composed
    (B) in excess
    (C) empty
    (D) full

22. The injuries sustained resulted in paralysis in two of the four *appendages*.

    (A) chambers
    (B) muscles
    (C) limbs
    (D) tubes

23. Security was *risked* to attain maximum career satisfaction.

    (A) ventured
    (B) squandered
    (C) exhausted
    (D) wasted

24. The fruit was *pared* and sliced for the salad.

    (A) divided
    (B) rinsed
    (C) peeled
    (D) sectioned

GO ON TO THE NEXT PAGE

25. Biogenesis is *a theory* that supports that living things can be produced only from other living things.

    (A) a principle
    (B) an opinion
    (C) a rationale
    (D) an experimentation

26. The introduction *delineates* the book's content and format.

    (A) discredits
    (B) describes
    (C) sanctions
    (D) endorses

27. The X ray clearly showed the torn *cartilage* in the knee.

    (A) tissue
    (B) ligament
    (C) tendon
    (D) membrane

28. The receptionist *confirmed* the appointment.

    (A) canceled
    (B) rescheduled
    (C) verified
    (D) recorded

29. Arthropod is the *phylum* that includes insects, spiders, centipedes, and surprisingly, shrimp.

    (A) the fifth highest taxonomical category of the animal kingdom
    (B) the second highest taxonomical category of the animal kingdom
    (C) the fourth highest taxonomical category of the animal kingdom
    (D) the third highest taxonomical category of the animal kingdom

30. If the engine was *malfunctioning* at the time, it was

    (A) operative.
    (B) operating incorrectly.
    (C) firing.
    (D) igniting.

31. The clients were shocked at the *fraudulent* practices of the contractors.

    (A) thorough
    (B) extensive
    (C) legal
    (D) deceitful

32. The employer questioned the *competence* of his staff. The employer was not sure about their

    (A) honesty.
    (B) punctuality.
    (C) credibility.
    (D) ability.

33. The reading list included an *anthology* by a famous author.

    (A) collection of literary selections
    (B) annotated bibliography
    (C) archaeological study
    (D) autobiography

34. Some bacteria are mobile because of their *flagellum*.

    (A) cili
    (B) bacilli
    (C) cytoplasm
    (D) tails

35. He smiled *wryly*.

    (A) deceptively
    (B) nastily
    (C) ironically
    (D) delightedly

PART B: ANTONYMS

40 QUESTIONS ■□ TIME—15 MINUTES

Directions: For each of the following test items, select the word that is opposite in meaning to the term printed in capital letters.

1. IMPERIOUS
   - (A) submissive
   - (B) valuable
   - (C) pointed
   - (D) positive

2. CAPRICIOUS
   - (A) whimsical
   - (B) judicious
   - (C) steadfast
   - (D) tranquil

3. CANTANKEROUS
   - (A) pleasant
   - (B) dubious
   - (C) effective
   - (D) awkward

4. FORBEARANCE
   - (A) indulgence
   - (B) pliancy
   - (C) politeness
   - (D) impatience

5. HAPHAZARD
   - (A) inefficient
   - (B) premeditated
   - (C) unsatisfactory
   - (D) blundering

6. INEFFABLE
   - (A) forgettable
   - (B) exquisite
   - (C) unorganized
   - (D) race

7. CHIMERICAL
   - (A) philosophical
   - (B) elite
   - (C) factual
   - (D) unimpressive

8. REPRESS
   - (A) reserve
   - (B) liberate
   - (C) thrust
   - (D) precipitate

9. ABOMINABLE
   - (A) agreeable
   - (B) loathsome
   - (C) sufficient
   - (D) degrading

10. UNETHICAL
    - (A) vulgar
    - (B) feasible
    - (C) pompous
    - (D) scrupulous

11. ANTECEDENT
    - (A) previous
    - (B) subsequent
    - (C) foregoing
    - (D) propitious

12. PONDEROUS
    - (A) delicate
    - (B) potent
    - (C) supportive
    - (D) massive

13. SUPPLICATION
    - (A) worship
    - (B) compassion
    - (C) entreaty
    - (D) disdain

14. POSITIVE
    - (A) negative
    - (B) sensitive
    - (C) diplomatic
    - (D) popular

15. RENEGADE
    - (A) constant
    - (B) extricate
    - (C) obedient
    - (D) heretical

GO ON TO THE NEXT PAGE

16. DISREGARD

(A) disown
(B) respond
(C) revoke
(D) recover

17. WRATH

(A) delight
(B) travail
(C) frivolity
(D) detriment

18. TEDIOUS

(A) ungainly
(B) imperative
(C) stimulating
(D) suitable

19. EMBODY

(A) impel
(B) fuse
(C) dissociate
(D) collect

20. DEFERRABLE

(A) urgent
(B) furtive
(C) inclined
(D) deniable

21. HOMOGENOUS

(A) invariable
(B) homosexual
(C) importunate
(D) heterogeneous

22. ADHERENT

(A) disciple
(B) repudiator
(C) soothsayer
(D) hypocrite

23. CRUDE

(A) barbarous
(B) refined
(C) obscure
(D) covetous

24. DAFT

(A) cynical
(B) sharp
(C) prevalent
(D) sensible

25. GRAPHIC

(A) vague
(B) illustrative
(C) forcible
(D) glacial

26. DEVASTATE

(A) tolerate
(B) obstruct
(C) renovate
(D) promote

27. STRINGENT

(A) exacting
(B) tough
(C) influential
(D) flexible

28. ACQUIESCE

(A) contest
(B) invest
(C) dismiss
(D) supply

29. BREVITY

(A) abbreviation
(B) length
(C) ramification
(D) delusion

30. FLAUNT

(A) disavow
(B) conserve
(C) blight
(D) astonish

31. CULTIVATE

(A) restore
(B) stifle
(C) reinstate
(D) nurture

32. DILATE

   (A) negate
   (B) abet
   (C) constrict
   (D) suspend

33. BEFITTING

   (A) enhancing
   (B) conciliatory
   (C) inappropriate
   (D) elegant

34. COHERENT

   (A) illogical
   (B) consecutive
   (C) cognizant
   (D) courtly

35. PALTRY

   (A) political
   (B) complaisant
   (C) clever
   (D) impressive

36. BUCOLIC

   (A) urbane
   (B) gallant
   (C) valiant
   (D) functional

37. EXTRAVAGANT

   (A) coarse
   (B) superior
   (C) frugal
   (D) typical

38. LENIENCY

   (A) indulgence
   (B) severity
   (C) embroilment
   (D) inequality

39. MANIFEST

   (A) latent
   (B) oblivious
   (C) terminal
   (D) languid

40. PLEBEIAN

   (A) congenial
   (B) ignoble
   (C) scientific
   (D) patrician

PART C: VERBAL ANALOGIES
25 QUESTIONS ▪▫ TIME—15 MINUTES

Directions: In the following questions, determine the relationship between the first pair of capitalized words and then decide which of the choices share a similar relationship with the third capitalized word.

1. CAT is to DOG as TIGER is to

   (A) wild
   (B) fur
   (C) wolf
   (D) bovine

2. SALINE is to SALT as SWEET is to

   (A) sugar
   (B) stale
   (C) bread
   (D) insipid

3. FLANNEL is to WOOL as LINEN is to

   (A) cotton
   (B) flax
   (C) silk
   (D) rayon

4. CONTEMPORARY is to PRESENT as POSTERITY is to

   (A) past
   (B) present
   (C) future
   (D) ancient

5. MOON is to EARTH as EARTH is to

   (A) space
   (B) moon
   (C) sky
   (D) sun

GO ON TO THE NEXT PAGE

6. ACUTE is to CHRONIC as INTENSE is to
   - (A) sardonic
   - (B) tonic
   - (C) persistent
   - (D) pretty

7. VALLEY is to GORGE as MOUNTAIN is to
   - (A) freshet
   - (B) cliff
   - (C) steep
   - (D) high

8. EAST is to WEST as NORTHWEST is to
   - (A) southeast
   - (B) southwest
   - (C) north
   - (D) northeast

9. GASOLINE is to PETROLEUM as SUGAR is to
   - (A) oil
   - (B) cane
   - (C) plant
   - (D) sweet

10. AGGRAVATE is to TEASE as FONDLE is to
    - (A) vex
    - (B) wound
    - (C) embrace
    - (D) pursuit

11. LATITUDE is to LONGITUDE as WARP is to
    - (A) weave
    - (B) woof
    - (C) thread
    - (D) line

12. EDGE is to CENTER as EFFUSIVE is to
    - (A) unemotional
    - (B) exuberant
    - (C) eclectic
    - (D) eccentricity

13. DISCIPLE is to MENTOR as PROSELYTE is to
    - (A) opinion
    - (B) expedition
    - (C) leader
    - (D) football

14. SOPHISTICATION is to FINESSE as INEPTITUDE is to
    - (A) inefficiency
    - (B) artistry
    - (C) trickiness
    - (D) insatiability

15. CAPTAIN is to STEAMSHIP as PRINCIPAL is to
    - (A) interest
    - (B) school
    - (C) agent
    - (D) concern

16. DIME is to SILVER as PENNY is to
    - (A) mint
    - (B) copper
    - (C) currency
    - (D) value

17. REVERT is to REVERSION as SYMPATHIZE is to
    - (A) sympathetic
    - (B) symposium
    - (C) sympathy
    - (D) sympathizer

18. REGRESSIVE is to REGRESS as STERILE is to
    - (A) sterilization
    - (B) sterilize
    - (C) sterility
    - (D) sterilizer

19. DOWN is to UP as AGE is to
    - (A) year
    - (B) youth
    - (C) snow
    - (D) date

20. I is to MINE as MAN is to
    - (A) men
    - (B) his
    - (C) man's
    - (D) mine

21. DISLOYAL is to FAITHLESS as IMPERFECTION is to

    (A) faithful
    (B) depression
    (C) foible
    (D) decrepitude

22. NECKLACE is to PEARLS as CHAIN is to

    (A) locket
    (B) prisoner
    (C) links
    (D) clasp

23. DRIFT is to SNOW as DUNE is to

    (A) hill
    (B) rain
    (C) sand
    (D) hail

24. DILIGENT is to UNREMITTING as COMPLETE is to

    (A) pretentious
    (B) diametric
    (C) adamant
    (D) dietetic

25. SCHOONER is to VESSEL as PERSIMMON is to

    (A) machine
    (B) fruit
    (C) engine
    (D) vehicle

STOP If you finish before time is called, you may check your work on this section only. Do not turn to any other section in the test.

ANSWER KEY

PART A: SYNONYMS

1. **B**	8. **B**	15. **D**	22. **C**	29. **B**
2. **C**	9. **A**	16. **C**	23. **A**	30. **B**
3. **B**	10. **A**	17. **D**	24. **C**	31. **D**
4. **A**	11. **D**	18. **A**	25. **A**	32. **D**
5. **D**	12. **D**	19. **B**	26. **B**	33. **A**
6. **D**	13. **B**	20. **D**	27. **A**	34. **D**
7. **D**	14. **C**	21. **C**	28. **C**	35. **C**

PART B: ANTONYMS

1. **A**	9. **A**	17. **A**	25. **A**	33. **C**
2. **C**	10. **D**	18. **C**	26. **C**	34. **A**
3. **A**	11. **B**	19. **C**	27. **D**	35. **D**
4. **D**	12. **A**	20. **A**	28. **A**	36. **A**
5. **B**	13. **D**	21. **D**	29. **B**	37. **C**
6. **A**	14. **A**	22. **B**	30. **A**	38. **B**
7. **C**	15. **C**	23. **B**	31. **B**	39. **A**
8. **B**	16. **B**	24. **D**	32. **C**	40. **D**

PART C: VERBAL ANALOGIES

1. **C**	6. **C**	11. **B**	16. **B**	21. **C**
2. **A**	7. **B**	12. **A**	17. **C**	22. **C**
3. **B**	8. **A**	13. **C**	18. **B**	23. **C**
4. **C**	9. **B**	14. **A**	19. **B**	24. **B**
5. **D**	10. **C**	15. **B**	20. **C**	25. **B**

MATHEMATICS

MATHEMATICS REVIEW

The review of mathematics in this section and the numerical ability tests include the following: basic quantitative problems involving addition, subtraction, multiplication, and division; calculations including decimals, fractions, percentages, and measurements; basic operations in algebra and geometry; and quantitative comparison questions. Throughout the exercises, emphasis is placed on verbal problems in order to prepare you for the interpretations and methods required for problem solving. The explanatory answers and problem solutions provide a variety of opportunities to review or to learn the numerical processes included on the pre-nursing examinations.

Study the guidelines listed below; they provide the major concepts needed for successful performance on your mathematics examination.

TIPS FOR STUDYING MATHEMATICS

In order to perform well on mathematics tests, it is important to be well prepared. To prepare, you must know what material will be covered on the test. The mathematics guidelines and practice exercises in this book provide a review of materials that are covered on the mathematics section of the nursing school entrance examination. You can maximize your performance on the test by following the steps below.

1. Choose a place to study where you won't be distracted.

2. Set aside adequate time to study. Try to set aside at least one hour for each study session. Study and practice each day if possible. Make a study schedule and stick to it.

3. Give your full focus and attention to your studies.

4. Read the explanatory material in your book before doing any practice tests. Make sure that you understand what you're reading. Review information that you don't understand, and use other references when necessary.

5. Take the practice tests under test conditions. Read the instructions carefully. Complete tests in the amount of time suggested. Use the problem-solving strategies below.

6. Compare your answers with those provided in the book. Carefully review answers to questions that you missed.

7. Seek help if you don't understand a problem after several tries.

8. Review regularly, and practice, practice, practice.

TEST-TAKING TIPS

There are four basic steps involved in solving mathematics problems. They are: Read the problem; plan how to solve the problem; solve the problem; and check your solution. These steps are explained in more detail in the tips given below.

- Read test instructions carefully. Note the amount of time allotted for completion of the test and pace yourself accordingly.

- Read each problem carefully for clarity and understanding. Make sure you understand the concepts and terms being used. Try to restate the problem in your own words.

- Simplify the problem by breaking it down into smaller parts.

- Determine what information is given and what is to be solved.

- Determine whether there is sufficient information given to solve the problem.

- Eliminate extraneous information.

- Choose a strategy for solving the problem.

- Express your answer in the number of units requested. You may be asked to express your answer in terms of minutes, feet, or hours, or you may be asked to write your answer as a decimal or fraction.

- Check your solution to determine if it is reasonable. Does your answer appear to be unreasonably large or small?

- Don't spend too much time on a question that you find difficult. Move on to the next question and return to the problem after you complete the other test questions.

- Try an alternative strategy if the one you used didn't work.

- Review your answers if you finish before time is up. Check your computations very carefully.

GUIDELINES FOR MATHEMATIC CALCULATIONS

I. **Whole Numbers and Fractions**

   A. **Whole Numbers**

      1. Whole numbers have **place-value** based on units of ten (decimal system). Therefore, it is important that all whole numbers, including zeros, are lined up correctly in columns when adding and subtracting.

Example: a) Place values for the whole number 5,264 are illustrated below.

$$5,264 = (5 \times 1,000) + (2 \times 100) + (6 \times 10) + (4 \times 1)$$

           b) Numbers are lined up according to place values in the following **addition** and **subtraction** examples.

```
  5,264      5,264
+   478    −   478
 ------     ------
  5,742      4,786
```

2. Use **multiplication** to determine the value of several quantities with the same value if the value of one quantity is given.

Example: If one loaf of bread costs $0.80, how much will three loaves of bread cost? Multiply 3 times $0.80: The answer is $2.40.

When multiplying, be certain to include all zeros and to keep the columns in line.

Example:

$$
\begin{array}{r}
3,600 \\
\times\ \ \ \ 507 \\
\hline
25,200 \\
0000 \\
18,000 \\
\hline
1,825,200
\end{array}
$$

3. Use **division** to determine the value of one quantity when the value of several quantities is given.

Example: Three loaves of bread cost $2.40. How much will one loaf cost? Divide 3 into $2.40. The answer is $0.80 (3 is the divisor, $2.40 is the dividend, and the quotient is $0.80).

Divisibility Rules

a)   If the last digit of a number is 0, 2, 4, 6, or 8, the number is divisible by 2.

b)   If the last digit of a number ends in 0 or 5, the number is divisible by 5.

c)   If the sum of the digits of a number is divisible by 3, the number is divisible by 3.

Example: The sum of the digits of 234 is $2 + 3 + 4 = 9$. Since 9 is divisible by 3, we know that 234 is also divisible by 3 ($234 \div 3 = 78$).

d)   If the sum of the digits of a number is divisible by 9, the number is divisible by 9. In the example above, it was shown that the sum of the digits of 234 is 9. By the above rule, we know that 234 is divisible by 9.

e)   If the number represented by the last two digits of a number is divisible by 4, the number is divisible by 4.

32 is the number represented by the last two digits of 232. Since 32 is divisible by 4, the number 232 is divisible by 4.

f)   Note that it is not possible to divide by zero.

4. A **prime number** is any whole number other than 0 or 1 that is only divisible by itself and by 1.

Example: 17 is a prime number since it is only divisible by 1 and 17. The whole numbers 2, 3, 5, 7, and 11 are the first five prime numbers.

Divisibility rules can be used to find the prime factors of whole numbers.

Example: 24 is divisible by 2 (last digit is 4) and is divisible by 3 (sum of digits is 6).

a) $24 = 2 \times 2 \times 2 \times 3$
    $= 2^3 \times 3$

b)

c)

Two methods for determining the prime factors of a number are illustrated in examples b and c. In each method, keep dividing until your quotient is a prime number.

5. The **average** of a set of numbers is the sum of the numbers divided by the number of numbers added.

Example: The average of the numbers 10, 14, 17, and 23 is $\dfrac{10 + 14 + 17 + 23}{4} = \dfrac{64}{4} = 16$.

6. The **square** of a number is the product obtained when a number is multiplied by itself.

Example: $4^2 = 4 \times 4 = 16$

7. The **square root** ($\sqrt{}$) of a given number is the number that yields the given number when multiplied by itself.

Example: $\sqrt{16} = 4$, since $4 \times 4 = 16$

8. The square of any whole number is called a **perfect square**. Conversely, the square root of a perfect square is a whole number.

Example: $4^2 = 16$ (a perfect square); thus $\sqrt{16} = 4$.

9. If a number is not a perfect square, you can **approximate the square root** of the number when a calculator is not available. One method of approximating the square root of a number is given below.

Example: Approximate the square root of 90 ($\sqrt{90}$).

a) Estimate the square root of the given number. Since 90 is between 81 and 100, the square root of 90 will be between 9 and 10. A possible estimate is 9.30.

b) Divide the given number by the estimated square root.

$90 \div 9.30 = 9.68$

c) Find the average of the resulting quotient and the estimated square root.

$$\frac{9.68 + 9.30}{2} = 9.49 \text{ (9.49 is the first approximation for } \sqrt{90})$$

d) Divide the given number by the average (first approximation) found above.

$$90 \div 9.49 = 9.48$$

e) Find the **average of the divisor** (first approximation) and the **quotient** found in step 4.

$$\frac{9.49 + 9.48}{2} = 9.485$$

The approximate square root of 90 is 9.485.

This process may be repeated to get a more accurate estimate of the square root of a number.

10. To add or subtract **radicals** (numbers expressed as square roots), the **radicands** (numbers under the radical) must be the same.

Example: $4\sqrt{12} + 3\sqrt{12} = 7\sqrt{12}$

Example: If the radicands are *not* the same, simplify the radicals and then see if they can be combined.

$$\begin{aligned}
3\sqrt{12} - 8\sqrt{3} &= 3(\sqrt{4} \times \sqrt{3}) - 8\sqrt{3} &&\text{(12 can be factored as } 4 \times 3) \\
&= 3 \times 2\sqrt{3} - 8\sqrt{3} &&\text{(take } \sqrt{4}, \text{ which equals 2)} \\
&= 6\sqrt{3} - 8\sqrt{3} \\
&= -2\sqrt{3}
\end{aligned}$$

B. Fractions

A fraction is a part of something. A fraction is expressed using two terms: a **numerator**, which is the number above the fraction line, and a **denominator**, which is the number below the fraction line.

In the fraction $\frac{3}{4}$, the numerator is 3 and the denominator is 4.

A **proper fraction** is one whose numerator is less than its denominator. An **improper fraction** has a numerator that is equal to or greater than its denominator.

$\frac{4}{5}$ is a proper fraction and $\frac{7}{3}$ is an improper fraction.

An improper fraction can be expressed as a **mixed number**, which has both a whole and a fractional part. (Divide the denominator into the numerator to get the whole part. The remainder will be the numerator and the divisor will be the denominator of the fractional part.)

Example: $\frac{7}{3} = 2\frac{1}{3}$

7 divided by 3 gives a quotient of 2 and a remainder of 1.

1. **Reducing Fractions**

   Factor the numerator and denominator into prime factors and divide the numerator and denominator by the common factors. (The value of a fraction is unchanged when the numerator and denominator are multiplied or divided by the same number.)

   Example: $\dfrac{35}{35} = \dfrac{7 \times 5}{11 \times 5} = \dfrac{7}{11}$

   Note that the numerator and denominator were divided by 5.

2. **Multiplying Fractions**

   To multiply two fractions, multiply the two numerators to get the numerator of the product of the two fractions, and multiply the two denominators to get the denominator of the product of the fractions. Then simplify the resulting fraction by reducing it to lowest terms and/or by changing it to a mixed number.

   Example: $\dfrac{6}{9} \times \dfrac{3}{8} = \dfrac{18}{72} = \dfrac{2 \times 3 \times 3}{2 \times 2 \times 2 \times 3 \times 3} = \dfrac{1}{4}$

3. **Dividing Fractions**

   To divide two fractions, invert the divisor, then multiply the two fractions and simplify.

   Examples: $\dfrac{9}{20} \div \dfrac{3}{4} = \dfrac{9}{20} \times \dfrac{4}{3} = \dfrac{36}{60} = \dfrac{2 \times 2 \times 3 \times 3}{2 \times 2 \times 3 \times 5} = \dfrac{3}{5}$

   $2\dfrac{2}{3} \div 4 = \dfrac{8}{3} \times \dfrac{1}{4} = \dfrac{8}{12} = \dfrac{2 \times 2 \times 2}{2 \times 2 \times 3} = \dfrac{2}{3}$

   Note that the mixed number $2\dfrac{2}{3}$ was changed to the improper fraction $\dfrac{8}{3}$, and the inversion of the whole number 4, which equals $\dfrac{4}{1}$, is $\dfrac{1}{4}$.

4. **Adding and Subtracting Fractions**

   a) To add or subtract fractions with the **same**, or common, denominator, keep the common denominator and add or subtract the numerators of the fractions.

   Examples: $\dfrac{7}{9} = \dfrac{4}{9} = \dfrac{11}{9} = 1\dfrac{2}{9}$

   $\dfrac{15}{32} - \dfrac{5}{32} = \dfrac{10}{32} = \dfrac{5}{16}$

   b) To add or subtract fractions with **different** denominators, express the fractions as equivalent fractions with a common denominator. The lowest common denominator is the smallest number that can be divided evenly by the denominators of the given fractions. To find the **lowest common denominator (LCD)** of two fractions, first express each denominator as a product of its prime factors. The lowest common denominator will be the number formed by multiplying each prime factor the largest number of times it occurs in the factorization of the denominators.

Examples: (1) $\dfrac{5}{9} + \dfrac{7}{12} = \dfrac{20}{36} + \dfrac{21}{36} = \dfrac{41}{36} = 1\dfrac{5}{36}$

Since $9 = 3 \times 3$ and $12 = 3 \times 4$, the lowest common denominator of 9 and 12 is $3 \times 3 \times 4 = 36$.

(2) $\dfrac{7}{24} - \dfrac{9}{150}$

$150 = 2 \times 3 \times 5 \times 5$
$24 = 2 \times 2 \times 2 \times 3$

The largest number of times that 2 appears as a factor is 3 and the largest number of times that 5 appears as a factor is 2. Three appears as a factor only once in each of the factorizations.

Thus, the lowest common denominator of the two fractions is 600.

$2 \times 2 \times 2 \times 3 \times 5 \times 5 = 600$

$\dfrac{7}{24} - \dfrac{9}{150} = \dfrac{7}{24} \times \dfrac{25}{25} - \dfrac{9}{150} \times \dfrac{4}{4} = \dfrac{175}{600} - \dfrac{36}{600} = \dfrac{139}{600}$

Thus $\dfrac{7}{24} - \dfrac{9}{150} = \dfrac{175}{600} - \dfrac{36}{600} = \dfrac{139}{600}$

(3) $4\dfrac{2}{3} - 1\dfrac{3}{4} = 4\dfrac{8}{12} - 1\dfrac{9}{12}$

Since $\dfrac{9}{12}$ is greater than $\dfrac{8}{12}$, $4\dfrac{8}{12}$ is changed to $3 + 1 + \dfrac{8}{12}$.

(note that $1 = \dfrac{12}{12}$)

$= 3 + \dfrac{12}{12} + \dfrac{8}{12}$

$= 3 + \dfrac{20}{12}$ or $3\dfrac{20}{12}$

then $4\dfrac{2}{3} - 1\dfrac{3}{4}$

$= 4\dfrac{8}{12} - 1\dfrac{9}{12}$

$= 3\dfrac{20}{12} - 1\dfrac{9}{12}$

$= 2\dfrac{11}{12}$

5. **Comparison of Fractions**

To determine which of two fractions is larger, change the two fractions to equivalent fractions by expressing them as fractions with a common denominator and then comparing the numerators of the fractions. The fraction with the larger numerator is the larger fraction.

Example: Which is larger, $\frac{5}{6}$ or $\frac{7}{8}$?

24 is a common denominator for the two fractions, hence $\frac{5}{6} = \frac{20}{24}$ and $\frac{7}{8} = \frac{21}{24}$. Since $\frac{21}{24}$ is larger than $\frac{20}{24}$, $\frac{7}{8}$ is larger than $\frac{5}{6}$.

II. Decimals and Percents

A. Decimals

A common fraction can be expressed as a decimal. For example: $\frac{1}{2} = \frac{5}{10} = .5$. Each common fraction has an equivalent decimal form.

1. To change a common fraction to a decimal, divide the numerator of the fraction by the denominator.

Example: $\frac{3}{8} = .375$

$$
\begin{array}{r}
.375 \\
8\overline{)3.000} \\
\underline{24} \\
60 \\
\underline{56} \\
40 \\
\underline{40} \\
\end{array}
$$

2. When a decimal is changed to a fraction, the digits after the decimal point become the numerator. The denominator is 1 followed by as many zeros as there are decimal places. (The denominator can also be determined by raising 10 to a power. The power is the number of decimal places in the number.)

An alternate method for changing a decimal to a common fraction is to count the number of decimal places in the decimal. One decimal place represents tenths; two decimal places, hundredths; three decimal places, thousandths; and so on. The numerical part of the decimal indicates how many tenths, hundredths, thousandths, etc., there are.

Examples: a) $0.540 = \dfrac{540}{1,000}$ (Note that $1,000 = 10^3$. There are 3 decimal places in the number so the power is 3.)

           b) $.48 = \dfrac{48}{100}$ (There are 48 hundredths.)

3. Adding and Subtracting Decimals

Arrange the decimals vertically with the decimal points aligned under each other. (Express whole numbers as decimals by appending a decimal point at the end of the number and adding as many zeros as desired, e.g., $23 = 23.0$.)

Examples: a) Subtract 2.715 from 4

$$
\begin{array}{r}
4.000 \\
-\ 2.715 \\
\hline
1.285
\end{array}
$$

b) Add $11.3 + .968 + .24 + 3$

$$
\begin{array}{r}
11.300 \\
.968 \\
.240 \\
3.000 \\
\hline
15.508
\end{array}
$$

4. Multiplying Decimals

To multiply decimals, multiply as you would with whole numbers. The number of decimal places in the product is the sum of the number of decimal places in the two numbers being multiplied.

Example: Multiply 2.47 times .315, that is,

$$
\begin{array}{r}
2.47 \\
\times\ .315 \\
\hline
.77805
\end{array}
$$

$$
\begin{array}{r}
2.47 \\
.315 \\
\hline
1235 \\
247 \\
741 \\
\hline
.77805
\end{array}
$$

There are 2 decimal places in 2.47 and 3 in .315; therefore, there are 5 decimal places in the product of the two numbers. The product is .77805.

5. Dividing Decimals

a) When a decimal is divided by a whole number, the decimal point in the quotient should be aligned with the decimal point in the dividend. Divide as you would with whole numbers.

Example: .264 divided by 12

$$
\begin{array}{r}
.022 \\
12\overline{)\ .264} \\
24 \\
\hline
24 \\
24 \\
\hline
0
\end{array}
$$

b) To divide by a decimal, multiply the divisor by the multiple of 10 that will make the divisor a whole number, then multiply the dividend by the same multiple of ten. Divide as you would with whole numbers.

Example: 2.752 divided by .16

$$.16\overline{)2.752}$$

Multiply the divisor and dividend by 100 to get a new divisor of 16 and dividend of 275.2.

```
        17.2
   16)275.2
       16
       ___
       115
       112
       ___
         32
         32
         ___
          0
```

B. Percents

Percent means "by the hundredths." The symbol "%" denotes a percent. A percent can be expressed as a fraction with a denominator of 100.

$$63\% = \frac{63}{100}$$

1. Converting decimals and fractions to percents and vice versa.

Examples: a) To convert a decimal to a percent, multiply the decimal by 100.

$$.134 = .134 \times 100 = 13.4\%$$

b) To convert a percent to a decimal, divide the percent by 100.

$$47\% = \frac{47}{100} = .47$$

2. To find a percent of a given number (the base), change the percent to a decimal and multiply the decimal times the base.

Examples: a) 35% of 80 = .35 × 80 = 28

b) The number of patients admitted to Get Well Hospital for drug overdoses was 24% higher in 1994 than in 1993. If 325 patients were admitted for drug overdoses in 1993, how many were admitted in 1994?

24% of 325 = .24 × 325 = 78

325 + 78 = 403

There were 78 more patients in 1994 than 1993, making a total of 403 admitted for drug overdoses in 1994.

3. To determine the base when the percent and percentage are known, change the percent to a decimal and divide the percentage by the result. (Note that "is" can be interpreted as = and "of" as multiplication.)

Example: 32 is 20% of what number?

$32 = .20 \times B$ (B represents the base, which is the unknown number, and 32 is the percentage)

$$\frac{32}{.20} = B$$

$$160 = B$$

32 is 20% of 160.

4. To determine what percent a given percentage is of a base, divide the percentage by the base and change the resulting decimal to a percent.

Examples: a) What percent of 60 is 15?

$15 = P \times 60$ (60 is the base and 15 is the percentage.)

$$\frac{15}{60} = \frac{1}{4} = .25 = 25\%$$

b) If a nurse with a salary of $40,000 receives a $2,000 bonus, what percent of his salary is his bonus? (That is, what percent of $40,000 is $2,000?)

$2,000 = P \times 40,000$

$$P = \frac{2,000}{40,000} = \frac{1}{20} = .05 \text{ or } 5\%$$

5. To find a percentage increase or percentage decrease in a verbal problem, write a fraction with the amount of increase or decrease as the numerator and the original amount as the denominator. Then change fraction to percentage.

Examples: A patient's prescription was decreased from 2 grams to 1.5 grams. What is the percent of decrease of the new prescription?

The amount of decrease was .5 grams. What percent of 2 grams is .5 grams?

$.5 = \underline{?}\%$ of 2

$$\frac{.5}{2} = .25 = 25\%$$

The dosage was decreased by 25%.

6. To determine discount in verbal problems, change the percentage to a fraction or decimal, multiply by the original cost, and deduct this amount from the original cost.

7. For verbal problems dealing with **commission and taxes,** multiply the total value of the goods or services by the percentage of tax or commission.

III. Ratios and Proportions

A. Ratios

A ratio is the comparison of two numerical quantities by division.

Example: A box contains 3 red balls and 2 blue balls. The ratio of blue to red balls in the box is 2 to 3 or $\frac{2}{3}$.

B. Proportions

A proportion is a statement that two ratios are equivalent.

Example: The ratio of 4 to x is equivalent to the ratio of 5 to 10.

$$\frac{4}{x} = \frac{5}{10}$$

C. Direct Proportions

In a direct proportion, one quantity increases ($\uparrow$) or decreases ($\downarrow$) as the other increases or decreases. In other words, the direction of the changes is the same for both factors. (x increases as y increases or x decreases as y decreases.)

Example: One orange sells for 15 cents. How much will six oranges cost?

$$\frac{1 \text{ orange}}{15\cancel{c}} = \frac{6 \text{ oranges}}{y\cancel{c}}$$

Cross multiply: $1y = 6 \times 15 \quad y = 90\cancel{c}$

The total cost increases as the number of oranges sold increases.

Example: Six oranges cost 90 cents. How much would one orange cost?

$$\frac{6 \text{ oranges}}{90\cancel{c}} = \frac{1 \text{ orange}}{y\cancel{c}}$$

Cross multiply: $6y = 90\cancel{c} \quad y = 15\cancel{c}$ (Divide both sides by 6.)

The cost decreases as the number of oranges purchased decreases.

D. Inverse Proportions

In an inverse proportion, one quantity increases ($\uparrow$) as the other decreases ($\downarrow$), and vice versa. In other words, the direction of the changes is opposite. (As x increases, y decreases; or as x decreases, y increases.)

Example: A 5-pound bag of dog food lasts one week when the dog is given 2 servings per day. How long would this bag last if the dog were to receive 3 servings per day?

$$\frac{3}{2} = \frac{7}{y}$$

$$3y = 14$$

$$y = 4.6$$

(As the number of meals increases, the number of days the dog food lasts decreases.)

IV. Algebra

Algebra involves the use of letters and symbols as well as numbers. Some of the introductory concepts of algebra are reviewed in this section.

A. Operations with signed numbers

For operations with signed numbers ($+$ or $-$):

1. **Addition**

    a) For numbers with the same sign, add and keep the same sign in the answer.

    b) For numbers with different signs, subtract and give the answer the sign of the higher number.

2. **Subtraction**

    Combine the two signs of the subtrahend, taking the subtraction sign as a negative sign, $[- \text{ times } - = +]$ $[- \text{ times } + = -]$. Then use the rules for addition.

    Examples: $-4 - (-2) = -4 + 2 = -2$
    $-4 - (+2) = -4 - 2 = -6$

3. **Multiplication**

    a) The product of an odd number of negative numbers is negative.

    b) The product of an even number of negative numbers is positive.

    Examples: $(-3)(-2)(-5) = -30$
    $(-4)(-2)(-3)(-5) = 120$

4. **Division**

    If the two numbers have the same sign, the quotient is positive; if otherwise, the quotient is negative.

B. Algebraic Expressions

Algebraic expressions consist of a combination of variables and numbers connected by addition and subtraction signs. The parts of algebraic expressions connected by plus and minus signs are called **terms.**

1. **Combining like terms**

    Like terms are terms that contain the same variables. These variables have the same exponents.

    $2xy^2$ and $5xy^2$ are like terms.

    $3xy$ and $4x^2y$ are not like terms. The variable x in the two terms has different exponents.

    Only like terms in an algebraic expression can be combined. To combine like terms, add their numerical coefficients.

    Examples: a) $7x - 4x + 2 + 3 = 3x + 5$
    b) $2xy + 7x^2y - 4xy + 6y = 7x^2y - 2xy + 6y$

C. Order of Operations

When simplifying an algebraic expression:

1. First remove grouping symbols (parentheses, brackets), starting with the innermost grouping symbols. (To remove grouping symbols, perform operations inside of symbols.)

2. Perform the operations of multiplication and division, moving from left to right.

3. Perform the operations of addition and subtraction, moving from left to right.

Example: $5x - 2[(3x - 1) + (4 - 2x)]$

$$= 5x - 2[3x - 1 + 4 - 2x]$$

$$= 5x - 2[x + 3] = 5x - 2x - 6$$

$$= 3x - 6$$

D. Evaluating Algebraic Expressions

Find the value of an algebraic expression for given values of the variable by substituting the value of the variables in the expression.

Evaluate the expression $2x^2y + 3xy$ when $x = 2$ and $y = 3$.

Example: $2x^2y + 3xy = 2(2)^2(3) + 3(2)(3)$

$$= 2(4)(3) + 3(2)(3)$$

$$= 2 \times 4 \times 3 + 3 \times 2 \times 3$$

$$= 24 + 18$$

$$= 42$$

E. Solving Equations with One Variable

An equation is a statement that two quantities are equal. An equation has one unknown if it has only one variable. Equations with one variable can be solved using inverse operations. One or more of the basic operations of addition, subtraction, multiplication, and division are used to solve equations.

Consider the equation $x - 7 = 3$.

7 has been subtracted from the variable; the inverse operation for subtraction is addition. To solve the equation, add 7 to both sides of the equation.

$$x - 7 = 3$$

$$x - 7 + 7 = 3 + 7$$

$$x = 10$$

Equivalent equations can be obtained by adding or subtracting the same number to both sides of the equation, or by multiplying or dividing both sides of the equation by the same number. (Do not divide by zero.)

Example:

1. $3x + 5 = 17$

$$3x + 5 - 5 = 17 - 5$$

$$3x = 12$$

$$\frac{3x}{3} = \frac{12}{3}$$

$$x = 4$$

Note that to solve an equation, it is necessary to get the variable on one side of the equation and the constant on the other side.

$$5x + 2 = x - 10$$

$$5x + 2 - 2 = x - 10 - 2$$

$$5x = x - 12$$

Example:

2. $5x - x = x - 12 - x$

$$4x = -12$$

$$\frac{4x}{4} = \frac{-12}{4}$$

$$x = 3$$

F.   Solving Verbal (Word) Problems

The above described methods can be used to solve verbal problems once they are translated into equations. The first step in translating a verbal problem into an equation is to represent the unknown quantity by a variable. Two equivalent algebraic expressions involving the variable are then written to represent information given in the problem. The two equivalent expressions form the equation.

Examples:

1.   When 3 times a number is increased by 4, the result is 19.

Let N represent the unknown number.

$3N$ represents 3 times the number.

$3N + 4$ represents 3 times the number increased by 4.

(To increase a number means to add to it.)

Since the result is 19, the desired equation is

$3N + 4 = 19$.

$3N = 15$ (4 was subtracted from both.)

$N = 5$ (Both sides were divided by 3.)

The solution to the problem is 5.

2. A number decreased by $\frac{1}{2}$ of itself equals $\frac{3}{4}$. What decimal is equivalent to the resulting fraction?

Let Y represent the unknown number.

$Y - \frac{1}{2}Y$ represents Y decreased by $\frac{1}{2}$ of itself.

The desired equation is

$$y - \frac{1}{2}y = \frac{3}{4}$$

$$\frac{1}{2}y = \frac{3}{4}$$

Multiply both sides of the equation by 4 to get

$$2y = 3$$

$$y = \frac{3}{2} = 1.5$$

The solution is 1.5.

G. Formulas

An equation in which a variable is expressed in terms of another variable is called a formula.

$I = PRT$ is a formula for finding interest.

   P represents the principal.
   R represents the rate.
   T represents the time.

$D = RT$ is the formula for finding distance.

   R is the rate or speed.
   T is the time.
   $F = \frac{9}{5}C + 32$ is the formula for changing a temperature from Celsius to Fahrenheit.
   C = Celsius
   F = Fahrenheit

Example: How long will it take to drive a distance of 330 miles traveling at a rate of 60 mph?

Substitute in the formula

$$D = R \times T$$

$$330 = 60 \times T$$

$$\frac{330}{60} = T$$

$$5\frac{1}{2} = T$$

It will take $5\frac{1}{2}$ hours to drive the 330 miles at a rate of 60 mph.

Example: If a temperature reading on the Celsius scale is 40 degrees, we substitute 40 for C in the temperature conversion formula to get

$$F = \frac{9}{5} \times 40 + 32$$

$$F = \frac{360}{5} + 32 = 72 + 32 = 104 \text{ degrees Fahrenheit}$$

H. Inequalities

The symbols "<" and ">" are used to represent the inequalities "less than" and "greater than." Various statements of inequality are expressed by the following:

Example:

1. $a < b$ means a is less than b.
   $7 < 12$ means   7 is less than 12.
2. $a \leq b$ means a is either less than or equal to b.
   $5 \leq 9$ means   5 is less than or equal to 9.
3. $a > b$ means a is greater than b.
   $18 > 14$ means   18 is greater than 14.
4. $a \geq b$ means a is either greater than or equal to b.
   $3 \geq 3$ means   3 is greater than or equal to 3.
5. $a < b \leq c$ means a is less than b, and b is less than or equal to c.
   $-1 < 3 \leq 5$ means -1 is less than 3, and 3 is less than or equal to 5.
   $2 \leq x < 5$ means x is greater than or equal to 2 and less than 5.

I. Defined Functions

Certain questions may include a special sign such as "*" or "#" that is defined for you. The sign tells you to perform a specific function or operation. This kind of problem tests your ability to learn and apply a new concept.

Example: For all numbers, $a * b = \frac{a}{b} + 2$. What is $6 * 3$?

$$6 * 3 = \frac{6}{3} + 2$$

$$= 2 + 2$$

$$= 4$$

V. Geometry

A. Standard Measurements

The following are some standard units of measurement.

Linear
inches
feet (1 ft. = 12 in.)
yard (1 yd. = 3 ft.)
gallon (1 gal. = 4 qts.)

Capacity
ounces
pints (16 oz. = pt.)
quart (1 qt. = 2 pts.)

Weight
ounces
pounds (1 lb. = 16 oz.)

Area is expressed in square units and volume is expressed in cubic units (square feet, cubic inches, etc.).

1. For **literal expressions** (problems with letters instead of numbers), use the same processes as you would for numbers.

Example: How many inches are in y yards and x feet?

$$y \text{ yd.} \times \frac{36 \text{ in.}}{\text{yd.}} = 36y \text{ in.} \qquad x \text{ ft.} \times \frac{12 \text{ in.}}{\text{ft.}} = 12x \text{ in.}$$

$$5 \text{ ft.} = 5 \times 12 = 60 \text{ in.}$$

B.   Metric Measurements

Metric measurements are based on powers of 10.

Problems involving metric measurements (other than conversions within the metric system) are solved using the same techniques as problems with English measurement units.

The basic metric units of measure are:

   Length—Meter
   Volume—Liter
   Weight—Gram
   Temperature—Celsius

Computations in the metric system involve multiplication and division by powers of 10. The chart below illustrates the relationship between metric units.

MILLI	CENTI	DECI	UNIT	DEKA	HECTO	KILO
.001	.01	.1	1	10	100	1000

Example: 1 gram = 1,000 milligrams
   2 liters = 2,000 meters
   1 hectometer = 100 meters

C.   Parallel and Perpendicular Lines

1. Parallel lines are two lines that do not intersect (have no points in common). The slopes of two parallel lines are equal.

2. Perpendicular lines are two lines that intersect at right angles. The slopes of two perpendicular lines have a product of -1.

D.   Polygons

A polygon is a simple closed plane figure made up of line segments.

1. Polygons with three sides are called **triangles.**

   a) If the lengths of two sides of a triangle are equal, the triangle is called an **isosceles** triangle.

   b) When all three sides of a triangle have the same length, the triangle is called an **equilateral** triangle.

2. Polygons with four sides are called quadrilaterals.

   a) A **square** is a quadrilateral with all four sides equal.

   b) A **rectangle** is a quadrilateral with opposite sides equal and parallel.

E. Perimeter

To find the **perimeter (P)** of a figure, add the lengths of all its sides.

Triangle P = sum of the three sides $P = a + b + c$

Rectangle $P = 2 \times$ Length $+ 2 \times$ Width $P = 2L + 2W$

Square $P = 4 \times S$, where S = length of each side.

Circle   The circumference (C) is the distance around a circle.

The circumference of a circle is equal to $\pi \times$ the diameter:

$$C = \pi \times d$$

Point O is the center of the given circle. Points P, R, and S are points on the circle.

A **chord** of a circle is any segment with its two end points on the circle. $\overline{MN}$ is a chord of the given circle.

A **radius** of a circle is a segment from the center of the circle to any point on the circle. $\overline{OP}$ is a radius of the circle.

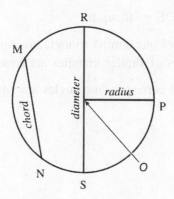

A **diameter** of a circle is a chord that passes through the center of a circle. $\overline{RS}$ is a diameter of the given circle.

All radii of a circle have the same length. A diameter of a given circle is always twice the radius of the circle.

Example: If the length of radius $\overline{OP}$ = 7 cm., the diameter $\overline{RS}$ = 14 cm.

F. Area

1. To find the **area (A) of plane figures:**

    Square $A = (\text{side})^2 A = S^2$

    Rectangle $A = \text{Base} \times \text{Height}$, or $A = L \times W$

    Triangle $A = \frac{1}{2} \text{Base} \times \text{Height}$, or $A = \frac{1}{2}bh$

    Circle $A = \pi \times (\text{radius})^2$ or $A = \pi r^2$

2. The **areas of other polygons** may be found by dividing the polygon into nonoverlapping triangles and/or quadrilaterals (squares, rectangles), and then adding the areas of the triangles and quadrilaterals.

Nonoverlapping triangles and quadrilaterals may be obtained by drawing diagonals of the polygon. A **diagonal** of a polygon is a line segment joining two nonconsecutive vertices of a polygon. BE is a diagonal of polygon ABCDE.

Example: Given polygon ABCDE with the measurements indicated, draw diagonal BE to divide the polygon into triangle BAE and rectangle BEDC.

Area of triangle BAE $= \dfrac{1}{2} \times 10 \times 4 = 20$ sq. in.

Area of rectangle BEDC $= 2 \times 10 = 20$ sq. in.

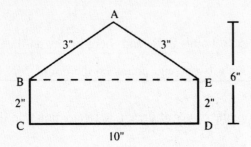

Since $20 + 20 = 40$, the area of polygon ABCDE $= 40$ sq. in.

G.   **Similar triangles** have the same shape. The angles of one similar triangle are equal to the angles of the other. The ratios of corresponding sides of similar triangles are equal.

Example: The two given triangles are similar (measures of corresponding angles are equal).

Therefore $\dfrac{8}{x} = \dfrac{y}{5}$

H.   **A right triangle** is a triangle with a right angle. The side of the triangle that is opposite the right angle is called the **hypotenuse**.

1.   **Pythagorean theorem:** The square of the hypotenuse of a triangle is equal to the sum of the squares of the other two sides.

$c^2 = a^2 + b^2$

Example: Find the hypotenuse of the right triangle given below:

The two sides of the triangle are 5 and 12. The hypotenuse (c) can be found with the use of the Pythagorean theorem.

$c^2 = 5^2 + 12^2 = 25 + 144 = 169$

$c^2 = 169$ (To find c, take the square root of 169.)

$c = 13$

I.   Units of measurement for angles are called **degrees.** An acute angle has a measure that is less than 90°.

A **right angle** has a measure of exactly 90°. (Perpendicular lines form right angles.)

An **obtuse angle** has a measure that is greater than 90° and less than 180°.

Two angles are **complementary** if the sum of their measures is 90°.

Two angles are **supplementary** if the sum of their measure is 180°.

If the exterior sides of a pair of adjacent angles form a straight line, the two adjacent angles are supplementary.

Example: If AB ⊥ DC (AB is perpendicular to DC), then

∠ABF and ∠FBC are complementary angles.

(The sum of the measures of ∠ABF and ∠FBC = 90°.)

∠EBD and ∠EBC are supplementary angles.

(The sum of ∠EBD and ∠EBC = 180°.)

∠FBC is an acute angle. ∠ABC is a right angle.

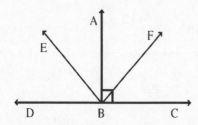

J.   The sum of the measures of the three angles of a triangle is 180°. If the measures of two angles of a triangle are given, the measure of the third angle can be found by subtracting the sum of the measures of the two known angles from 180°.

Example: If m∠A = 40° and m∠B = 60°, then

$$m\angle C = 180 - (m\angle A + m\angle B)$$
$$= 180° - (40° + 60°)$$
$$= 180° - (100°)$$
$$= 80°$$

K.   The total degree measure of a circle is 360°.

1.   A **central angle** of a circle is an angle whose vertex is the center of the circle. If a central angle represents $\frac{1}{n}$ of a circle, the measure of the central angle is $\frac{1}{n} \times 360°$.

Angle ∠AOB is a central angle in the circle below.

2.   A **minor arc** of a circle consists of two points A and B, where the sides of a central angle intersect the circle, plus all points of the circle that lie in the interior of the central angle.

The minor arc $\overparen{AB}$ is indicated in the given circle.

3.   A **major arc** of a circle consists of points A and B and all points on the circle that lie in the exterior of the central angle.

The major arc $\overparen{AB}$ is indicated in the circle below.

4.   An **inscribed angle** of a circle is an angle whose vertex is on the circle and whose rays intersect the circle in two points different from the vertex. The measure of an inscribed angle equals one-half the measure of its intercepted arc.

∠ACB is an inscribed angle of the given circle. The measure of ∠ACB is one half the measure of the central angle, ∠AOB.

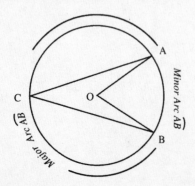

L. An exterior angle of a triangle is formed by a side of a triangle and by the extension of another side of the triangle.

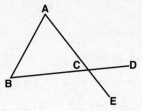

∠ACD is an exterior angle of ∠ABC.

∠BCE is also an exterior angle of ∠ABC.

Every triangle has 6 exterior angles.

1. An exterior angle of a triangle is greater than either of the remote interior angles. Angles A and B are the remote interior angles for the exterior angle ∠ACD.

2. An exterior angle of a triangle equals the sum of the remote interior angles (m∠ACD = m∠A + m∠B).

3. m∠ACD + m∠ACB = 180°.

ANSWER SHEET

Test 1

1. Ⓐ Ⓑ Ⓒ Ⓓ	5. Ⓐ Ⓑ Ⓒ Ⓓ	9. Ⓐ Ⓑ Ⓒ Ⓓ	13. Ⓐ Ⓑ Ⓒ Ⓓ	17. Ⓐ Ⓑ Ⓒ Ⓓ
2. Ⓐ Ⓑ Ⓒ Ⓓ	6. Ⓐ Ⓑ Ⓒ Ⓓ	10. Ⓐ Ⓑ Ⓒ Ⓓ	14. Ⓐ Ⓑ Ⓒ Ⓓ	18. Ⓐ Ⓑ Ⓒ Ⓓ
3. Ⓐ Ⓑ Ⓒ Ⓓ	7. Ⓐ Ⓑ Ⓒ Ⓓ	11. Ⓐ Ⓑ Ⓒ Ⓓ	15. Ⓐ Ⓑ Ⓒ Ⓓ	19. Ⓐ Ⓑ Ⓒ Ⓓ
4. Ⓐ Ⓑ Ⓒ Ⓓ	8. Ⓐ Ⓑ Ⓒ Ⓓ	12. Ⓐ Ⓑ Ⓒ Ⓓ	16. Ⓐ Ⓑ Ⓒ Ⓓ	20. Ⓐ Ⓑ Ⓒ Ⓓ

Test 2

1. Ⓐ Ⓑ Ⓒ Ⓓ	5. Ⓐ Ⓑ Ⓒ Ⓓ	9. Ⓐ Ⓑ Ⓒ Ⓓ	13. Ⓐ Ⓑ Ⓒ Ⓓ	17. Ⓐ Ⓑ Ⓒ Ⓓ
2. Ⓐ Ⓑ Ⓒ Ⓓ	6. Ⓐ Ⓑ Ⓒ Ⓓ	10. Ⓐ Ⓑ Ⓒ Ⓓ	14. Ⓐ Ⓑ Ⓒ Ⓓ	18. Ⓐ Ⓑ Ⓒ Ⓓ
3. Ⓐ Ⓑ Ⓒ Ⓓ	7. Ⓐ Ⓑ Ⓒ Ⓓ	11. Ⓐ Ⓑ Ⓒ Ⓓ	15. Ⓐ Ⓑ Ⓒ Ⓓ	19. Ⓐ Ⓑ Ⓒ Ⓓ
4. Ⓐ Ⓑ Ⓒ Ⓓ	8. Ⓐ Ⓑ Ⓒ Ⓓ	12. Ⓐ Ⓑ Ⓒ Ⓓ	16. Ⓐ Ⓑ Ⓒ Ⓓ	20. Ⓐ Ⓑ Ⓒ Ⓓ

Test 3

1. Ⓐ Ⓑ Ⓒ Ⓓ	5. Ⓐ Ⓑ Ⓒ Ⓓ	9. Ⓐ Ⓑ Ⓒ Ⓓ	13. Ⓐ Ⓑ Ⓒ Ⓓ	17. Ⓐ Ⓑ Ⓒ Ⓓ
2. Ⓐ Ⓑ Ⓒ Ⓓ	6. Ⓐ Ⓑ Ⓒ Ⓓ	10. Ⓐ Ⓑ Ⓒ Ⓓ	14. Ⓐ Ⓑ Ⓒ Ⓓ	18. Ⓐ Ⓑ Ⓒ Ⓓ
3. Ⓐ Ⓑ Ⓒ Ⓓ	7. Ⓐ Ⓑ Ⓒ Ⓓ	11. Ⓐ Ⓑ Ⓒ Ⓓ	15. Ⓐ Ⓑ Ⓒ Ⓓ	19. Ⓐ Ⓑ Ⓒ Ⓓ
4. Ⓐ Ⓑ Ⓒ Ⓓ	8. Ⓐ Ⓑ Ⓒ Ⓓ	12. Ⓐ Ⓑ Ⓒ Ⓓ	16. Ⓐ Ⓑ Ⓒ Ⓓ	20. Ⓐ Ⓑ Ⓒ Ⓓ

Test 4

1. Ⓐ Ⓑ Ⓒ Ⓓ	8. Ⓐ Ⓑ Ⓒ Ⓓ	14. Ⓐ Ⓑ Ⓒ Ⓓ	20. Ⓐ Ⓑ Ⓒ Ⓓ	26. Ⓐ Ⓑ Ⓒ Ⓓ
2. Ⓐ Ⓑ Ⓒ Ⓓ	9. Ⓐ Ⓑ Ⓒ Ⓓ	15. Ⓐ Ⓑ Ⓒ Ⓓ	21. Ⓐ Ⓑ Ⓒ Ⓓ	27. Ⓐ Ⓑ Ⓒ Ⓓ
3. Ⓐ Ⓑ Ⓒ Ⓓ	10. Ⓐ Ⓑ Ⓒ Ⓓ	16. Ⓐ Ⓑ Ⓒ Ⓓ	22. Ⓐ Ⓑ Ⓒ Ⓓ	28. Ⓐ Ⓑ Ⓒ Ⓓ
4. Ⓐ Ⓑ Ⓒ Ⓓ	11. Ⓐ Ⓑ Ⓒ Ⓓ	17. Ⓐ Ⓑ Ⓒ Ⓓ	23. Ⓐ Ⓑ Ⓒ Ⓓ	29. Ⓐ Ⓑ Ⓒ Ⓓ
5. Ⓐ Ⓑ Ⓒ Ⓓ	12. Ⓐ Ⓑ Ⓒ Ⓓ	18. Ⓐ Ⓑ Ⓒ Ⓓ	24. Ⓐ Ⓑ Ⓒ Ⓓ	30. Ⓐ Ⓑ Ⓒ Ⓓ
6. Ⓐ Ⓑ Ⓒ Ⓓ	13. Ⓐ Ⓑ Ⓒ Ⓓ	19. Ⓐ Ⓑ Ⓒ Ⓓ	25. Ⓐ Ⓑ Ⓒ Ⓓ	31. Ⓐ Ⓑ Ⓒ Ⓓ
7. Ⓐ Ⓑ Ⓒ Ⓓ				

QUANTITATIVE COMPARISONS

TEST 5

1. Ⓐ Ⓑ Ⓒ Ⓓ
2. Ⓐ Ⓑ Ⓒ Ⓓ
3. Ⓐ Ⓑ Ⓒ Ⓓ
4. Ⓐ Ⓑ Ⓒ Ⓓ
5. Ⓐ Ⓑ Ⓒ Ⓓ
6. Ⓐ Ⓑ Ⓒ Ⓓ

7. Ⓐ Ⓑ Ⓒ Ⓓ
8. Ⓐ Ⓑ Ⓒ Ⓓ
9. Ⓐ Ⓑ Ⓒ Ⓓ
10. Ⓐ Ⓑ Ⓒ Ⓓ
11. Ⓐ Ⓑ Ⓒ Ⓓ
12. Ⓐ Ⓑ Ⓒ Ⓓ

13. Ⓐ Ⓑ Ⓒ Ⓓ
14. Ⓐ Ⓑ Ⓒ Ⓓ
15. Ⓐ Ⓑ Ⓒ Ⓓ
16. Ⓐ Ⓑ Ⓒ Ⓓ
17. Ⓐ Ⓑ Ⓒ Ⓓ
18. Ⓐ Ⓑ Ⓒ Ⓓ

19. Ⓐ Ⓑ Ⓒ Ⓓ
20. Ⓐ Ⓑ Ⓒ Ⓓ
21. Ⓐ Ⓑ Ⓒ Ⓓ
22. Ⓐ Ⓑ Ⓒ Ⓓ
23. Ⓐ Ⓑ Ⓒ Ⓓ

24. Ⓐ Ⓑ Ⓒ Ⓓ
25. Ⓐ Ⓑ Ⓒ Ⓓ
26. Ⓐ Ⓑ Ⓒ Ⓓ
27. Ⓐ Ⓑ Ⓒ Ⓓ
28. Ⓐ Ⓑ Ⓒ Ⓓ

TEST 6

1. Ⓐ Ⓑ Ⓒ Ⓓ
2. Ⓐ Ⓑ Ⓒ Ⓓ
3. Ⓐ Ⓑ Ⓒ Ⓓ

4. Ⓐ Ⓑ Ⓒ Ⓓ
5. Ⓐ Ⓑ Ⓒ Ⓓ
6. Ⓐ Ⓑ Ⓒ Ⓓ

7. Ⓐ Ⓑ Ⓒ Ⓓ
8. Ⓐ Ⓑ Ⓒ Ⓓ
9. Ⓐ Ⓑ Ⓒ Ⓓ

10. Ⓐ Ⓑ Ⓒ Ⓓ
11. Ⓐ Ⓑ Ⓒ Ⓓ
12. Ⓐ Ⓑ Ⓒ Ⓓ

FINAL MATHEMATICS EXAMINATION

PART 1: GENERAL MATHEMATICS

1. Ⓐ Ⓑ Ⓒ Ⓓ
2. Ⓐ Ⓑ Ⓒ Ⓓ
3. Ⓐ Ⓑ Ⓒ Ⓓ
4. Ⓐ Ⓑ Ⓒ Ⓓ
5. Ⓐ Ⓑ Ⓒ Ⓓ
6. Ⓐ Ⓑ Ⓒ Ⓓ
7. Ⓐ Ⓑ Ⓒ Ⓓ
8. Ⓐ Ⓑ Ⓒ Ⓓ
9. Ⓐ Ⓑ Ⓒ Ⓓ

10. Ⓐ Ⓑ Ⓒ Ⓓ
11. Ⓐ Ⓑ Ⓒ Ⓓ
12. Ⓐ Ⓑ Ⓒ Ⓓ
13. Ⓐ Ⓑ Ⓒ Ⓓ
14. Ⓐ Ⓑ Ⓒ Ⓓ
15. Ⓐ Ⓑ Ⓒ Ⓓ
16. Ⓐ Ⓑ Ⓒ Ⓓ
17. Ⓐ Ⓑ Ⓒ Ⓓ
18. Ⓐ Ⓑ Ⓒ Ⓓ

19. Ⓐ Ⓑ Ⓒ Ⓓ
20. Ⓐ Ⓑ Ⓒ Ⓓ
21. Ⓐ Ⓑ Ⓒ Ⓓ
22. Ⓐ Ⓑ Ⓒ Ⓓ
23. Ⓐ Ⓑ Ⓒ Ⓓ
24. Ⓐ Ⓑ Ⓒ Ⓓ
25. Ⓐ Ⓑ Ⓒ Ⓓ
26. Ⓐ Ⓑ Ⓒ Ⓓ

27. Ⓐ Ⓑ Ⓒ Ⓓ
28. Ⓐ Ⓑ Ⓒ Ⓓ
29. Ⓐ Ⓑ Ⓒ Ⓓ
30. Ⓐ Ⓑ Ⓒ Ⓓ
31. Ⓐ Ⓑ Ⓒ Ⓓ
32. Ⓐ Ⓑ Ⓒ Ⓓ
33. Ⓐ Ⓑ Ⓒ Ⓓ
34. Ⓐ Ⓑ Ⓒ Ⓓ

35. Ⓐ Ⓑ Ⓒ Ⓓ
36. Ⓐ Ⓑ Ⓒ Ⓓ
37. Ⓐ Ⓑ Ⓒ Ⓓ
38. Ⓐ Ⓑ Ⓒ Ⓓ
39. Ⓐ Ⓑ Ⓒ Ⓓ
40. Ⓐ Ⓑ Ⓒ Ⓓ
41. Ⓐ Ⓑ Ⓒ Ⓓ
42. Ⓐ Ⓑ Ⓒ Ⓓ

PART 2: QUANTITATIVE COMPARISONS

1. Ⓐ Ⓑ Ⓒ Ⓓ
2. Ⓐ Ⓑ Ⓒ Ⓓ
3. Ⓐ Ⓑ Ⓒ Ⓓ

4. Ⓐ Ⓑ Ⓒ Ⓓ
5. Ⓐ Ⓑ Ⓒ Ⓓ
6. Ⓐ Ⓑ Ⓒ Ⓓ

7. Ⓐ Ⓑ Ⓒ Ⓓ
8. Ⓐ Ⓑ Ⓒ Ⓓ
9. Ⓐ Ⓑ Ⓒ Ⓓ

10. Ⓐ Ⓑ Ⓒ Ⓓ
11. Ⓐ Ⓑ Ⓒ Ⓓ
12. Ⓐ Ⓑ Ⓒ Ⓓ

TEST 1

20 QUESTIONS ■ TIME—15 MINUTES

Directions: Each problem on this test requires logical reasoning and thinking, besides simple computations, to find the solution. Read each problem carefully and choose the correct answer from the four choices that follow. Fill in the corresponding space on your answer sheet.

1. Find the interest on $25,800 for 144 days at six percent per annum. Base your calculations on a 360-day year.

   (A) $619.20
   (B) $619.02
   (C) $691.02
   (D) $691.20

2. Arthur can shovel snow from a sidewalk in 60 minutes and Jack can do it in 30 minutes. How many minutes will it take them to do the job together?

   (A) 90
   (B) 15
   (C) 30
   (D) 20

3. The visitors' section of a courtroom seats 105 people. The court is in session six hours per day. On one particular day, 485 people visited the court and were given seats. What is the average length of time spent by each visitor in the court? Assume that as soon as a person leaves his seat it is immediately filled and that at no time during the day is one of the 105 seats vacant. Express your answer in hours and minutes.

   (A) 1 hour 20 minutes
   (B) 1 hour 18 minutes
   (C) 1 hour 30 minutes
   (D) 2 hours

4. If copy paper costs $14.50 per ream and a five percent discount is allowed for cash, how many reams can be purchased for $690 cash? Do not round off cents in your calculations.

   (A) 49 reams
   (B) 60 reams
   (C) 50 reams
   (D) 53 reams

5. How many hours are there between 8:30 A.M. today and 3:15 A.M. tomorrow?

   (A) $17\frac{3}{4}$ hours
   (B) $18\frac{3}{4}$ hours
   (C) $18\frac{2}{3}$ hours
   (D) $18\frac{1}{2}$ hours

6. How many days are there from September 19 to December 25 (*inclusive*)?

   (A) 98 days
   (B) 96 days
   (C) 89 days
   (D) 90 days

7. A clerk is requested to file 800 cards. If he can file cards at the rate of 80 cards per hour, the number of cards remaining to be filed after seven hours of work is

   (A) 40
   (B) 240
   (C) 140
   (D) 260

8. If your monthly electricity bill increases from $80 to $90, the percentage of increase is, most nearly,

   (A) 10 percent.

   (B) $11\frac{1}{9}$ percent.

   (C) $12\frac{1}{2}$ percent.

   (D) $14\frac{1}{7}$ percent.

9. Fifteen nurses who work the morning shift at Get Well Hospital are responsible for 135 patients. The average number of patients served by each nurse is

   (A) 120

   (B) 10

   (C) 9

   (D) 140

10. If a nursing exam contained 80 questions and you answered 72 of them correctly, what percent of the questions did you answer correctly?

    (A) 90 percent

    (B) 72 percent

    (C) 8 percent

    (D) 28 percent

11. If a patient is required to get 45 minutes of exercise each day, how many hours of exercise does he get in a week?

    (A) 315 hours

    (B) 5.25 hours

    (C) 52 hours

    (D) 6.4 hours

12. If a hospital has 120 nurses on duty during the afternoon shift and one half as many on duty for the night shift, what is the total number of nurses on duty for the two shifts?

    (A) 60

    (B) 180

    (C) 90

    (D) 120.5

13. If an inspector issued 182 summonses in the course of seven hours, his hourly average of summonses issued was

    (A) 23 summonses.

    (B) 26 summonses.

    (C) 25 summonses.

    (D) 28 summonses.

14. Last week 23 of the 76 patients admitted to Emergency Hospital had been in accidents. How many of the admitted patients had not been in accidents?

    (A) 23

    (B) 99

    (C) 53

    (D) 76

15. A truck going at a rate of 40 miles per hour will reach a town 80 miles away in how many hours?

    (A) 1 hour

    (B) 3 hours

    (C) 2 hours

    (D) 4 hours

16. If a barrel has a capacity of 100 gallons, how many gallons will it contain when it is two-fifths full?

    (A) 20 gallons

    (B) 60 gallons

    (C) 40 gallons

    (D) 80 gallons

17. If a monthly salary of $3,000 is subject to a 20 percent tax, the net salary is

    (A) $2,000

    (B) $2,400

    (C) $2,500

    (D) $2,600

18. If $1,000 is the cost of repairing 100 square yards of pavement, the cost of repairing one square yard is

    (A) $10

    (B) $150

    (C) $100

    (D) $300

GO ON TO THE NEXT PAGE

19. If an employee's base pay is $3,000 per month, and it is increased by a monthly bonus of $350 and a seniority increment of $250 this month, her total salary for the month is

(A) $3,600
(B) $3,500
(C) $3,000
(D) $3,700

20. If an annual salary of $21,600 is increased by a bonus of $7,200 and by a service increment of $1,200, the total pay rate is

(A) $29,600
(B) $39,600
(C) $26,900
(D) $30,000

STOP   If you finish before time is called, you may check your work on this section only. Do not turn to any other section in the test.

TEST 2

20 QUESTIONS ▪▫ TIME—15 MINUTES

Directions: Each problem on this test requires logical reasoning and thinking, besides simple computations, to find the solution. Read each problem carefully and choose the correct answer from the four choices that follow. Fill in the corresponding space on your answer sheet.

1. An emergency medical technician was standing 40 feet behind his vehicle when a second emergency medical vehicle arrived and parked 90 feet from the first vehicle. If the emergency medical technician is standing between the two vehicles, how much closer is he to the first vehicle than to the second?

   (A) 30 feet
   (B) 50 feet
   (C) 10 feet
   (D) 70 feet

2. If an IV bag has a capacity of 1,260 milliliters, how many milliliters does it contain when it's two-thirds full?

   (A) 809 ml.
   (B) 750 ml.
   (C) 630 ml.
   (D) 840 ml.

3. If an employee's salary is $2,500 a month and there are 23 working days in the month, he earns approximately how much for each day he works that month?

   (A) $108.70
   (B) $150.00
   (C) $112.50
   (D) $186.70

4. A nursing home assistant earns $360.00 a week and has deductions of $18.00 for her retirement fund, $15.00 for medical insurance, $21.00 for social security, and $72.00 for withholding taxes. How much is her take home pay?

   (A) $488.00
   (B) $296.00
   (C) $234.00
   (D) $288.00

5. A company uses 40 thirty-three-cent stamps, 25 twenty-cent stamps, and 320 sixty-cent stamps each day. The total cost of stamps used by the company in a five-day period is

   (A) $1,051.00
   (B) $210.20
   (C) $21,000.00
   (D) $105,100.00

6. A city department issued 12,000 applications in 1979. The number of applications that the department issued in 1977 was 25 percent greater than the number it issued in 1979. If the department issued 10 percent fewer applications in 1975 than it did in 1977, the number it issued in 1975 was

   (A) 16,500
   (B) 13,500
   (C) 9,900
   (D) 8,100

7. A secretary can add 40 columns of figures in an hour by using a calculator and 20 columns of figures an hour without using a calculator. The total number of hours it would take him to add 200 columns if he does three fifths of the work by machine and the rest without the machine is

   (A) 6
   (B) 7
   (C) 8
   (D) 9

GO ON TO THE NEXT PAGE ➤

8. In 1995, a medical office bought 500 dozen rubber gloves at a price of $2.60 per dozen. In 1998, 25 percent fewer gloves were bought than in 1995, but the price per dozen was 20 percent higher than the price in 1995. The total cost of the gloves bought in 1998 was

   (A) $1,560.00
   (B) $1,170.00
   (C) $975.00
   (D) $1,040.00

9. A nurse is assigned to check the accuracy of the entries on 490 forms. He checks 40 forms per hour. After working one hour on this task, he is joined by another nurse, who checks these forms at the rate of 35 per hour. The total number of hours required to do the entire assignment is

   (A) 5
   (B) 6
   (C) 7
   (D) 8

10. Assume there is a total of 420 employees in a medical care building. Thirty percent of the employees are doctors and one seventh are nurses. The difference between the number of nurses and the doctors is

    (A) 60
    (B) 66
    (C) 186
    (D) 360

11. Assume that a duplicating machine produces copies of a bulletin at a cost of 12 cents per copy. The machine produces 120 copies of the bulletin per minute. If the cost of producing a certain number of copies was $36, how many minutes did it take the machine to produce this number of copies?

    (A) 10 minutes
    (B) 6 minutes
    (C) 2.5 minutes
    (D) 1.2 minutes

12. The average number of medical records filed per day by a filing clerk during a five-day week was 720. She filed 610 records the first day, 720 records the second day, 740 records the third day, and 755 records the fourth day. The number of records she filed the fifth day was

    (A) 748
    (B) 165
    (C) 775
    (D) 565

13. A city department employs 1,400 people, of whom 35 percent are clerks and one eighth are stenographers. The number of employees in the department who are neither clerks nor stenographers is

    (A) 640
    (B) 665
    (C) 735
    (D) 750

14. Two nurses were assigned to take blood pressure readings at a health fair. They took the blood pressure of 190 people. If Nurse A took 40 more blood pressures than Nurse B, then the number of blood pressures taken by Nurse A was

    (A) 75
    (B) 110
    (C) 115
    (D) 150

15. A stock clerk had on hand the following items:

    500 pads, worth $0.04 each

    130 pencils, worth $0.03 each

    50 dozen rubber bands, worth $0.02 a dozen

    If, from this stock, he issued 125 pads, 45 pencils, and 48 rubber bands, the value of the remaining stock would be

    (A) $6.43
    (B) $8.95
    (C) $17.63
    (D) $18.47

16. Joe can paint a fence in three hours and his friend can paint the fence in four hours. How long will it take them to do the job if they work together?

(A) 7 hours

(B) $\frac{15}{7}$ hours

(C) $1\frac{5}{7}$ hours

(D) 2 hours

17. A department head hired a total of 60 temporary employees to handle a seasonal increase in the department's workload.

The following lists the number of temporary employees hired, their rates of pay, and the duration of their employment:

One third of the total were hired as clerks, each at the rate of $9,750 per year, for two months.

30 percent of the total were hired as office machine operators, each at the rate of $11,500 per year, for four months.

22 stenographers were hired, each at the rate of $10,200 per year, for three months.

The total amount paid to these temporary employees was approximately

(A) $178,000

(B) $157,600

(C) $52,200

(D) $48,500

18. Assume that there are 2,300 employees in a city agency. Also assume that five percent of these employees are accountants; that 80 percent of the accountants have college degrees; and that one half of the accountants who have college degrees have five years of experience. Then the number of employees in the agency who are accountants with college degrees and five years of experience is

(A) 46

(B) 51

(C) 460

(D) 920

19. If a monthly salary of $3,000 is subject to a $425 tax deduction, the net salary is

(A) $2,557.00

(B) $2,755.00

(C) $2,575.00

(D) $2,555.00

20. A sanitation worker who reports 45 minutes early for 8:00 A.M. duty will report at

(A) 7:00 A.M.

(B) 7:30 A.M.

(C) 6:15 A.M.

(D) 7:15 A.M.

STOP If you finish before time is called, you may check your work on this section only. Do not turn to any other section in the test.

TEST 3

20 QUESTIONS ▪▭ TIME—15 MINUTES

Directions: Each problem on this test requires logical reasoning and thinking, besides simple computations, to find the solution. Read each problem carefully and choose the correct answer from the four choices that follow. Fill in the corresponding space on your answer sheet.

1. If the average cost of sweeping a square foot of a small town's street is $0.75, the cost of sweeping 100 square feet is

    (A) $7.50
    (B) $750
    (C) $75
    (D) $70

2. After his car broke down on the way to a conference, a nurse had the car towed home 90 miles away. If the car was towed at a rate of 36 miles per hour, how many hours did it take to tow his car home?

    (A) .4 hours
    (B) 54 hours
    (C) 2.5 hours
    (D) 25 hours

3. A man is standing between a bank and a drugstore. He is 60 feet away from the bank and the drugstore is 100 feet away from the bank. How many feet nearer is the man to the bank than the drugstore is to the bank?

    (A) 60 feet
    (B) 40 feet
    (C) 50 feet
    (D) 20 feet

4. A clerk divided his 35-hour work week as follows:

    One fifth of his time in sorting mail; one half of his time in filing letters; and one seventh of his time in reception work.

    The rest of his time was devoted to messenger work. The percentage of time spent on messenger work by the clerk during the week was nearly

    (A) 6 percent.
    (B) 10 percent.
    (C) 14 percent.
    (D) 16 percent.

5. A city department has set up a computing unit and rented five computing machines at a yearly rental of $1,400 per machine. In addition, the cost to the department for the maintenance and repair of each of these machines is $100 per year. Five computing machine operators, each receiving an annual salary of $30,000 and a supervisor, who receives $38,000 a year, have been assigned to the unit. This unit will perform the work previously performed by 10 employees whose combined salary was $324,000 per year. On the basis of these facts, the savings that will result from the operation of this computing unit for five years will be nearly

    (A) $500,000
    (B) $947,500
    (C) $640,000
    (D) $950,000

6. Joe can do a certain job in eight days. After working alone for four days, he is joined by Mary, and together they finish the work in two more days. How long would it take Mary alone?

   (A) Five days
   (B) Six days
   (C) Seven days
   (D) Eight days

7. Eighty dozen pairs of rubber gloves were purchased for a medical facility. If the gloves are used at a rate of 32 pairs per day, what is the maximum number of days the gloves will last?

   (A) Two and a half days
   (B) Forty-eight days
   (C) Thirty days
   (D) 360 days

8. At a certain health-care facility, the average cost of providing care for 3 patients for five days is $7,200.00. What is the average cost of providing care for 24 patients for five days?

   (A) $43,200.00
   (B) $36,000.00
   (C) $34,560.00
   (D) $57,600.00

9. Typist A can do a job in 3 hours. Typist B can do the same job in 5 hours. How long would it take both, working together, to do the job?

   (A) 5 hours

   (B) $3\frac{1}{2}$ hours

   (C) $1\frac{7}{8}$ hours

   (D) $1\frac{5}{8}$ hours

10. After gaining 50 percent of his original capital, a person had capital of $18,000. Find the original capital.

    (A) $12,200.00
    (B) $13,100.00
    (C) $12,000.00
    (D) $12,025.00

11. To work off 60 calories, Brenda needs to walk on the treadmill for 15 minutes. How long will it take her to work off 100 calories?

    (A) 25 minutes
    (B) 55 minutes
    (C) 40 minutes
    (D) 45 minutes

12. A student worked thirty days at a part-time job. He paid two fifths of his earnings for room and board and had $81 left. What was his daily wage?

    (A) $4.50
    (B) $5.00
    (C) $5.50
    (D) $6.25

13. A dealer bought motorcycles for $4,000. He sold them for $6,200, making $50 on each motorcycle. How many motorcycles were there?

    (A) 40
    (B) 38
    (C) 43
    (D) 44

14. An organization had one fourth of its capital invested in goods, two thirds in land, and the remaining $1,224 in cash. What was the capital of the firm?

    (A) $4,986.00
    (B) $4,698.00
    (C) $4,896.00
    (D) $4,869.00

15. A and B together earn $2,100. If B is paid one fourth more than A, how many dollars should B receive?

    (A) $1,166.66
    (B) $1,162.66
    (C) $1,617.66
    (D) $1,167.66

GO ON TO THE NEXT PAGE

16. If a boat is purchased for $21,500 and sold for $23,650, what is the percentage of gain?

    (A) 8 percent
    (B) 15 percent
    (C) 20 percent
    (D) 10 percent

17. A person owned five sixths of a piece of property and sold three fourths of her share for $1,800. What was the value of the property?

    (A) $2,808.00
    (B) $2,880.00
    (C) $2,088.00
    (D) $2,880.80

18. A lot costing $21,250 leases for $1,900 per year. The taxes and other expenses are $300 per year. Find the percentage of net income on the investment.

    (A) $7\frac{1}{2}$ percent
    (B) 6 percent
    (C) 4 percent
    (D) 10 percent

19. B owned 75 shares of stock in a building association worth $50 each. The association declared a dividend of 8 percent, payable in stock. How many shares did he own then?

    (A) 81 shares
    (B) 80 shares
    (C) 90 shares
    (D) 85 shares

20. It requires 4 men three days to take an inventory; the weekly salary of each is as follows:

    A—$250, B—$130, C—$120, D—$90.

    Calculate the cost of taking the inventory, assuming that there are five full working days in a week.

    (A) $119.00
    (B) $196.00
    (C) $354.00
    (D) $588.00

STOP   If you finish before time is called, you may check your work on this section only. Do not turn to any other section in the test.

TEST 4

31 QUESTIONS ▪▫ TIME—22 MINUTES

Directions: Each problem on this test requires logical reasoning and thinking, besides simple computations, to find the solution. Read each problem carefully and choose the correct answer from the choices that follow. Fill in the corresponding space on your answer sheet.

1. In simplest form, $-11 - (-2)$ is
   - (A) 7
   - (B) 9
   - (C) -11
   - (D) -9

2. Find the average of 6.47, 5.89, 3.42, 0.65, and 7.09.
   - (A) 5.812
   - (B) 4.704
   - (C) 3.920
   - (D) 4.705

3. $\dfrac{456.3}{0.89}$ equals
   - (A) $513\dfrac{13}{89}$
   - (B) 512.70
   - (C) 513.89
   - (D) $512\dfrac{59}{89}$

4. Add 5 hours 13 minutes; 3 hours 49 minutes; and 24 minutes. The sum is
   - (A) 9 hours 26 minutes.
   - (B) 8 hours 16 minutes.
   - (C) 9 hours 76 minutes.
   - (D) 8 hours 6 minutes.

5. Two numbers are in the ratio of 18:47. If the smaller number is 126, the larger number is
   - (A) 376
   - (B) 144
   - (C) 235
   - (D) 329

6. Change 0.3125 to a fraction.
   - (A) $\dfrac{3}{64}$
   - (B) $\dfrac{1}{16}$
   - (C) $\dfrac{1}{64}$
   - (D) $\dfrac{5}{16}$

7. Divide $\dfrac{7}{8}$ by $\dfrac{7}{8}$.
   - (A) 1
   - (B) 0
   - (C) $\dfrac{7}{8}$
   - (D) $\dfrac{49}{64}$

8. In the series 5, 8, 13, 20, the next number should be
   - (A) 23
   - (B) 26
   - (C) 29
   - (D) 32

9. What is the interest on $300 at 6 percent for ten days? (Assume year = 360 days.)
   - (A) $0.50
   - (B) $1.50
   - (C) $2.50
   - (D) $5.50

GO ON TO THE NEXT PAGE

10. If the scale on a map indicates that one and one-half inches equals 500 miles, then 5 inches on the map will represent approximately

    (A) 1,800 miles.
    (B) 1,700 miles.
    (C) 1,300 miles.
    (D) 700 miles

11. $\frac{1}{2}$ percent equals

    (A) 0.002
    (B) 0.020
    (C) 0.005
    (D) 0.050

12. If 20 percent of an employee's bonus was $260.00, what was her entire bonus?

    (A) $2,300
    (B) $2,600
    (C) $1,600
    (D) $1,300

13. If a kilogram equals about 35 ounces, the number of grams in 1 ounce is approximately

    (A) 29
    (B) 30
    (C) 31
    (D) 32

14. An IV pump delivers medication at a constant rate of 24 milligrams per hour. How long does it take to deliver 90 milligrams?

    (A) 3 hours 15 minutes
    (B) 3 hours 45 minutes
    (C) 3 hours 75 minutes
    (D) 4 hours 15 minutes

15. If sound travels at the rate of 1,100 feet per second, in one-half minute it will travel about

    (A) 6 miles.
    (B) 8 miles.
    (C) 10 miles.
    (D) 3 miles.

16. If a kilometer is about five eighths of a mile, 2 miles is about

    (A) 1.6 kilometers.
    (B) 3.2 kilometers.
    (C) 2.4 kilometers.
    (D) 3.75 kilometers.

17. A lecture hall that is 25 feet wide and 75 feet long has a perimeter equal to

    (A) 1,750 feet.
    (B) 200 yards.
    (C) $66\frac{2}{3}$ yards.
    (D) 1,875 feet.

18. After deducting a discount of $16\frac{2}{3}$ percent, the price of a blouse was $35. The list price was

    (A) $37.50
    (B) $38
    (C) $41.75
    (D) $42

19. The number of decimal places in the product of 0.4266 and 0.3333 is

    (A) 8
    (B) 4
    (C) 14
    (D) None of the above

20. What is the cost of 5,500 bandages at $50 per thousand?

    (A) $385
    (B) $550
    (C) $275
    (D) $285

21. 572 divided by 0.52 is

    (A) 1,100
    (B) 110
    (C) 11.10
    (D) 11,000

22. 200 percent of 800 equals

 (A) 2,500
 (B) 16
 (C) 1,600
 (D) 4

23. A seventh-grade baseball team won ten games and lost five. Their average is

 (A) 0.667
 (B) 0.500
 (C) 0.333
 (D) 0.200

24. The number of cubic feet of soil needed for a flower box 3 feet long, 8 inches wide, and 1 foot deep is

 (A) 24
 (B) 12
 (C) $4\frac{2}{3}$
 (D) 2

25. At $1,250 per hundred, 228 watches will cost

 (A) $2,850
 (B) $36,000
 (C) $2,880
 (D) $360

26. The area of the shaded portion of the rectangle below is

 (A) 54 square inches.
 (B) 90 square inches.
 (C) 45 square inches.
 (D) 36 square inches.

27. On February 12, 1989, the age of a boy who was born on March 15, 1979, will be

 (A) 10 years, 10 months, and 3 days.
 (B) 9 years, 9 months, and 27 days.
 (C) 10 years, 1 month, and 3 days.
 (D) 9 years, 10 months, and 27 days.

Questions 28–31 are based on the following graph.

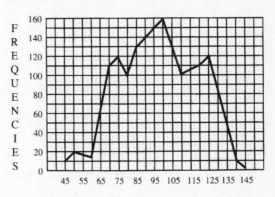

INTELLIGENCE QUOTIENTS (IQs)

28. The number of pupils having the highest IQ is about

 (A) 5
 (B) 160
 (C) 145
 (D) 20

29. The number of pupils having an IQ of 75 is about

 (A) 130
 (B) 100
 (C) 120
 (D) 110

GO ON TO THE NEXT PAGE

30. The number of pupils having an IQ of 80 is identical to the number of pupils having an IQ of
   (A) 100
   (B) 68
   (C) 110
   (D) 128

31. The IQ that has the greatest frequency is
   (A) 100
   (B) 95
   (C) 105
   (D) 160

STOP If you finish before time is called, you may check your work on this section only. Do not turn to any other section in the test.

QUANTITATIVE COMPARISONS
TEST 5

28 QUESTIONS ▪▫ TIME—35 MINUTES

Common Information: In each question, information concerning one or both of the quantities to be compared is given in the ITEM column. A symbol that appears in any column represents the same thing in Column A as it does in Column B.

Figures: Assume that the position of points, angles, regions, and so forth, are in the order shown; that the lines shown as straight are indeed straight; that figures lie in a plane unless otherwise indicated. Figures accompanying questions are intended to provide information you can use in answering the questions. However, unless a note states that a figure is drawn to scale, you should solve the problems by using your knowledge of mathematics, NOT by estimating sizes by sight or by measurement.

Directions: For each of the following questions, two quantities are given: one in Column A and one in Column B. Compare the two quantities and mark your answer sheet with the correct, lettered conclusion. These are your options:

  A   if the quantity in Column A is the greater;
  B   if the quantity in Column B is the greater;
  C   if the two quantities are equal;
  D   if the relationship cannot be determined from the information given.

Column A	Column B		Column A	Column B

1.

Isosceles triangle ABC
∠CAB = ∠ACB

$\angle x$	$\angle y$

2.

Parallelogram ABCD
E is a point on AB

Area of Δ DEC	Area of Δ AED + Area of Δ EBC

GO ON TO THE NEXT PAGE ➤

SUMMARY DIRECTIONS

Select: A if Column A is greater;
  B if Column B is greater;
  C if the two columns are equal;
  D if the relationship cannot be determined from the information given.

| Column A | Column B | Column A | Column B |

3. $x = -1$

| $x^3 + x^2 - x + 1$ | $x^3 - x^2 + x - 1$ |

6. x is a given number.

| Area of a circle radius = x^3 | Area of a circle radius = $3x$ |

4.

| The edge of a cube whose volume is 27 | The edge of a cube whose total surface area is 54 |

7.

| $\left(\dfrac{1}{4}\right)^{-2}$ | 4^2 |

5.

| $\dfrac{\dfrac{1}{2} + \dfrac{1}{3}}{\dfrac{2}{3}}$ | $\dfrac{\dfrac{2}{3}}{\dfrac{1}{2} + \dfrac{1}{3}}$ |

8.

| 0.02 | $\sqrt{0.02}$ |

SUMMARY DIRECTIONS

Select: A   if Column A is greater;
         B   if Column B is greater;
         C   if the two columns are equal;
         D   if the relationship cannot be determined from the information given.

Column A	Column B

9.

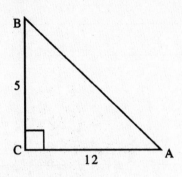

Right △ABC

$(AB)^2$	$(AC)^2 + 5(CB)$

Column A	Column B

11.

∠ADE > ∠AED

∠B	∠C

10.

Area of circle with radius 7	Area of equilateral triangle with side 14

12.

Area of shaded portion	Area of small circle

GO ON TO THE NEXT PAGE

SUMMARY DIRECTIONS

Select: A   if Column A is greater;
           B   if Column B is greater;
           C   if the two columns are equal;
           D   if the relationship cannot be determined from the information given.

Column A	**Column B**

13.

m ‖ n ‖ o ‖ p and q ‖ r

∠x	∠y

14. $a < 0 < b$

a^2	$\dfrac{b}{2}$

Column A	**Column B**

15. $t < 0 < r$

t^2	r

Diagram for problems 16–20

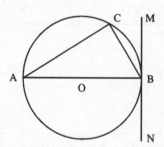

MN tangent to circle O at point B and ∠A = 30°

Column A	**Column B**

16. | m∠ACB | m∠NBO |

SUMMARY DIRECTIONS

Select: A   if Column A is greater;
          B   if Column B is greater;
          C   if the two columns are equal;
          D   if the relationship cannot be determined from the information given.

Column A	**Column B**
17. $\overset{\frown}{CB}$	$\overset{\frown}{AB}$
18. m∠CBM	m∠CAB
19. m∠CBA	m∠CBM
20. $\overline{AO} + \overline{AC}$	$\overline{BO} + \overline{BC}$

Diagram for problems 21–25

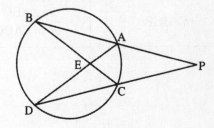

$$\overline{AB} + \overline{CD}$$

$$\overset{\frown}{BD} = 160°$$

$$\overset{\frown}{AC} = 40°$$

Column A	**Column B**
21. m∠APC	m∠ABC
22. m∠BED	m∠BEA
23. m∠BAD	m∠DCB

GO ON TO THE NEXT PAGE ➤

SUMMARY DIRECTIONS

Select: A if Column A is greater;
         B if Column B is greater;
         C if the two columns are equal;
         D if the relationship cannot be determined from the information given.

Column A	Column B
24. m∠BCP	m∠AEC + m∠ADC

Column A	Column B
27. 4% of 0.003	3% of 0.004

Column A	Column B
25. $\overset{\frown}{DC} + \overset{\frown}{AC}$	$\overset{\frown}{BD}$

28.

Intersecting straight lines; AB ⊥ CB, CD = ED

∠BCA	∠FEG

Column A	Column B
26. 75% of $\dfrac{3}{4}$	0.09 × 6

STOP   If you finish before time is called, you may check your work on this section only. Do not turn to any other section in the test.

TEST 6

12 QUESTIONS ▬ TIME—15 MINUTES

Common Information: In each question, information concerning one or both of the quantities to be compared is given in the ITEM column. A symbol that appears in any column represents the same thing in Column A as it does in Column B.

Figures: Assume that the position of points, angles, regions, and so forth, are in the order shown; that the lines shown as straight are indeed straight; that figures lie in a plane unless otherwise indicated. Figures accompanying questions are intended to provide information you can use in answering the questions. However, unless a note states that a figure is drawn to scale, you should solve the problems by using your knowledge of mathematics, and NOT by estimating sizes by sight or by measurement.

Directions: For each of the following questions, two quantities are given: one in Column A and one in Column B. Compare the two quantities and mark your answer sheet with the correct lettered conclusion. These are your options:

    A   if the quantity in Column A is the greater;
    B   if the quantity in Column B is the greater;
    C   if the two quantities are equal;
    D   if the relationship cannot be determined from the information given.

Column A	Column B
1. $a > 0; x > 0$	
$a + x$	$a - x$
2. The average of: 17, 19, 21, 23, 25	The average of: 16, 18, 20, 22, 24

Column A	Column B
3.	
$2x$	y

GO ON TO THE NEXT PAGE ▶

SUMMARY DIRECTIONS

Select: A if Column A is greater;
            B if Column B is greater;
            C if the two columns are equal;
            D if the relationship cannot be determined from the information given.

Column A	**Column B**

4. $0 < a < 12;\ 0 < b < 12$

a	b

5. $4a - 4b = 20$

a	b

6.

$\angle A$	$\angle B$

Column A	**Column B**

7. $\dfrac{a}{9} = b^2$

a	b

8.

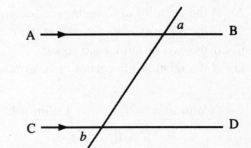

AB ‖ CD

a	b

SUMMARY DIRECTIONS

Select: A   if Column A is greater;
          B   if Column B is greater;
          C   if the two columns are equal;
          D   if the relationship cannot be determined from the information given.

Column A	**Column B**

9.

$3 + 24(3 - 2)$	$27 + 5(0)(5)$

11.

Column A	**Column B**

$\angle B > \angle A; \angle ACB < \angle A + \angle B$

$\angle A + \angle B$	$\angle ACD$

10.

$\angle 1 > \angle 2$

$\overline{AM}$	$\overline{BM}$

12.

$\left(\dfrac{2}{3}\right)^2 (3)^3$	$(3)^2 \left(\dfrac{2}{3}\right)^3$

STOP   If you finish before time is called, you may check your work on this section only. Do not turn to any other section in the test.

FINAL MATHEMATICS EXAMINATION PART 1: GENERAL MATHEMATICS

42 QUESTIONS • TIME—40 MINUTES

Directions: Each problem on this test requires logical reasoning and thinking, besides simple computations, to find the solution. Read each problem carefully and choose the correct answer from the choices that follow. Fill in the corresponding space on your answer sheet.

1. Jane Doe borrowed $225,000 for five years at $13\frac{1}{2}$ percent. The annual interest charge was
   - **(A)** $1,667
   - **(B)** $6,000
   - **(C)** $30,375
   - **(D)** $39,375

2. A junior salesman gets a commission of 14 percent on his sales. If he wants his commission to amount to $140, he will have to sell merchandise totaling
   - **(A)** $1,960
   - **(B)** $10
   - **(C)** $1,000
   - **(D)** $100

3. On a list price of $200, the difference between a single discount of 25 percent and successive discounts of 20 percent and 5 percent is
   - **(A)** $0
   - **(B)** $48
   - **(C)** $8
   - **(D)** $2

4. *A* worked five days on overhauling an old car. *B* worked four days more to finish the job. After the sale of the car, the net profit was $243. They wanted to divide the profit on the basis of the time spent by each. *A*'s share of the profit was
   - **(A)** $108
   - **(B)** $135
   - **(C)** $127
   - **(D)** $143

5. If cloth costs $42\frac{1}{2}$ cents per yard, how many yards can be purchased for $76.50?
   - **(A)** 220
   - **(B)** 180
   - **(C)** 190
   - **(D)** 230

6. A fashionable dress shop offers a 20 percent discount on selected items. For a dress marked at $280, what is the discount price?
   - **(A)** $224.00
   - **(B)** $232.00
   - **(C)** $248.00
   - **(D)** $261.00

7. If *A* takes six days to do a task and *B* takes three days to do the same task, working together they should do the same task in
   - **(A)** $2\frac{2}{3}$ days.
   - **(B)** 2 days.
   - **(C)** $2\frac{1}{3}$ days.
   - **(D)** $2\frac{1}{2}$ days.

8. The area of a mirror 40 inches long and 20 inches wide is approximately
   - **(A)** 8.5 square feet.
   - **(B)** 5.5 square feet.
   - **(C)** 8.0 square feet.
   - **(D)** 2.5 square feet.

9. $\frac{2}{3}$ plus $\frac{1}{8}$ equals

(A) $\frac{37}{72}$

(B) $\frac{82}{72}$

(C) $\frac{3}{11}$

(D) $\frac{19}{24}$

10. A student has received two grades of 90 and two grades of 80 in an English course. Assuming the grades are weighted equally, what is the student's average for the course?

(A) 90
(B) 87
(C) 85
(D) 84

11. If a man has only quarters and dimes totaling $2.00, the number of quarters CANNOT be

(A) 2
(B) 4
(C) 6
(D) 3

12. The number that increased by one sixth of itself and yields 182 is

(A) 156
(B) 176
(C) 148
(D) 160

13. $0.16\frac{3}{4}$ written as a percent is

(A) $16\frac{3}{74}$ percent.

(B) $16.\frac{3}{4}$ percent.

(C) $0.016\frac{3}{4}$ percent.

(D) $0.0016\frac{3}{4}$ percent.

14. If 4 ounces of protein provide 448 calories, how much protein is needed to provide 392 calories?

(A) 2.8 ounces
(B) 3.5 ounces
(C) 4.57 ounces
(D) 56 ounces

15. $1,296.53 minus $264.87 is

(A) $1,232.76
(B) $1,032.76
(C) $1,031.66
(D) $1,132.53

16. $12\frac{1}{2}$ minus $6\frac{1}{4}$ is

(A) $5\frac{3}{4}$

(B) $6\frac{1}{4}$

(C) $6\frac{1}{2}$

(D) $5\frac{1}{2}$

17. Men's handkerchiefs cost $1.29 for three. The cost per dozen handkerchiefs is

(A) $7.74
(B) $3.87
(C) $14.48
(D) $5.16

18. Add: $\frac{1}{4}$, $\frac{7}{12}$, $\frac{3}{8}$, $\frac{1}{2}$, and $\frac{5}{6}$.

(A) $2\frac{1}{2}$

(B) $2\frac{13}{24}$

(C) $2\frac{3}{4}$

(D) $2\frac{15}{24}$

GO ON TO THE NEXT PAGE

19. A floor is 25 feet wide by 36 feet long. To cover this floor with carpet will require
    - **(A)** 100 square yards.
    - **(B)** 300 square yards.
    - **(C)** 900 square yards.
    - **(D)** 25 square yards.

20. 72 divided by 0.0009 is
    - **(A)** 0.125
    - **(B)** 800
    - **(C)** 80,000
    - **(D)** 80

21. 345 safety pins at $4.15 per hundred will cost
    - **(A)** $0.1432
    - **(B)** $1.4320
    - **(C)** $14.32
    - **(D)** $143.20

22. The number that decreased by one fifth of itself yields 132 is
    - **(A)** 165
    - **(B)** 198
    - **(C)** 98
    - **(D)** 88

23. 285 is 5 percent of
    - **(A)** 1,700
    - **(B)** 7,350
    - **(C)** 1,750
    - **(D)** 5,700

24. A store sold jackets for $65 each. The jackets cost the store $50 each. The percentage of increase of selling price over cost is
    - **(A)** 40 percent.
    - **(B)** $33\frac{1}{2}$ percent.
    - **(C)** $33\frac{1}{3}$ percent.
    - **(D)** 30 percent.

25. The denominator of a fraction is 20 more than the numerator. What is the numerator if the fraction is equivalent to $\frac{3}{5}$?
    - **(A)** 12
    - **(B)** 30
    - **(C)** −50
    - **(D)** 10

26. Which statement below is true about the inequality of $2 < x \le 7$?
    - **(A)** $x < 2$
    - **(B)** $x = 2$
    - **(C)** x is greater than 7
    - **(D)** $x > 2$

27. $\frac{x}{5} - 4 = 11$. Find the value of x.
    - **(A)** 75
    - **(B)** 3
    - **(C)** 35
    - **(D)** 59

28. A punch recipe for a half gallon (64 ounces) of punch requires one pint (16 ounces) of grape juice. How many quarts (1 quart = 32 ounces) of grape juice are required for $2\frac{1}{2}$ gallons of the punch?
    - **(A)** 5 quarts
    - **(B)** 10 quarts
    - **(C)** $1\frac{1}{4}$ quarts
    - **(D)** $2\frac{1}{2}$ quarts

29. Mrs. Bowler got up at 7:00 A.M. last Wednesday morning and went to bed at 11:00 P.M. Wednesday night. During the time that she was up, she spent $\frac{1}{2}$ of her time at work, $\frac{1}{8}$ of her time bowling with friends, and $\frac{1}{4}$ of her time with her family. How much time did she have left for other activities?
    - **(A)** 2 hours
    - **(B)** 4 hours
    - **(C)** 1 hour
    - **(D)** 8 hours

30. If 24 percent of the students who enrolled in an algebra class of 50 students dropped the course before the semester ended, how many students remained in the class?

   (A) 27
   (B) 76
   (C) 12
   (D) 38

31. How many $\frac{3}{4}$ gram tablets are needed for a dosage of $4\frac{1}{2}$ grams?

   (A) 3.75
   (B) 1.5
   (C) 6
   (D) 3

32. $3.6 - 1.2(.8 - .3) + 8 \div .4 =$

   (A) 23
   (B) 20.5
   (C) 50
   (D) 3.2

33. Find .2 percent of 400.

   (A) 80
   (B) 800
   (C) .8
   (D) 2000

34. An 8-ounce bottle of fruit juice provides 200 calories. What percent of the 200 calories is provided by 3 ounces of the fruit juice?

   (A) 12.5 percent
   (B) 22.5 percent
   (C) 37.5 percent
   (D) 75 percent

35. Find the length of the hypotenuse in the triangle below.

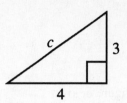

   (A) 7
   (B) 5
   (C) 25
   (D) 6

36. What is the width of a rectangle with an area of 63 square feet and a length of 9 feet?

   (A) 22.5 feet
   (B) 7 feet
   (C) 567 feet
   (D) 144 feet

37. If the triangles below are similar, find the length of side x.

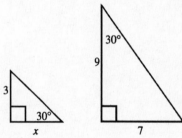

   (A) 21 inches
   (B) 11 inches
   (C) 13 inches
   (D) $3\frac{6}{7}$ inches

38. If two lines are parallel, which of the following statements is true?

   (A) The two lines have equal slopes.
   (B) The two lines have one point in common.
   (C) The product of the slopes of the lines is -1.
   (D) The two lines form right angles.

GO ON TO THE NEXT PAGE

39. If the area of a square is 144 m², what is the length of a side of the square?

(A) 12m

(B) 12m²

(C) 72m

(D) 72m²

40. Find the area of the figure below.

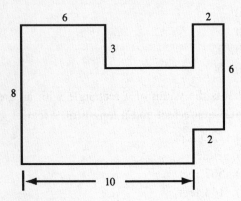

(A) 40m

(B) 46m

(C) 80m²

(D) 96m²

41. Consider the circle with central angles shown below:

What percent of the circle does the central angle of 60° represent? (Give answer to the nearest degree.)

(A) 6 percent

(B) 60 percent

(C) 17 percent

(D) 25 percent

42. If $\frac{1}{12}$ of a family's weekly budget is spent on entertainment and $\frac{1}{8}$ of the budget is spent on gasoline, which central angle represents the total spent on entertainment and gasoline?

(A) 20

(B) 45

(C) 90

(D) 75

STOP If you finish before time is called, you may check your work on this section only. Do not turn to any other section in the test.

PART 2: QUANTITATIVE COMPARISONS

12 QUESTIONS ▭ TIME—20 MINUTES

Common Information: In each question, information concerning one or both of the quantities to be compared is given in the ITEM column. A symbol that appears in any column represents the same thing in column A as it does in column B.

Figures: Assume that the position of points, angles, regions, and so forth, are in the order shown; that the lines shown as straight are indeed straight; that figures lie in a plane unless otherwise indicated. Figures accompanying questions are intended to provide information you can use in answering the questions. However, unless a note states that a figure is drawn to scale, you should solve the problems by using your knowledge of mathematics, and NOT by estimating sizes by sight or by measurement.

Directions: For each of the following questions, two quantities are given: one in Column A and one in Column B. Compare the two quantities and mark your answer sheet with the correct, lettered conclusion. These are your options:

- A   if the quantity in Column A is the greater;
- B   if the quantity in Column B is the greater;
- C   if the two quantities are equal;
- D   if the relationship cannot be determined from the information given.

Column A	Column B

1. $n < 0; a < 0$

$n + a$	$n - a$

Column A	Column B

3.

$\angle N - \angle C$	$90°$

2.

The average of: 22, 24, 26, 28, 30	The average of: 17, 19, 21, 23, 25, 27, 29, 31, 33

GO ON TO THE NEXT PAGE ▶

SUMMARY DIRECTIONS

Select: A if Column A is greater;
         B if Column B is greater;
         C if the two columns are equal;
         D if the relationship cannot be determined from the information given.

Column A	**Column B**

4. $0 < y < 5; 0 < n < 7$

y	n

Column A	**Column B**

7. $\dfrac{m}{2} = c^2$

m	c

5. $5n - 5a = 25$

n	a

8.

c	a

6.   In isosceles $\triangle NCY$:

$\angle C$	$\angle Y$

SUMMARY DIRECTIONS

Select: A   if Column A is greater;
          B   if Column B is greater;
          C   if the two columns are equal;
          D   if the relationship cannot be determined from the information given.

Column A	Column B

9.

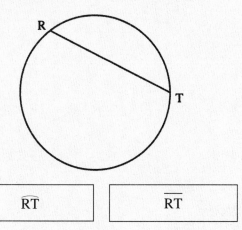

$\overparen{RT}$	$\overline{RT}$

11.

Column A	Column B
$8[2x - 3$ $(4x - 6) - 9]$	$6[3x - 2$ $(6x - 3) + 2]$

12.

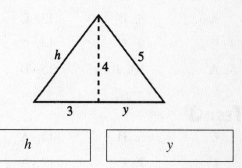

h	y

10.

$5 + 16(3 - 2)$	$21 + 5 -$ $[3 (4 - 3)(0)]$

S T O P   If you finish before time is called, you may check your work on this section only. Do not turn to any other section in the test.

ANSWER KEY

TEST 1

1. A	6. A	11. B	16. C
2. D	7. B	12. B	17. B
3. B	8. C	13. B	18. A
4. C	9. C	14. C	19. A
5. B	10. A	15. C	20. D

TEST 2

1. C	6. B	11. C	16. C
2. D	7. B	12. C	17. B
3. A	8. B	13. C	18. A
4. C	9. C	14. C	19. C
5. A	10. B	15. D	20. D

TEST 3

1. C	6. D	11. A	16. D
2. C	7. C	12. A	17. B
3. B	8. D	13. D	18. A
4. D	9. C	14. C	19. A
5. C	10. C	15. A	20. C

TEST 4

1. D	9. A	17. C	25. A
2. B	10. B	18. D	26. A
3. B	11. C	19. A	27. D
4. A	12. D	20. C	28. A
5. D	13. A	21. A	29. C
6. D	14. B	22. C	30. C
7. A	15. A	23. A	31. A
8. C	16. B	24. D	

QUANTITATIVE COMPARISONS

TEST 5

1. D	8. B	15. D	22. A
2. C	9. C	16. C	23. C
3. A	10. A	17. B	24. B
4. C	11. D	18. C	25. B
5. A	12. A	19. A	26. A
6. D	13. D	20. A	27. C
7. C	14. D	21. A	28. C

TEST 6

1. A	4. D	7. D	10. B
2. A	5. A	8. C	11. C
3. B	6. C	9. C	12. A

FINAL MATHEMATICS

PART 1: GENERAL MATHEMATICS

1. C	12. A	23. D	33. C
2. C	13. A	24. D	34. C
3. D	14. B	25. B	35. B
4. B	15. C	26. D	36. B
5. B	16. B	27. A	37. D
6. A	17. D	28. D	38. A
7. B	18. B	29. A	39. A
8. B	19. A	30. D	40. C
9. D	20. C	31. C	41. C
10. C	21. C	32. A	42. D
11. D	22. A		

PART 2: QUANTITATIVE COMPARISONS

1. B	4. D	7. D	10. B
2. A	5. A	8. A	11. D
3. C	6. D	9. A	12. A

EXPLANATORY ANSWERS

TEST 1

1. **The correct answer is (A).**

   Interest = Principal × Rate × Time

   Note: 6% = 0.06

   144 days = $\dfrac{144}{360}$ year

   $I = P \times R \times T$

   $= \$25,800 \times 0.06 \times \dfrac{144}{360}$

   $= \dfrac{\$222,912}{360}$

   $= \$619.20$

2. **The correct answer is (D).** Let n = number of minutes in which they can do the job together. Arthur can do $\dfrac{1}{6}$ of the job in one minute, so in n minutes he can do $\dfrac{n}{60}$ of the job. Jack can do $\dfrac{1}{30}$ of the job in one minute and $\dfrac{n}{30}$ of the job in n minutes. Together, in n minutes they can do the complete job.

   $\dfrac{n}{60} + \dfrac{n}{30} = 1$

   $n + 2n = 60$ (multiplying both sides by 60, the lowest common denominator)

   $3n = 60$ (combine like terms)

   $n = 20$ (divide by 3)

   They can do the job together in 20 minutes.

3. **The correct answer is (B).** Total seats = 105

   Total time = 6 hours

   Total people involved = 486

   105 seats × 6 hours = 630 seating hours

   To find the average seating time, divide

   $\quad$ 630 ÷ 485 = 1.3 hours

   Now change the 0.3 hours to minutes

   $\quad$ (1 hour = 60 minutes)

   $\quad$ .03 hour × $\dfrac{60 \text{ minutes}}{1 \text{ hour}}$ = 18 minutes

   The amount is 1 hour 18 minutes.

4. **The correct answer is (C).** Paper per ream = $14.50

   Discount = 5% or 0.05

   Total cash = $690.00

   First, find the discount on the paper per ream when paying cash.

   $\quad$ $14.50 × 0.05 = $0.725

   Our price per ream is $14.50 − $0.725 = $13.775. Given $690 to spend, divide to find how much paper can be purchased.

   $\quad$ $690.00 ÷ $13.775/ream = 50

   50 reams for $688.75

5. **The correct answer is (B).** Use simple logic on this problem.

From	*To*	
8:30 A.M. →	8:30 P.M. =	12 hours
8:30 P.M. →	3:30 A.M. =	7 hours

   Total = 19 hours,

   but this is 15 minutes too much.

   Note: Change one of the hours to minutes (1 hour = 60 minutes).

   $\quad$ 45 minutes = $\dfrac{45}{60}$ hours or $\dfrac{3}{4}$ hours

   $\quad\quad$ 18 hours 60 minutes

   $\quad\quad\quad$ − 15 minutes

   $\quad\quad$ ─────────────

   $\quad\quad$ 18 hours 45 minutes

   $18\dfrac{3}{4}$ is the total number of hours.

6. **The correct answer is (A).** Again, use logic.

Month	*Number of days/month*	
September	from 19 to 30	12 days
October	31 days	31 days
November	30 days	30 days
December	from 1 to 25	25 days
		─────
		98 days

   Note: Remember that 19 September and 25 December are included.

   Total = 98 days inclusive

7. **The correct answer is (B).**

Total to be filed = 800 cards
Rate cards can be filed = 80 cards per hour

How many cards were filed in the first 7 hours?

$$7 \times 80 = 560 \text{ cards were filed}$$

Subtract to find the remaining cards to be filed.

$$800 - 560 = 240$$

240 cards remain unfiled

8. **The correct answer is (C).** From $80 to $90, there is a $10 increase; the percentage of increase is found by dividing the amount of increase by the original amount:

$$10 \div 80 = 0.125 \text{ or } 12\frac{1}{2}\%$$

Note: $0.125 = 12.5\%$ or $12\frac{1}{2}\%$

Percentage of increase = $12\frac{1}{2}\%$

9. **The correct answer is (C).** To find the *average* number of patients served by each nurse, divide 135 patients by 15 nurses to get 9 patients per nurse.

10. **The correct answer is (A).** To find the percent of correct answers on the test, divide the number of correct answers by the total number of items on the test.

$$\frac{72}{80} = .90$$

Change .90 to a percent.

$$.90 = 90\%$$

90% of the test items were correct.

11. **The correct answer is (B).** To find the number of hours of exercise the patient gets in a week, multiply

45 min. × 7 days = 315 minutes

Convert the minutes to hours by dividing by 60 since there are 60 minutes in an hour.

$$\frac{315}{60} = 5.25 \text{ hours per week}$$

12. **The correct answer is (B).** To find the number of nurses on duty for the two shifts, determine the total number of nurses who worked on the night shift by finding one half of the number who worked the afternoon shift.

$$120 \times \frac{1}{2} = 60$$

Add the number who worked the afternoon shift to the number who worked the night shift.

$$120 + 60 = 180$$

180 nurses worked on the two shifts.

13. **The correct answer is (B).** Total summonses in seven hours = 182

To find the *average* number of summonses per hour, divide:

$$182 \text{ summonses} \div 7 \text{ hours} = 26$$

Average = 26 summonses/hour

14. **The correct answer is (C).** To find the number of admitted patients who weren't in accidents, subtract the number of patients who were in accidents from the total number of patients.

$$76 - 23 = 53$$

53 of the admitted patients had not been in accidents.

15. **The correct answer is (C).** If it takes one truck one hour to go 40 miles, it will take two hours to go 80 miles.

$$2 \text{ hours} \times 40 \frac{\text{miles}}{\text{hour}} = 80 \text{ miles}$$

16. **The correct answer is (C).** If the total capacity is 100 gallons, then

$$\frac{2}{5} \text{ of } 100 = \frac{2}{5} \times 100$$

$$= \frac{200}{5}$$

$$= 40 \text{ gallons}$$

17. **The correct answer is (B).** Total salary = $3,000

Tax = 20% or .20

Find the amount of 20% tax by multiplying:

$$\$3,000 \times .20 = \$600$$

Subtract the tax from the salary to find the net:

$$\$3,000 - \$600 = \$2,400$$

$2,400 = net pay

18. **The correct answer is (A).**

Total cost = $1,000

Total square yards = 100

Find the cost per square yard by dividing:

$1,000 ÷ 100 square yards = $10

$10/square yard

19. **The correct answer is (A).**

Base pay	$3,000
Bonus	+ 350
Serv. Increment	+ 250
Total pay	$3,600

20. **The correct answer is (D).**

Annual salary	$21,600
Bonus	+ 7,200
Increment	+ 1,200
Total pay	$30,000

TEST 2

1. **The correct answer is (C).**

The second vehicle is 90 feet − 40 feet = 50 feet from the emergency medical technician (EMT). The first vehicle is 40 feet from the EMT. The first vehicle is 50 feet − 40 feet = 10 feet closer than the second vehicle.

2. **The correct answer is (D).** To find the number of milliliters the IV bag has when it's two-thirds full, multiply $1{,}260 \text{ milliliters} \times \frac{2}{3} = 840 \text{ milliliters}$

There are 840 milliliters in the IV bag when it's two-thirds full.

3. **The correct answer is (A).**

Salary per month = $2,500
Days worked = 23

To find the earnings per day, divide:

$$\frac{\$2{,}500}{\text{month}} \div \frac{23 \text{ days}}{\text{month}} = \frac{\$108.70}{\text{day}}$$

or

$$\frac{\$2{,}500}{\text{month}} \div \frac{23 \text{ days}}{\text{month}}$$

$$= \frac{\$2{,}500}{\text{month}} \times \frac{\text{month}}{23 \text{ days}}$$

$$= \frac{\$2{,}500}{23 \text{ days}} = \frac{\$108.70}{\text{day}}$$

4. **The correct answer is (C).** To find the take-home pay of the nursing home assistant, subtract the total amount of her deductions from her weekly salary.

Total deductions	= $18.00 + $15.00 + $21.00 + $72.00 = $126.00
Weekly salary	= $360.00
Salary − deductions	= $360.00 − $126.00 = $234.00
Take-home pay	= $234.00

5. **The correct answer is (A).**

Stamps per day	*Cost per day*
$\dfrac{40}{\text{day}} \times \$0.33$	= 13.20
$\dfrac{25}{\text{day}} \times \$0.20$	= 5.00
$\dfrac{320}{\text{day}} \times \$0.60$	= 192.00
Total cost/day	$210.20

For five days, 5 × $210.20 = $1,051.00

Total cost = $1,051.00

6. **The correct answer is (B).** Number of applications issued in 1979 = 12,000

In 1977, 25 percent more were issued, or 0.25 × 12,000 = 3,000 more in 1977.

So there were 3000 + 12,000 = 15,000 issued in 1977.

In 1975, 10 percent fewer were issued than in 1977, or 0.10 × 15,000 = 1,500 fewer were issued in 1975.

The number issued in 1975 is

15,000 − 1,500 = 13,500.

13,500 issued

7. **The correct answer is (B).** If three fifths of the 200 are done by calculator, then:

$$\frac{3}{5} \times 200 = \frac{600}{5} = 120$$

columns will be done by the machine. To find the number done by hand, subtract:

$$200 - 120 = 80 \text{ will be done by hand.}$$

To find the time it takes to do the 120 columns by machine and the 80 columns by hand, divide:

$$120 \text{ columns} \div 40 \text{ columns per hour} = 3 \text{ hours}$$
$$80 \text{ columns} \div 20 \text{ columns per hour} = 4 \text{ hours}$$

Total time = 7 hours

8. **The correct answer is (B).** To find the total cost of the rubber gloves bought in 1998, first determine the amount of the 20% increase for a dozen gloves in 1998.

$$.20 \times \$2.60 = 0.52$$

Add the cost in 1995 to the amount of the increase to get the cost of the gloves in 1998.

$$\$2.60 + 0.52 = \$3.12$$

In 1998 a dozen gloves cost \$3.12.

The number of gloves purchased in 1998 was 25% less than the number purchased in 1995.

To find how many dozens of gloves were purchased in 1999, find 25% of 500 dozen and subtract the result from 500 dozen.

$$500 \text{ dozen} - .25 \times 500 \text{ dozen}$$
$$= 500 \text{ dozen} - 125 \text{ dozen} = 375 \text{ dozen}$$

375 dozen gloves were purchased in 1998.

Multiply the price per dozen $\$3.12 \times 375$ dozen = \$1,170.00.

The total cost of the gloves bought in 1998 was \$1,170.00.

9. **The correct answer is (C).** During the first hour, 40 forms were checked, leaving 450 to be checked:

$$490 - 40 = 450$$

The two nurses working together can check 75 forms.

Now find the time it takes to do the 450 forms. Do this by dividing:

$$450 \text{ forms} \div 75 \text{ forms/hour} = 6 \text{ hours}$$

It takes 6 hours to do the 450 and 1 hour for the first 40 forms:

$$6 \text{ hours} + 1 \text{ hour} = 7 \text{ hours to do the job.}$$

A total of 7 hours is needed.

10. **The correct answer is (B).** Total employed = 420

If 30 percent are nurses,

$$420 \times 0.30 = 126 \text{ nurses}$$

$\frac{1}{7}$ are doctors:

$$420 \times \frac{1}{7} = 60 \text{ doctors}$$

The difference is $126 - 60 = 66$.

11. **The correct answer is (C).** Cost = \$0.12 per copy

Time = 120 copies per minute

To find the number of copies produced, divide:

$$36 \div \$0.12 = 300 \text{ copies}$$

To find the number of minutes, divide:

$$300 \text{ copies} \div 120 \text{ copies/minute} = 2.5 \text{ minutes}$$

12. **The correct answer is (C).** If the average number of medical records filed for five days was 720, then 5 days $\times$ 720 records/day = 3,600 records for the five-day period.

For four days:

$$610 + 720 + 740 + 755 = 2,825 \text{ medical records were filed}$$

Subtract:

$$3600 - 2,825 = 775 \text{ need to be filed the fifth day to get an average of 720 for the five-day period}$$

13. **The correct answer is (C).** Total employees = 1,400

    35% clerks = 1,400 × .35 = 490 clerks

    $\frac{1}{8}$ stenos = 1,400 × $\frac{1}{8}$ = 175 stenos

    Together (490 + 175 = 665), there are 665 clerks and stenographers. To find how many employees are neither, subtract:

    1,400 − 665 = 735

    Answer = 735 other employees

14. **The correct answer is (C).** If Nurse A takes 40 more blood pressure readings than Nurse B, let x represent the number of blood pressure readings taken by Nurse B. Then $x + 40$ = the number of blood pressure readings taken by Nurse A. Add the number taken by Nurse A to the number taken by Nurse B to get the total number of blood pressure readings taken.

    $x + x + 40 = 190$

    $2x + 40 = 190$

    $2x = 150$

    $x = 75$, the number of blood pressure readings taken by Nurse B

    $x + 40 = 75 + 40 = 115$, the number of blood pressure readings taken by Nurse A

15. **The correct answer is (D).** Stock on hand and cost per item:

	Cost
500 pads × $0.04/pad	= $20.00
130 pencils × $0.03/pencil	= $3.90
50 dozen rubber bands × $0.02/dozen	= $1.00
value of stock on hand	= $24.90

    If we issue the items below,

125 pads × $0.04	= $5.00
45 pencils × $0.03	= $1.35
48 rubber bands or 4 dozen × $0.02	= $0.08
	$6.43

    To find the value of the remaining stock, subtract:

    $24.90 − $6.43 = $18.47

    Value = $18.47

16. **The correct answer is (C).** Let t be the amount of time for both to do the job. If Joe does $\frac{t}{3}$ part of the job, and his friend does $\frac{t}{4}$ part of the job, then $\frac{t}{3} + \frac{t}{4} = 1$ (the whole job).

    $4t + 3t = 12$ (multiply lowest common denominator by 12)

    $7t$ = combine like terms

    $t = \frac{12}{7}$ divide by 7

    t $1\frac{5}{7}$ hours

17. **The correct answer is (B).** Total employees = 60

    $\frac{1}{3} \times 60 = 20$ clerks

    30% × 60, or .30 × 60 = 18 office machine operators (OMOs)

    60 − 38 = 22 stenos

    To find their *rate per month*, divide their monthly salaries by 12, because there are 12 months in a year:

    clerks $\frac{\$9,750}{12}$ = $812.50 per month

    OMOs $\frac{\$11,500}{12}$ = $958.33 per month

    stenos $\frac{\$10,200}{12}$ = $850.00 per month

    Now find the salary for all employees for the time they worked:

    If 20 clerks worked two months, total pay equals:

    20 × 2 × $812.50 = $32,500.00

    If 18 OMOs worked four months, total pay equals:

    18 × 4 × $958.33 = $68,999.76

    If 22 stenos worked three months, total pay equals:

    22 × 3 × $850.00 = $56,100.00

    Total salaries = $68,999.76 + $32,500.00 + $56,100.00 = $157,599.76. This amount can be rounded off to $157,600.00.

18. **The correct answer is (A).** 5 percent of 2,300 are accountants:

$$0.05 \times 2{,}300 = 115$$

80 percent of the 115 accountants have college degrees:

$$0.80 \times 115 = 92$$

One half of the 92 have five years' experience:

$$\frac{1}{2} \times 92 = 46$$

46 employees have all three qualifications.

19. **The correct answer is (C).** $3,000 is subject to $425 tax. The net can be found by subtracting:

$$\$3{,}000 - \$425 = \$2{,}575$$

20. **The correct answer is (D).** A sanitation worker who reports 45 minutes early for 8:00 A.M. duty reports

$$\begin{array}{r} 7 \text{ hours } 60 \text{ minutes} \\ - \ 45 \text{ minutes} \\ \hline 7 \text{ hours } 15 \text{ minutes} \end{array}$$

Note: 1 hour = 60 minutes

8 hours = 7 hours 60 minutes

This worker reports at 7:15 A.M.

TEST 3

1. **The correct answer is (C).** If it costs $0.75 to sweep one square foot, to find the cost for 100 square feet, multiply 100 square feet × 0.75 square foot = $75.

Total cost = $75

2. **The correct answer is (C).** To determine how many hours it will take to tow the car 90 miles at a rate of 36 mph, divide

$$90 \div 32 = 2.5$$

It will take 2.5 hours = $2\frac{1}{2}$ hours to tow the car 90 miles.

3. **The correct answer is (B).** To determine how many feet nearer the man is to the bank than the drugstore is to the bank, use the following diagram:

The total distance from the bank to the drugstore is 100 feet. Subtract to find the distance from the man to the drugstore.

$$100 \text{ feet} - 60 \text{ feet} = 40 \text{ feet}$$

The man is 40 feet nearer to the bank than the drug store is to the bank.

4. **The correct answer is (D).** A clerk works 35 hours per week. $\frac{1}{5}$ of his time is used to sort mail:

$$\frac{1}{5} \times 35 = 7 \text{ hours}$$

$\frac{1}{2}$ of his time is used to file letters:

$$\frac{1}{2} \times 35 = 17\frac{1}{2} \text{ hours}$$

$\frac{1}{7}$ of his time is used for reception work.

$$\frac{1}{7} \times 35 = 5 \text{ hours}$$

Total = $29\frac{1}{2}$ hours

$29\frac{1}{2}$ were used for the above. To find the time left for messenger work, subtract

$$35 - 29\frac{1}{2} = 5\frac{1}{2} \text{ hours}$$

Now to find what percentage of 35 is $5\frac{1}{2}$, divide:

$$5.5 \div 35 = 0.16 \text{ or } 16\%$$

Note: $5\frac{1}{2} = 5.5$

16% remains for messenger work.

5. **The correct answer is (C).**

Item

5 machines
$1,400/year   5 × 1,400 $7,000

Maintenance, repairs
$100/machine   5 × 100 $500

5 operators' annual salaries
$30,000   5 × $30,000 $150,000

Supervisor's annual salary
$38,000   1 × $38,000 $38,000

Total cost $195,500

If 10 employees were paid a total of $324,000, find the savings by subtracting:

$324,000 − $195,500 = $128,500 one year's savings

To find the savings for five years, multiply:

$128,500 × 5 = $642,500

This amount *rounds off* to (or, is nearest to) $640,000.

6. **The correct answer is (D).** If Joe can do the job alone in eight days, then he can do $\frac{1}{8}$ in one day and $\frac{6}{8}$ or $\frac{3}{4}$ in six days.

Let n be the number of days it would take Mary to do the job alone. Then:

$\frac{1}{n}$ is the part of the job she can do in one day,

and $\frac{2}{n}$ is the part of the job she can do in the two days she works with Joe.

Now, the sum of parts done by Joe and Mary equals one whole job:

$$\frac{3}{4} + \frac{2}{n} = 1$$

$3n + 8 = 4n$ (multiply by the lowest common denominator, 4n)

$8 = 4n − 3n$ (subtract 3n from both sides of the equation)

$8 = n$ (subtract like term)

$n = 8$

Mary alone could do the job in eight days.

7. **The correct answer is (C).**

Eighty dozen = 80 × 12 = 960

960 pairs of gloves were purchased.

To find the maximum number of days the gloves will last, divide 960 ÷ 32 = 30

If the gloves are being used at a rate of 32 pairs per day, they will last thirty days.

8. **The correct answer is (D).** To determine the cost of caring for 24 patients for five days, find the cost of caring for 1 patient by dividing.

$7,200.00 ÷ 3 = $ 2,400.00

To get the cost for caring for 24 patients, multiply

24 × $2,400.00 = $57,600.00

The cost for caring for 24 patients is $57,600.00.

9. **The correct answer is (C).** A can do one third of the job in 1 hour. B can do one fifth of the job in 1 hour. Together they can do $\frac{1}{3} + \frac{1}{5}$ of the job in 1 hour. Let t be the time it takes for both to do the job. Together, they can do $\frac{1}{t}$ of the job in 1 hour. Thus:

$$\frac{1}{3} + \frac{1}{5} = \frac{1}{t}$$

$5t + 3t = 15$ (multiply lowest common denominator by the 15t or 3 × 5 × t)

$8t = 15$ (add like terms)

$t = \frac{15}{8}$ (divide both sides by 8 hours)

$t = 1\frac{7}{8}$

10. **The correct answer is (C).** Let x be the unknown original capital and $0.50x$ be 50 percent of the unknown capital.

$x + .50x = $18,000$

$1.50x = $18,000$ (add like terms)

$\frac{150x}{1.50} = \frac{$18,000}{1.50}$ (divide both sides by 1.50)

$x = $12,000$

$12,000 is the original amount of the capital.

11. **The correct answer is (A).** Let x represent the amount of time it takes to walk off 100 calories.

The ratio of the amount of time it takes to work off 60 calories equal the ratio of the amount of time it takes to work off 100 calories:

$$\frac{15 \text{ minutes}}{60 \text{ calories}} = \frac{x \text{ minutes}}{100 \text{ calories}}$$

$$60x = 15 \times 100$$
$$60x = 1{,}500$$
$$x = 25 \text{ minutes}$$

It will take 25 minutes on the treadmill to work off 100 calories.

12. **The correct answer is (A).** If two fifths of his salary was used, then three fifths was left; three fifths of his salary is $81. Now, since his salary is unknown, let x represent it:

$$\frac{3}{5} \times x = \$81$$

$$x = \$81 \div \frac{3}{5} \quad \left(\text{divide both sides by } \frac{3}{5}\right)$$

$$x = \$81 \times \frac{5}{3} \quad (\text{invert and multiply})$$

$$x = \$135$$

His salary is $135 for 30 days of work. To find the *daily wage*, divide the salary by 30:

$$\$135 \div 30 \text{ days} = \$4.50/\text{day}$$

Daily wage = $4.50

13. **The correct answer is (D).** To find the number of motorcycles purchased, first subtract his original purchase price from the selling price:

$$\$6{,}200 - \$4{,}000 = \$2{,}200 \text{ profit}$$

Since the profit was $2,200, and the profit on each motorcycle was $50, the number of motorcycles sold is:

$$\$2{,}200 \text{ profit} \div 50 \text{ profit/motorcycle} = 44$$
motorcycles sold

14. **The correct answer is (C).** $\frac{1}{4}$ in *goods* (given)

$\frac{2}{3} \times \frac{3}{4} = \frac{1}{2}$ in *land* (because $\frac{3}{4}$ is the remainder after the goods are invested), $\frac{1}{4}$ is left in *cash*, because if $\frac{1}{4}$ is in goods, $+\frac{1}{2}$ is in land, $\frac{3}{4}$ is invested, leaving $\frac{1}{4}$ for cash

If $\frac{1}{4}$, which is the cash, is valued at $1,224,

$$\frac{1}{4} \text{ in goods} = \$1{,}224.$$

$\frac{1}{2}$ is twice as much as $\frac{1}{4}$

$$\frac{1}{2} \text{ in land} = \$2{,}448$$

$$\frac{1}{4} \text{ in cash} = \frac{\$1{,}224}{\$4{,}896}$$

Total capital = $4,896

15. **The correct answer is (A).** Let A equal the amount A earned, and B equal the amount B earned.

Together, they earned $A + B = \$2{,}100$.

If B is paid $\frac{1}{4}$ more than A, then A's salary plus $\frac{1}{4}$ of A's salary is equal to B's salary.

Express this as follows:

$$B = A + \frac{1}{4}A$$

$$4B = 4A + A \quad (\text{multiply by 4})$$

$$-5A + 4B = 0 \quad (\text{transpose the } A \text{ terms})$$

Now you have two equations with two unknowns. Use the elimination method to find B's salary:

$$A + B = \$2{,}100$$
$$-5A + 4B = 0$$
$$5A + 5B = \$10{,}500 \quad \begin{array}{l}(\text{multiply the first} \\ \text{equation by 5})\end{array}$$
$$-5A + 4B = 0$$
$$9B = \$10{,}500 \quad (\text{add the two equations})$$
$$B = \$1{,}166.67 \quad (\text{now divide by 9})$$

or $1,166$\frac{2}{3}$

Note: $0.67 = \frac{2}{3}$

16. **The correct answer is (D).** The boat costs $21,500 and was sold for $23,650. Subtract:

$$\$23,650 - \$21,500 = \$2,150$$

$2,150 was gained. To find the percentage gained, divide the amount gained by the original amount:

$$\$2,150 \div \$21,500 = 0.10 \text{ or } 10\%$$

Percentage gained = 10%

17. **The correct answer is (B).** $\frac{5}{6} \times \frac{3}{4} = \frac{5}{8}$ of the property costs $1,800

Then, letting y represent the value of the property,

$$\frac{5}{8} \times y = \$1,800$$

$$y = \$1,800 \div \frac{5}{8} \quad \left(\text{divide both side by } \frac{5}{8}\right)$$

$$y = \$1,800 \times \frac{8}{5} \quad \text{(invert and multiply)}$$

Therefore, $2,880 is the price of the property.

18. **The correct answer is (A).** A lot costs $21,250.

$1,900	is received for lease
− 300	is deducted for expenses
$1,600	is net income

To find what percentage $1,600 is of the cost of the lot, divide:

$$1,600 \div 21,250 = 0.075 \text{ or } 7\frac{1}{2}\%$$

$7\frac{1}{2}\%$ = percentage of cost

19. **The correct answer is (A).** Total shares currently owned = 75

Values per share = $50

To find the value of the stock, multiply

$$75 \times \$50 = \$3,750$$

To find 8%, multiply the stock value by 0.08

$3,750 × 0.08 = $300 (dividend)

Given $300, divide by $50 to see how many additional shares of stock can be purchased:

$$\$300 \div 50 = 6 \text{ shares}$$

Therefore, he now owns 75 + 6 = 81 shares.

20. **The correct answer is (C).** First, find the salary each man is paid for one day. To do so, divide their salaries by 5 days:

		salary/day	salary/3 days
A	$\frac{\$250}{5} =$	$50.00 × 3=	$150
B	$\frac{\$130}{5} =$	$26.00 × 3 =	$78
C	$\frac{\$120}{5} =$	$24.00 × 3 =	$72
D	$\frac{\$90}{5} =$	$18.00 × 3 =	$54

Total salaries for 3 days = $354

TEST 4

1. **The correct answer is (D).**

$$-11 - (-2)$$
$$= -11 + 2$$
$$= -9$$

2. **The correct answer is (B).** 6.47 + 5.89 + 3.42 + .65 + 7.09 = 23.52

To find the average, divide the sum by 5 (the number of terms involved)

$$23.52 \div 5 = 4.704$$

Average = 4.704

3. **The correct answer is (B).**

$$
\begin{array}{r}
512.69\frac{59}{89} \\
.89\overline{)456.30.00} \\
445 \\
\hline
113 \\
89 \\
\hline
240 \\
178 \\
\hline
620 \\
534 \\
\hline
860 \\
801 \\
\hline
59 \quad \text{remainder}
\end{array}
$$

$512.69\frac{59}{89}$ rounds off to 512.70.

4. **The correct answer is (A).**

    $$\begin{array}{r} 5 \text{ hours } 13 \text{ minutes} \\ 3 \text{ hours } 49 \text{ minutes} \\ + \ 24 \text{ minutes} \\ \hline 8 \text{ hours } 86 \text{ minutes} \end{array}$$

    Since there are 60 minutes in one hour, then 86 minutes = 60 minutes + 26 minutes or 1 hour and 26 minutes.

    So, 8 hours and 86 minutes = 9 hours and 26 minutes.

5. **The correct answer is (D).** $\dfrac{18}{47} = \dfrac{126}{x}$

    $18x = 47(126)$ (cross multiply)

    $18x = 5,922$

    $x = 329$ (divide by 18)

6. **The correct answer is (D).** $0.3125 = \dfrac{3,125}{10,000} = \dfrac{5}{16}$

7. **The correct answer is (A).** $\dfrac{7}{8} \div \dfrac{7}{8}$

    $= \dfrac{7}{8} \times \dfrac{8}{7}$ (invert the second term and multiply)

    $= 1$

8. **The correct answer is (C).** 5, 8, 13, 20. To each number, add the next odd number to determine the next number in the series.

    Series   Odd Number

5	+	3	=	8
8	+	5	=	13
13	+	7	=	20
20	+	9	=	29

    29 will be the next number.

9. **The correct answer is (A).** *Interest = Principal ×* *Rate × Time*

    $= \$300 \times 0.06 \times \dfrac{10}{360}$

    $= \dfrac{\$180}{360} = \dfrac{\$1}{2}$

    $= \$.50$

10. **The correct answer is (B).** First, find the number of $1\dfrac{1}{2}$ inch units there are in 5 inches. Do this by dividing:

    $5 \div 1\dfrac{1}{2}$

    $= 5 \div \dfrac{3}{2}$ $\left(\text{change } 1\dfrac{1}{2} \text{ to } \dfrac{3}{2}\right)$

    $= 5 \times \dfrac{2}{3}$ (invert and multiply)

    $= \dfrac{10}{3}$

    Now find the total miles by multiplying:

    $500 \times \dfrac{10}{3} = 1,666.67$

    Five inches represents approximately 1,700 miles.

11. **The correct answer is (C).** $\dfrac{1}{2}\% = 0.5\%$ or $\dfrac{0.5}{100} = 0.005$

12. **The correct answer is (D).** $260 is 20% of the bonus. Write this in equation form. Let the bonus be x.

    $\$260 = .20x$

    $\dfrac{260}{.20} = \dfrac{.20x}{.20}$ (divide by 0.20)

    $\$1,300 = x$

    Her entire bonus was $1,300.

13. **The correct answer is (A).** 1 kilogram = 35 ounces

    Find how many grams there are in 1 ounce.

    Note: 1 kilogram = 1,000 grams

    1,000 grams = 35 ounces

    $1 \text{ ounce} \times \dfrac{1,000 \text{ grams}}{35 \text{ ounces}}$

    $= \dfrac{1,000 \text{ grams}}{35}$

    = 28.6 or 29 grams in 1 ounce

14. **The correct answer is (B).** To find the amount of time it takes to deliver the 90 milligrams at a rate of 24 milligrams per hour, divide

    amount of time = 90 milligrams
    $\div$ 24 milligrams per hour = 3.75 hours

    3.75 hours $= 3\dfrac{3}{4}$ hours = 3 hours and 45 minutes

15. **The correct answer is (A).** First, find the number of seconds there are in one-half minute:

$$\frac{1}{2} \times 60 \text{ sec/min} = 30 \text{ seconds}$$

Since sound travels 1,100 feet per second, it will travel:

30 sec. × 1,100 ft. = 33,000 ft.

Change the 33,000 feet to miles (1 mile = 5,280 feet)

$$33,000 \text{ feet} \times \frac{1 \text{ mile}}{5,280 \text{ feet}} = \frac{33,000}{5,280}$$

$$= 6.25$$

Round off: 6.25 miles = about 6 miles

16. **The correct answer is (B).** 1 kilometer = $\frac{5}{8}$ mile

x kilometer = 2 miles

$$\frac{1 \text{ kilometer}}{\frac{5}{8} \text{ mile}} = \frac{x}{2}$$

$$\frac{5}{8}x = 2$$

$$5x = 16$$

$$x = 3.2$$

2 miles = about 3.2 kilometers

17. **The correct answer is (C).** Perimeter of a rectangle (the hall is shaped like a rectangle) is:

Perimeter = 2 *length* + 2 *width*

$$= 2(75) + 2(25)$$

$$= 150 + 50$$

$$= 200 \text{ feet}$$

The perimeter is 200 feet.

Now change 200 feet to yards (3 feet = 1 yard).

$$200 \text{ feet} \times \frac{1 \text{ yard}}{3 \text{ feet}} = 66\frac{2}{3} \text{ yards}$$

18. **The correct answer is (D).** Let the price of a blouse be x. Then:

$$x - 16\frac{2}{3}\% = 35$$

$$\frac{2}{3} = 0.67, \text{ so } 16.6770\% = 0.1667$$

$$x - 0.1667x = \$35 \quad \text{(change the percent to a decimal)}$$

$$0.8333x = \$35 \quad \text{(combine like terms)}$$

$$x = \$42 \quad \text{(divide by 0.8333)}$$

The list price was $42.

19. **The correct answer is (A).** To find the number of decimal places in the product of two numbers, find the sum of the number of digits to the right of the decimal of each number.

0.4266 has 4 digits to the right.
0.3333 has 4 digits to the right.

There should be 8 digits in the product.

20. **The correct answer is (C).** 5.5 thousand × $50 thousand = $275

21. **The correct answer is (A).**

```
        1100.
 .52.)572.00.
      52
      ──
      52
      52
      ──
      00
      00
      ──
```

Answer: 1,100

22. **The correct answer is (C).** 200 percent of 800

$$2.00 \times 800 = 1,600$$

23. **The correct answer is (A).** The total games played was 15. To find their average, divide games won by total played:

$$10 \div 15 = 0.667$$

Their average is 0.667.

24. The correct answer is (D). To find the soil needed, first change the 8 inches to feet, so all units will be the same.

$$8 \text{ inches} \times \frac{1 \text{ foot}}{12 \text{ inches}} = 0.67 \text{ feet}$$

Now multiply all units.

$$3 \text{ feet} \times 0.67 \text{ feet} \times 1 \text{ foot} = 2 \text{ cubic feet}$$

2 cubic feet of soil will be needed to fill the box.

25. The correct answer is (A). Find the price for one watch by dividing:

$$\$1{,}250 \text{ (per hundred)} \div 100 = \$12.50 \text{ (price of one watch)}$$

To find the cost of 228, multiply the number of watches by the price per watch.

$$228 \text{ watches} \times \$12.50 \text{ per watch} = \$2{,}850$$

The cost of the watches will be $2,850.

26. The correct answer is (A). Find the area of the small rectangle and subtract its area from the large rectangle to determine the shaded area.

Large rectangle
$$A = length \times width$$
$$= 6 \times 15$$
$$= 90 \text{ square inches}$$

Small rectangle
$$A = length \times width$$
$$= 4 \times 9$$
$$= 36 \text{ square inches}$$

$$90 - 36 = 54 \text{ square inches}$$

The area of the shaded area is 54 square inches.

27. The correct answer is (D).

From	To	Time
March 15, 1979	March 15, 1988	9 years
March 15, 1988	Jan. 15, 1989	10 months
Jan. 15, 1989	Feb. 12, 1989	27 days

His age will be 9 years, 10 months, 27 days.

28. The correct answer is (A). On the chart, each line represents 10 units. The highest IQ is about halfway on the first line, which is half of 10.

So the answer is 5.

29. The correct answer is (C). Locate IQ on base and trace to horizontal intersection.

30. The correct answer is (C). There are 100 students with an IQ of 80. Looking across the chart we see that there are also 100 students with an IQ of 110.

31. The correct answer is (A). Highest point on the graph, an IQ of 100

QUANTITATIVE COMPARISONS

Test 5

1. The correct answer is (D). The value of $\angle x$ or $\angle y$ cannot be determined unless the measure of at least one angle is known.

2. The correct answer is (C).

Area of $\triangle DEC = \frac{1}{2}$ base $\times$ height

Area of parallelogram $=$ base $+$ height

Area of $\triangle ADE + \triangle EBC =$ (area of the whole parallelogram $-$ area of $\triangle DEC$)

$$= (\text{base} \times \text{height} - \frac{1}{2} \text{ base} \times \text{height})$$
$$= \frac{1}{2} \text{ base} \times \text{height}$$

3. The correct answer is (A).

$$x^3 + x^2 - x + 1 = (-1)^3 + (-1)^2 - (-1) + 1$$
$$= -1 + 1 + 1 + 1$$
$$= 2$$

$$x^3 - x^2 + x - 1 = (-1)^3 - (-1)^2 + (-1) - 1$$
$$= -1 - 1 - 1 - 1$$
$$= -4$$

4. The correct answer is (C). A cube has six surfaces, each one's area e^2:

$$e^3 = 27$$
$$e = 3$$
$$6e^2 = 54$$
$$e^2 = 9$$
$$e = 3$$

5. **The correct answer is (A).**

$$\frac{\frac{1}{2}+\frac{1}{3}}{\frac{2}{3}}=\frac{\frac{3}{6}+\frac{2}{6}}{\frac{4}{6}}=\frac{\frac{5}{6}}{\frac{4}{6}}=\frac{5}{6}\times\frac{6}{4}=\frac{5}{4}$$

$$\frac{\frac{2}{3}}{\frac{1}{2}+\frac{1}{3}}=\frac{\frac{4}{6}}{\frac{3}{6}+\frac{2}{6}}=\frac{\frac{4}{6}}{\frac{5}{6}}=\frac{4}{6}\times\frac{6}{5}=\frac{4}{5}$$

$$\frac{5}{4}=\frac{5}{4}\times\frac{5}{5}=\frac{25}{20}$$

$$\frac{4}{5}=\frac{4}{5}\times\frac{4}{4}=\frac{16}{20}$$

$$\frac{25}{20}>\frac{16}{20}$$

6. **The correct answer is (D).** Area of circle with radius x^3:

$$A=\pi r^2=\pi(x^3)^2=\pi x^6$$
$$=3.14x^6$$

Area of circle radius $3x$:

$$A=\pi r^2=\pi(3x)^2=\pi(9x^2)=3.14(9x^2)$$
$$=28.26x^2$$

We cannot know whether $3.14x^6$ or $28.26x^2$ is larger unless we know the value of x.

$$\left(\frac{1}{4}\right)^{-2}=\frac{1}{\left(\frac{1}{4}\right)^2}\quad\text{(Note that }4^2=16.)$$

7. **The correct answer is (C).**

$$=\frac{1}{\frac{1}{16}}$$
$$=16$$

8. **The correct answer is (B).** $0.02=\sqrt{0.0004}$

$$\sqrt{0.02}>\sqrt{0.0004}$$

9. **The correct answer is (C).** By the Pythagorean theorem, $(AB)^2=(AC)^2+(BC)^2$

However, $(BC)^2=5^2=25$ and $5CB=5\times5=25$

Therefore, $(BC)^2=5CB$

$(AB)^2=(AC)^2+5CB$ [substituting $5CB$ for $(BC)^2$ in the Pythagorean theorem]

10. **The correct answer is (A).** Area of circle with radius

$$A=\pi r^2=3.14\times7^2$$
$$=3.14\times49=153.86$$

Note: $\pi\approx3.14$

Area of equilateral Δ with side of 14:

A line from one vertex to the mid-point of the opposite side is perpendicular to the opposite side. It is, therefore, the height of the triangle.

Let the length of this line be h. Then, by the Pythagorean theorem, $7^2+h^2=14^2$.

$$h^2=14^2-7^2=147$$
$$h^2=3\times7\times7$$
$$h=7\sqrt{3}$$

Area of $\Delta=\frac{1}{2}$ base $\times$ height

$$=\frac{1}{2}(14)(7\sqrt{3})\quad\textit{Note: }\sqrt{3}\approx1.732$$

Area of $\Delta=(7)7\sqrt{3}$
$$=49\sqrt{3}$$
$$=49\times1.732=84.87$$

$153.86>84.87$

Thus, area of circle is greater than area of the triangle.

11. **The correct answer is (D).** Not enough information is given to determine the values of the angles.

12. **The correct answer is (A).** (Area of shaded portion) = (Area of larger circle) − (Area of smaller circle)

Area of larger circle $=\pi r^2=\pi\times10^2$
$$=3.14\times10^2$$
$$=3.14\times100$$
$$=314$$

Area of smaller circle $=\pi r^2=\pi\times7^2$
$$=3.14\times7^2$$
$$=3.14\times49$$
$$=153.85$$

Area of shaded region $=314-153.86=160.14$

$160.14>153.86$

13. **The correct answer is (D).**

All that can be determined is that *x* and *y* are supplementary.

14. **The correct answer is (D).** There is insufficient information to determine an answer.

15. **The correct answer is (D).** There is insufficient information to determine an answer.

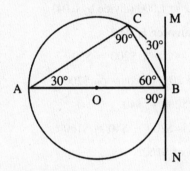

16. **The correct answer is (C).** m∠ACB = 90°

m∠NBO = 90°

A tangent to a circle is perpendicular to the radius of the circle at their point of contact. An inscribed angle is equal to one-half its intercepted arc. Therefore, m∠ACB = 90°.

17. **The correct answer is (B).**

$\overarc{AC}$ = 120° $\overarc{CB}$ = 60°

An inscribed angle is equal to one half its intercepted arc.

18. **The correct answer is (C).**

m∠CBM = 30°   m∠CAB = 30°

19. **The correct answer is (A).**

m∠CBA = 60°   m∠CBM = 30°

20. **The correct answer is (A).** $\overline{AO} = \overline{BO}$; all radii in the same circle are equal.

$\overline{AC} > \overline{BC}$; in a triangle, the greater side lies opposite the greater angle.

$$\overline{AO} + \overline{AC} > \overline{BO} + \overline{BC}$$

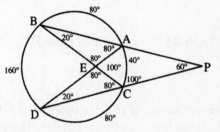

21. **The correct answer is (A).**

m∠APC = 60°   m∠ABC = 20°

22. **The correct answer is (A).**

m∠BED = 100°   m∠BEA = 80°

23. **The correct answer is (C).**

m∠BAD = 80°   m∠DCB = 80°

24. **The correct answer is (B).** m∠BCP = 100°

m∠AEC + m∠ADC = 100° + 20° = 120°

25. **The correct answer is (B).**

$\overarc{DC} + \overarc{AC}$ = 80° + 40° = 120°

$\overarc{BD}$ = 160°

26. **The correct answer is (A).**

75% of $\frac{3}{4}$ = .75 × .75   .09 × 6 = .54

= .5625

27. **The correct answer is (C).**

4% of 0.003 = 0.04 × .003

= 0.00012

3% of 0.004 = 0.03 × 0.004

= 0.00012

28. **The correct answer is (C).**

∠BCA = 45°   ∠FEG = 45°

TEST 6

1. **The correct answer is (A).** The statement $a > 0$ and $x > 0$ implies both a and x are positive. The sum of two positive numbers is always greater than their difference.

2. **The correct answer is (A).** The averages of Column A and Column B are 21 and 20, respectively.

3. **The correct answer is (B).** ∠ABC = x (vertical angles are equal). Since ∠C = 90°, ∠A + ∠ABC = 90° (180° in a triangle). Therefore, $2x = 90°$, and $x = 45°$. ∠ABC and ∠y are supplementary; hence, $y = 135°$. Therefore, $y > 2x$.

4. **The correct answer is (D).** Impossible to determine because a could be any number between 0 and 12 and b, any number between 0 and 10.

5. **The correct answer is (A).** $4a - 4b = 20$

    $a - b = 5$
    $a - 5 = b$

    For all values of a and b, $a > b$.

6. **The correct answer is (C).** Angles opposite equal sides of a triangle are equal.

7. **The correct answer is (D).** Impossible to determine because b could be positive or negative.

8. **The correct answer is (C).** If two parallel lines are cut by a transversal, the alternate exterior angles are equal.

9. **The correct answer is (C).** Column A and Column B both equal 27.

10. **The correct answer is (B).** The greater side lies opposite the greater angle.

11. **The correct answer is (C).** The exterior angle of a triangle is equal to the two interior nonadjacent angles.

12. **The correct answer is (A).** The value of Column A is 12, and the value of Column B is $2\frac{2}{3}$. Therefore, A > B.

FINAL MATHEMATICS EXAMINATION

PART 1: GENERAL MATHEMATICS

1. **The correct answer is (C).** $I = P \times R \times T$

    $= \$225,000 \times 0.135 \times 1$ (year)
    $= \$30,375$

2. **The correct answer is (C).** 14% of $x = \$140$ (Let x be the total sales.)

    $0.04 \times x = \$140$
    $x = 1,000$ (divide by 0.04)

3. **The correct answer is (D).**

    25% of $\$200 = .25 \times \$200 = \$50$

    Next, find the 20% discount on $200:

    $0.20 \times \$200 = \$40$

    The list price is $\$200 - \$40 = \$160$

    Now take 5% of $160:

    $0.05 \times \$160 = \$8$

    The discount is $48 when taken at 20% and 5% successively.

    $\$50 - \$48 = \$2$

4. **The correct answer is (B).** The job took nine days to complete.

    A worked five days: he completed $\frac{5}{9}$ of the work.

    B worked four days: he completed $\frac{4}{9}$ of the work.

    If the net profit was $243, then A received $\frac{5}{9} \times \$243 = \$135$

5. **The correct answer is (B).** $\$76.50 \div 42\frac{1}{2}¢$/yard

    $\left(42\frac{1}{2}¢ = \$0.425\right)$

    $= \$76.50 \div \$0.425$/yard
    $= 180$ yards

6. **The correct answer is (A).**

    Discount = 20%
    Sale price = 80%

    $$0.80 \times \$280.00 = \$224.00$$

7. **The correct answer is (B).** $\dfrac{n}{6} + \dfrac{n}{3} = 1$

    $n + 2n = 6$ (multiply by 6)
    $3n = 6$ (combine like terms)
    $n = 2$ (divide by 3)

8. **The correct answer is (B).** Area of a rectangle is

    $A = length \times width$
      $= 40$ inches $\times 20$ inches
      $= 800$ square inches

    Note: 1 square foot = 144 square inches

    $$\frac{800 \text{ square inches}}{144 \text{ square inches}} = 5.5 \text{ square feet}$$

9. **The correct answer is (D).**

    $\dfrac{2}{3} \times \dfrac{8}{8} = \dfrac{16}{24}$ (lowest common denominator
                  is 24

    $+\dfrac{1}{8} \times \dfrac{3}{3} = \dfrac{3}{24}$

             $= \dfrac{19}{24}$

10. **The correct answer is (C).** To arrive at the average, add all numbers and divide by total number of grades.

        80
        80
        90
    $+90$
    $\overline{340 \div 4 = 85}$

11. **The correct answer is (D).** The number of quarters must be even; otherwise, adding dimes will not give $2.00 *exactly*. So the answer cannot be 3, choice (D).

    $3 \times 25¢ = 75¢$ or 0.75
    $\$2.00 - 0.75 = \$1.25$

    $1.25 cannot be changed to all dimes.

12. **The correct answer is (A).** Let the *number* be x. A *number* increased by $\dfrac{1}{6}$ of itself is 182. To put this in equation form:

    $$x + \frac{1}{6} = 182$$
    $6x + x = 1,092$ (multiple each term by 6)
    $7x = 1,092$ (combine like terms)
    $x = 156$ (divide by 7)

13. **The correct answer is (A).** $.16\dfrac{3}{4} = 16\dfrac{3}{4}\%$

    When changing decimals to percents, move the decimal to the right two places.

14. **The correct answer is (B).** Let p represent the amount of protein needed for 392 calories. Use a proportion

    $$\frac{4 \text{ ounces}}{448 \text{ calories}} = \frac{p \text{ ounces}}{392 \text{ calories}}$$
    $448p = 4 \times 392$
    $448p = 1,568$
    $p = 3.5$ ounces of protein

    3.5 ounces of protein are needed for 392 calories.

15. **The correct answer is (C).**

    $\$1,296.53$
    $\underline{-246.87}$
    $\$1,031.66$

16. **The correct answer is (B).**

    $12\dfrac{1}{2} = 12\dfrac{2}{4}$

    $\underline{-6\dfrac{1}{4} = -6\dfrac{1}{4}}$

            $6\dfrac{1}{4}$

    Note: $\dfrac{1}{2} \times \dfrac{2}{2} = \dfrac{2}{4}$

17. **The correct answer is (D).** Price per dozen can be found by multiplying the $1.29 by 4. (There are 4 groups of 3 in a dozen.)

    $$\$1.25 \times 4 = \$5.16$$

18. **The correct answer is (B).** $\frac{1}{4} + \frac{7}{12} + \frac{3}{8} + \frac{1}{2} + \frac{5}{6} =$

$\frac{6}{24} + \frac{14}{24} + \frac{9}{24} + \frac{12}{24} + \frac{20}{24}$

Note: The lowest common denominator is 24. Each fraction needs to be rewritten to an equivalent fraction, so the denominator will be 24.

$$= \frac{6 + 14 + 9 + 12 + 20}{24} = \frac{61}{24}$$

Divide:

$$24\overline{)61} = 2\frac{13}{24}$$
$$\underline{48}$$
$$13$$

19. **The correct answer is (A).** 25 feet × 36 feet = 900 square feet

Now change 900 square feet to square yards.

Note: 9 square feet = 1 square yard

$$900 \text{ square feet} \times \frac{1 \text{ square yard}}{9 \text{ square feet}}$$

$$= 100 \text{ square yards}$$

20. **The correct answer is (C).**

$$.0009\overline{)72.0000} \text{ or } 80,000$$
$$80000.$$

21. **The correct answer is (C).** One safety pin costs:

$$\$4.15 \div 100 = \$.0415$$

So 345 safety pins cost:

$$345 \times 0.0415 = \$14.32$$

22. **The correct answer is (A).** A number, x, that decreased by $\frac{1}{5}$ of itself equals 132, can be expressed as:

$$x - \frac{1x}{5} = 132.$$

$5x - x = 660$ (multiply each term by 5)
$4x = 660$ (combine like terms)
$x = 165$ (divide by 4)

23. **The correct answer is (D).** $285 = 0.05y$ (y is the unknown value)

$5,700 = y$ (divide by 0.05)

24. **The correct answer is (D).** $\$65 - \$50 = \$15$ is the increase, but to find the percentage of increase, we divide the increase by the original amount:

$$\$15 \div \$50 = 0.30 \text{ or } 30\%$$

25. **The correct answer is (B).** Let x represent the numerator of the fraction, then the denominator will be $x + 20$.

Since the fraction is equivalent to $\frac{3}{5}$, we get

$$\frac{x}{x + 20} = \frac{3}{5}$$
$$5x = 3(x + 20)$$
$$5x = 3x + 60$$
$$2x = 60$$
$$x = 30$$

26. **The correct answer is (D).** $2 < x \leq 7$ means that x is greater than 2 and it is less than or equal to 7.

27. **The correct answer is (A).**

$$\frac{x}{5} - 4 = 11$$
$$\frac{x}{5} - 4 + 4 = 11 + 4$$
$$\frac{x}{5} = 15$$
$$5 \times \frac{x}{5} = 5 \times 15$$
$$x = 75$$

28. **The correct answer is (D).** Note that one gallon of punch contains 128 ounces (one-half gallon contains 64 ounces; hence, $2\frac{1}{2}$ gallons equals 320 ounces). A direct proportion can be used to solve the problem.

Let x = the number of ounces of grape juice needed.

$$\frac{16 \text{ ounces grape}}{64 \text{ ounces punch}} = \frac{x}{320 \text{ ounces punch}}$$
$$\frac{1}{4} = \frac{x}{320}$$
$$4x = 320$$
$$x = 80 \text{ ounces grape juice}$$

Since the answer is to be given in quarts, change 80 ounces to quarts by dividing 80 by 32. (There are 32 ounces in a quart.)

$80 \div 32 = 2.5$; thus, 2.5 quarts of grape juice are needed to make $2\frac{1}{2}$ gallons of punch.

29. **The correct answer is (A).** There are 16 hours from 7:00 A.M. until 11:00 P.M. Hence, Mrs. Bowler was up 16 hours.

Let x = the time Mrs. Bowler had left for other activities, then

$$\frac{1}{2}(16) + \frac{1}{8}(16) + \frac{1}{4}(16) + x = 16$$
$$8 + 2 + 4 + x = 16$$
$$14 + x = 16$$
$$x = 2$$

30. **The correct answer is (D).** 24 percent of the 50 students dropped the class.

$$24 \text{ percent of } 50 = .24 \times 50 = 12$$

Since 12 students dropped, $50 - 12$, or 38 students remained in the class.

31. **The correct answer is (C).** Divide $4\frac{1}{2}$ by $\frac{3}{4}$. (First change $4\frac{1}{2}$ to $\frac{9}{2}$.)

$$4\frac{1}{2} \div \frac{3}{4} = \frac{9}{2} \times \frac{4}{3} = \frac{36}{6} = 6$$

32. **The correct answer is (A).** $3.6 - 1.2(.8 - .3) + 8 \div .4$

$$= 3.6 - 1.2(.5) + 8 \div 4$$
$$= 3.6 - .6 + 8 \div .4$$
$$= 3.6 - .6 + 20$$
$$= 3 + 30$$
$$= 23$$

Note: Operations must be performed in the correct order. (Parentheses first, then multiplication and division before addition and subtraction.)

33. **The correct answer is (C).** Change .2 percent to a decimal and multiply .2 percent by 400.

$$.002 \times 400 = .800 \text{ or } .8$$

34. **The correct answer is (C).** Find the number of calories provided by 3 ounces of fruit juice.

$$\frac{8}{200} = \frac{3}{c}$$
$$8c = 600$$
$$c = 75$$

75 calories are provided by 3 ounces of fruit juice.

Now determine what percent 75 is of 200.

$$n\% \text{ of } 200 = 75$$
$$200n = 75$$
$$n = .375 = 37.5\%,$$

Three ounces of the fruit juice provide 37.5% of the calories in the 8 ounces.

35. **The correct answer is (B).** Use the Pythagorean theorem.

$$c^2 = a^2 + b^2$$
$$c^2 = 3^2 + 4^2$$
$$c^2 = 9 + 16$$
$$c^2 = 25$$
$$c = \sqrt{25}$$
$$c = 5$$

36. **The correct answer is (B).** The formula for the area of a rectangle is $A = LW$. We know the area of the rectangle is 63 and the length is 9 feet. Thus,

$$63 \text{ square feet} = 9W \text{ feet}$$
$$\frac{63 \text{ square feet}}{9 \text{ feet}} = \frac{9W \text{ feet}}{9 \text{ feet}}$$
$$7 \text{ feet} = W$$

37. **The correct answer is (D).** The corresponding sides of similar triangles are proportional. Therefore,

$$\frac{3}{7} = \frac{x}{9}$$
$$7x = 27$$
$$x = 3\frac{6}{7}$$

38. **The correct answer is (A).** Parallel lines have equal slopes; they do not intersect.

39. **The correct answer is (A).** The area of a square is found by squaring a side of the square.

If $A = 144m^2$

$$144m^2 = s^2 \text{ where } s \text{ is a side of the square}$$
$$\sqrt{144m^2} = s$$
$$12m = s$$

40. **The correct answer is (C).** Divide the figure into nonoverlapping rectangles. Find the area of each rectangle. Add the areas of the rectangles to get the total area of the figure.

$$A = 48m^2 + 20m^2 + 12m^2 = 80m^2$$

41. **The correct answer is (C).** The entire circle contains 360°. The central angle of 60° represents $\frac{60}{360} = \frac{1}{6}$. Change $\frac{1}{6}$ to a percent by dividing the denominator into the numerator. Thus, $\frac{1}{6} = 16\frac{2}{3}\%$. We get 17 when we express $16\frac{2}{3}$ to the nearest whole percent.

42. **The correct answer is (D).** The weekly budget is represented by the entire circle; $\frac{1}{12}$ of the circle represents $\frac{1}{12} \times 360 = 30°$, which is the measure of the central angle for the amount spent on entertainment. $\frac{1}{8}$ of the circle represents $\frac{1}{8} \times 360 = 45°$, which is the measure of the central angle for the amount spent on gasoline. A central angle that represents the total spent on entertainment and gasoline is 30° + 45° = 75°. (Alternatively, $\frac{1}{8} + \frac{1}{12} = \frac{5}{24}$ and $\frac{5}{24} \times 360° = 75°$.)

PART 2: QUANTITATIVE COMPARISONS

1. **The correct answer is (B).** Both n and a are negative because they are both less than 0. Hence $(n - a)$ must be greater than $(n + a)$ because a negative minus a negative is greater than a negative plus a negative.

$-a > +a$ ($-a$ = positive, $+a$ = negative)

$n - a > n + a$ (adding n to both sides)

2. **The correct answer is (A).** The average of Column A is 26, while the average of Column B is 25.

3. **The correct answer is (C).**

∠N = ∠C + 90°　　An exterior angle is equal to the sum of the interior remote angles.

∠N − ∠C = 90°　　When equals are subtracted from equals, the differences are equal.

4. **The correct answer is (D).** It is impossible to determine because y could be any number from 0 to 5 and n any number from 0 to 7.

5. **The correct answer is (A).** $5n - 5a = 25$

$n - a = 5$　(equals divided by equals are equals)

$n = a + 5$ (equals plus equals are equal)

n is 5 greater than a.

6. **The correct answer is (D).** An isosceles triangle has two equal angles, but from the information given, it is impossible to determine which two angles are actually equal.

7. **The correct answer is (D).** There is insufficient information to determine whether m or c is the greater. By substituting numbers for m and c, we see that either quantity could be greater—for example

(1) $m = 2$, $c = 1$;

(2) $m = \frac{1}{8}$, $c = \frac{1}{4}$.

8. **The correct answer is (A).**

$\angle c = 120°$ and $\angle a = \angle a_1$ since all vertical angles are equal.

$\angle c + \angle a_1 = 180°$ since the two interior angles on the same side of a transversal are supplementary.

$\angle a_1 = 60°$

$\angle a = 60° < \angle c = 120°$

9. **The correct answer is (A).** The shortest distance between two points is a straight line. Therefore, the chord, a straight line, must be shorter than the arc.

10. **The correct answer is (B).**

$$5 + 16 \, (3 - 2) = 5 + 16(1)$$
$$= 5 + 16$$
$$= 21$$

$$21 + 5 - [3(4 - 3)(0)] = 21 + 5 - 0$$
$$= 26$$

11. **The correct answer is (D).** Since the value of x cannot be determined, the values of Columns A and B remain unknown.

12. **The correct answer is (A).** It can be readily seen that the figure consists of two 3-4-5 right triangles. Therefore, $h = 5$ and $y = 3$.

SCIENCE

INTRODUCTION

Living organisms used to be placed into either a plant kingdom or animal kingdom. However, modern classification systems are more sophisticated, and more than two kingdoms are now recognized. The most widely accepted classification system includes five kingdoms of organisms, as presented below:

Monera

Prokaryotic (cells without a nucleus bounded by a membrane, or true, membrane-bounded organelles in the cytoplasm), unicellular or colonial, autotrophic or saprotrophic.

Includes bacteria and cyanobacteria (formerly called "blue-green algae").

Protista

Eukaryotic (cells with a nucleus bounded by a membrane and with membrane-bound organelles, such as mitochondria or chloroplasts, in the cytoplasm); unicellular or with a simple multicellular body lacking distinct tissues; autotrophic, saprotrophic, or phagotrophic.

Includes amoebae, flagellates, ciliates, algae (except cyanobacteria), and slime molds.

Fungi

Eukaryotic, usually with a simple multicellular body in the form of a mass of slender filaments (mycelium); sometimes unicellular (e.g., yeasts); lacking chlorophyll; saprophytic; often parasitic.

Includes mushrooms and many types of molds.

Animalia

Eukaryotic; multicellular; body usually complex and with many types of true tissues; phagotrophic; sometimes parasitic; usually motile; cells lacking a cell wall.

Includes all types of animals such as sponges, worms, arthropods, and vertebrates.

Plantae

Eukaryotic; multicellular; body usually complex and usually with many types of true tissues; possessing chlorophyll; autotrophic; rarely parasitic; never motile; cells always surrounded by a cell wall made of cellulose.

Includes flowering plants, conifers, ferns, and mosses.

CHARACTERISTICS OF ORGANISMS

Regardless of the kingdom in which organisms are classified, all living things have certain characteristics in common. These characteristics sometimes are used to describe life: We can say that any object that exhibits all of these characteristics is alive. Organisms are always made of cells; they respond to stimuli; they reproduce; they exhibit growth and development; they obtain food and metabolize it for the generation of energy and the synthesis of materials for growth and life; they possess nucleic acid(s); and they exhibit some adaptation to environmental conditions.

Organisms are interdependent. This can be exhibited by an indirect relationship, in which two species are adapted to occupying the same habitat, or a direct relationship, such as predation or symbiosis. In addition, organisms may have an effect on the environment, and the environment, in turn, can affect the organisms and the species that are able to live within it.

Organisms are composed of matter; all matter, whether organic or inorganic, obeys certain physical and chemical laws. Thus, the life sciences include Biology, Chemistry, Physics, Anatomy and Physiology, and general science content.

The outline below indicates some of the basic principles of the sciences with special emphasis on the descriptions of the "activities or characteristics of life" as related to humans.

I. The cell is the basic structural and functional unit of an organism.
  A. All cells have cytoplasm and a cell membrane.
    1. *Prokaryotic cells* lack a nuclear membrane surrounding the DNA.
    2. *Eukaryotic cells* possess a nuclear membrane that surrounds the DNA and separates it from the cytoplasm, creating a well-defined nucleus.
    3. Some types of eukaryotic cells, such as red blood cells of humans, lack a nucleus at maturity for functional reasons; however, these cells always possess a nucleus during their development.
  B. Typical plant cells lack a centriole, but have plastids and a cell wall, while typical animal cells lack a cell wall and plastids, but possess a centriole.
  C. Reproduction of cells normally involves mitosis, a nuclear process during which nuclear materials, including DNA, are distributed equally to daughter nuclei.
    1. Mitosis may occur without division of the cell, leading to a multinucleate cell.
    2. DNA replicates itself during interphase, before the nucleus enters the mitotic process.
  D. The sum total of cellular functions comprises the functions of the tissues or organ.
    1. The cellular functions are accomplished by one or more parts, or *organelles*, of the cell.
      a) The cell membrane is differentially permeable and functions in regulating the passage of materials into and out of the cell.
        (1) Materials may pass through the membrane by osmosis, by diffusion, by active transport, or by some other mechanism.
      b) *Mitochondria* are cellular organelles in which food is oxidized for the release of energy.
      c) *Plastids* (in plants) are of different types and vary in function.
        (1) *Chloroplasts* are green plastids in which photosynthesis occurs.
        (2) *Chromoplasts* and *leucoplasts* function in storage and other processes.
      d) The *endoplasmic reticulum* is a network of branching tubules composed of membrane that functions as an intracellular transport system for many types of materials. It extends throughout the cytoplasm of the cell.
      e) *Ribosomes* are organelles in which protein synthesis occurs. They are typically associated with the rough endoplasmic reticulum of the cell; RNA passes over the ribosomes to "line up" the amino acids to form the protein.
      f) The *Golgi apparatus* functions in collecting and preparing secretions of the cell for export outside the cell.

    g) *Contractile vacuoles* are membranous sacs that maintain a proper concentration of water inside the cell by draining excess water from the cytoplasm and expelling it. They are found in many protists and some animal cells.

    h) *Cilia and flagella* are slender projections of the cell used for movement. Flagella are longer than cilia, but both have the same internal arrangement of microtubules, the 9 + 2 pattern, and are formed by the same kind of organelle, a *kinetosome*.

    i) *Centrioles* are tiny, barrel-shaped organelles similar to kinetosomes that form the *spindle apparatus* that pulls chromosomes to opposite poles of the cell during mitosis or meiosis.

    j) *Phagocytic vacuoles*, also called *food vacuoles*, are membranous sacs used by some types of cells to engulf and digest food material. Cells form similar organelles called *autophagic vacuoles* to engulf, digest, and recycle worn-out cytoplasmic organelles.

    k) The *nucleus* is the control center of the cell; the nuclear membrane is porous, and materials pass into and out of the nucleus through the nuclear membrane.

       (1) In eukaryotes, DNA is stored in the nucleus.

       (2) *Transcription*, or the biosynthesis of RNA from the DNA, occurs within the nucleus; the RNA travels to the ribosomes where *translation*, or the synthesis of a polypeptide, occurs.

       (3) The *nucleolus*, located within the nucleus, is the site where RNA is manufactured.

II. Animals and plants exhibit organizational levels.

  A. Unicellular organisms are composed of one cell, which accomplishes all of the functions necessary for life.

    1. Unicellular organisms may be prokaryotic, as with bacteria, or eukaryotic, as with protistans.

      a) The first indication of "division of labor" is seen in some colonial unicellular forms, in which specific cells are concerned with the specific functions.

  B. Organisms at the tissue level of organization have well-developed tissues, some of which may be specialized for certain functions, but do not have well-developed organs.

  C. The organ level of organization indicates the presence of well-developed organs.

  D. Most animals, from round and segmented worms to vertebrates, are characterized by the system level of organization in which organs are arranged to accomplish a multiphase process.

III. All organisms exhibit response to stimuli.

  A. Response involves reception of a stimulus, transmission of the impulse, and reaction to the stimulus.

    1. In higher animals, such as humans, well-developed sense organs may be involved in the reception of stimuli; these include the skin, eye, and ear.

      a) Primitive sense organs may be seen in lower animals; in some lower animals, the sense organs may be well developed.

      b) Sensory organelles may be seen in some unicellular forms, such as the eyespot of *Euglena*.

    2. The transmission of impulses involves nerves or nerve fibers; in humans and other animals, a nervous system is involved in the transmission of impulses.

a) Transmission of nerve impulses is electrical, and involves a difference in the concentration of certain ions, especially potassium and sodium, along the nerve fibers.

b) Nerve impulses are transmitted from one nerve fiber to another across a tiny gap, called a *synapse*, that separates the two cells. Passage of a nerve impulse along the presynaptic fiber causes it to release a substance called a *neurotransmitter* into the synaptic space that either stimulates or blocks the generation of a nerve impulse in the postsynaptic neuron. This enables synapses to function as points of control in nerve pathways.

3. Reaction to stimuli may involve a change in position, in movement, and in secretory activities. Thus, the skeletal system, muscle system, endocrine glands, and digestive glands may be involved in reactions, as exhibited by humans and other higher animals.

a) Other systems that may be indirectly involved in reactions are the circulatory system, the respiratory system, and the excretory system.

IV. All organisms exhibit reproduction; this maintains continuity of the species or population extant.

Reproduction may be sexual or asexual.

A. Asexual reproduction occurs by means of mitosis and does not involve a union of reproductive cells (gametes) or gametic nuclei.

1. The following are types of asexual reproduction:

a) *Sporulation* involves the production of asexual reproductive cells (or multicellular units) called spores; these spores develop directly into new individuals.

b) *Binary fission* involves the division of the organism (usually unicellular) into two organisms. In the case of unicellular eukaryotes, binary fission usually involves mitosis.

c) *Multiple fission*, or *fragmentation*, as seen in lower organisms, such as filamentous algae, involves the breaking of the organism into smaller units, each of which can develop into a new organism.

d) *Budding* involves the production of an outgrowth or miniature organism that breaks away from the parent and develops into a new adult.

B. Sexual reproduction involves meiosis followed by fertilization, meaning the union of the nuclei of reproductive cells.

1. Several types of sexual reproduction may be described, depending on the morphology of the gametes.

a) *Isogamy* is reproduction involving fusion of morphologically identical gametes; this is more common among lower plants.

b) *Heterogamy* is sexual reproduction involving fusion of gametes that differ in size and/or structure.

(1) One type of heterogamy involves motile gametes differing only in size; this is *anisogamy*.

(2) The other type of heterogamy involves gametes differing in size and in structure: this is *oogamy*.

(a) Oogamy is exhibited by humans; the gamete produced by the male is the spermatozoon; the gamete produced by the female is the ovum or egg.

       (b)   In animals such as humans, gametes are produced in gonads: the male gonads are the testes; the female gonads are the ovaries.

           i.   Gonads in higher animals, such as humans, also have an endocrine function, producing hormones involved with the appearance of secondary sex characteristics and with reproductive cycles.

       (c)   *Conjugation* is sexual reproduction involving a temporary union of cells for exchange or transmission of nuclei or DNA.

2. Meiosis is involved in the production of gametes or of spores in the case of most plants.

   a)   Gametes are haploid, having one-half the chromosome number characteristic of the zygote of the species.

   b)   The diploid number is restored to the zygote (the cells resulting from gametic union, or *syngamy*) when fertilization occurs.

   c)   The zygote typically develops mitotically into the embryo; thus, there is no further change in chromosome number.

   d)   Because of meiosis and syngamy, the individual developing from the zygote receives one-half of its DNA from each parent; thus, the chromosome number for the species remains constant.

   e)   Sexual reproduction allows for the spread of changes through a population.

V. Growth and development allow for the characteristic size range of a species to be maintained and for the differentiation of organs and tissues to be accomplished.

   A.   In multicellular organisms, growth may involve an increase in the number of cells, an increase in the size of cells, or both.

   B.   The zygote develops mitotically into a multicellular organism. In humans and other multicellular organisms, development or differentiation, accompanies growth.

   C.   In higher animals, such as humans, the basic development patterns are similar.

     1.   The zygote undergoes cleavage to produce a cluster of cells known as a *morula*.

     2.   The morula develops into a *blastula* or *blastocyst*; this is a hollow ball of cells with a cavity known as a *blastocoel*.

     3.   The blastula develops into a two-layered *gastrula* with a cavity known as a *gastrocoel* or *archenteron*.

        a)   The outer germ layer of the gastrula is the *ectoderm*.

        b)   The inner germ layer of the gastrula is the *endoderm*.

        c)   The third germ layer, *mesoderm*, develops between the ectoderm and the endoderm.

     4.   Each germ layer gives rise to definite body structures and tissues.

        a)   From the ectoderm develops the nervous system, some sense organs, such as the eye, and the outer skin.

        b)   From the mesoderm develops the muscle system, skeletal system, muscle of the viscera, mesenteries, and circulatory system.

        c)   From the endoderm develops the lining of the digestive tract, the lungs, much of the liver and pancreas, the thyroid, parathyroid, and thymus glands.

VI. Nutritional processes, involving obtaining and utilizing food, are exhibited by all organisms.

    A. Food may be defined as any substance that can be used by the organism as a source of energy and as a source of materials for growth and maintenance of the body.

        1. Most food is organic; the process involving the conversion of inorganic materials into organic foods is photosynthesis.

            a) This process occurs only in green plants, in the presence of the chlorophylls, and in the presence of light as an energy source.

                (1) The chloroplast is the cellular organelle in which photosynthesis occurs.

            b) All organisms (except for a few algae and prokaryotes that may exhibit similar processes) depend directly or indirectly on photosynthesis for food.

        2. Some food consists of inorganic minerals necessary for the maintenance of bodily processes. Examples of essential minerals are sodium, potassium, iron, calcium, zinc, and cobalt.

    B. Organisms must obtain food to live.

        1. *Autotrophs*, such as green plants, manufacture food within their bodies from inorganic environmental materials.

        2. *Heterotrophs* receive organic food from the environment.

            a) *Saprotrophs* digest food externally and absorb the digested food into the body; most bacteria and fungi are saprotrophs.

            b) *Parasites* live on and at the expense of a host.

            c) *Phagotrophs*, such as humans and most animals, ingest solid food into a digestive cavity of some sort.

                (1) The digestive cavity of phagotrophic protozoa may be a *food vacuole*; this is characteristic of the cellular level of organization.

                (2) The digestive cavity of simple animals, such as coelenterates and flatworms, consists of a *gastro vascular cavity* with a mouth as its only opening; this is characteristic of the tissue level of organization or simpler versions of the system level.

                (3) The digestive cavity of humans and most other animals is a complete *digestive tract* (digestive system), with a mouth at one end and an anus at the other end; this is characteristic of the system level of organization.

    C. Food that has been obtained must be digested—changed into a usable, absorbable state. This occurs in the digestive system in humans.

        1. In lower animals, as in protozoa, digestion occurs in a food vacuole—a gastrovascular cavity, or a simple gut.

    D. The digested food is distributed throughout the body to the cells.

        1. In humans, the circulatory or vascular system distributes the food to the cells.

    E. Utilization of food, or *metabolism*, occurs in the cells.

        1. Oxidation of glucose within the cells (in the mitochondria) yields energy for life and for life's activities.

            a) Aerobic oxidation is most common, involving the use of free, molecular oxygen. Enzymes control each step of oxidation.

                (1) Oxygen is made available by means of respiratory organs, or, in the case of humans, the respiratory system.

(2) Oxygen is absorbed from air inhaled into the lungs of humans and transported to the cells by means of the circulatory system.

(a) In humans, oxygen is transported in combination with hemoglobin of the red blood cells.

(3) Carbon dioxide, resulting from the oxidation of glucose, is transported by the blood stream to the lungs for elimination through exhalation.

(4) As a result of oxidation of glucose, the energy transporting substance, adenosine triphosphate (ATP), is formed. ATP transfers energy to the areas that need it or to specialized areas and compounds for energy storage.

(5) Liquid waste from metabolism is collected, concentrated, and eliminated by the excretory system.

2. The synthesis of other compounds, proteins, and secretory products occurs in the cell.

F. Solid indigestible wastes are eliminated from the digestive system; in humans, elimination occurs through the anus.

VII. Organisms must adapt to the environment in which they live in order to survive.

A. Organisms may possess or develop certain traits that enable them to live or thrive in a specific environment.

1. Changes may originate in and spread throughout populations, making survival and thriving a greater possibility.

a) Changes that are conducive to survival are conserved, accumulate, and may eventually lead to a new variety or race.

B. Organisms, by their presence and exploitation of an environment, may change the environment to the extent that it becomes suitable for a different group or species. Thus, succession occurs as the environment continues to change under the influence of different species, causing other species to adapt to or invade the environment.

VIII. Two types of nucleic acids are known; all organisms possess one or both types. Most organisms possess both.

A. Deoxyribonucleic acid (DNA) functions as the genetic information of an individual. Different parts of the genetic information contained in the structure of DNA can be used for the following purposes: day to day regulation of cellular processes (metabolism), development of a new individual (heredity), or manufacture of ribonucleic acid (RNA). DNA is contained within the nucleus of eukaryotic cells and is attached to the inner side of the cell membrane in prokaryotic cells.

1. DNA is a long, double-stranded, chain-like molecule that is twisted into the form of a helix (double helix). Each strand is a chain of "building units," which are smaller molecules called nucleotides.

a) A nucleotide consists of a sugar (deoxyribose), a phosphate, and a purine or pyrimidine base.

(1) The purine bases are guanine and adenine.

(2) The pyrimidine bases are cytosine and thymine.

2. DNA is the pattern or template from which complementary RNA (ribonucleic acid) is synthesized.

a) RNA is similar in structure to DNA except that it is much smaller and consists of only one strand. Like DNA, the single strand of RNA is a chain of nucleotides.

(1) The purine bases of RNA nucleotides are guanine and adenine.

(2) The pyrimidine bases of RNA nucleotides are cytosine and uracil.

b) There are three types of RNA and all of them play essential roles in protein synthesis. Together, DNA and RNA form a system for the storage and use of information needed to make the proper structure of each of the many different types of proteins used by an individual organism.

   (1) Messenger RNA serves as the actual pattern or template for the sequential arrangement of amino acids into a chain to make a protein. The information in a molecule of messenger RNA is copied from part of a DNA molecule (transcription); this information is equivalent to a *gene* or a group of related genes.

   (2) Transfer RNA carries amino acids to specific complementary spots on the messenger RNA template, ensuring that amino acids are placed in the correct sequence for a particular protein (translation).

   (3) Ribosomal RNA is the key component of ribosomes, which are the cellular sites for the synthesis of proteins.

Of major concern in the health sciences is an understanding of how humans function biologically, psychologically, and socially. Human behavior is influenced by environment; thus, the "laws of nature" apply to humans as well as to other organisms and to the matter making up their environment. It is necessary, therefore, for a person involved in the health sciences to have knowledge of the physical sciences as well as the life sciences.

CONCEPTS RELATED TO HEALTH SCIENCES

Concepts	Related Topics
I. Concepts about humans	Cell structure
A. Develops from a single cell (zygote)	Similarities and differences in animal and plant cellular activities
1. Reproduction is a basic function of life.	Animal cell division
a) Humans reproduce by sexual reproduction (mating), the union of male and female sex cells.	
b) Humans transmit like characteristics to offspring.	Plant cell division
2. Heredity, the transmission of traits, can be explained in terms of	Mutations
a) Mendel's Law.	Dominant and recessive genes
b) Gene theory.	Hybrids
c) Blending.	Punnett Square
d) Meiosis.	
e) Chromosomal influence in sex determination.	Role of RNA and DNA
3. Deoxyribonucleic acid (DNA) is the only known type of self-duplicating molecule that plays a central role in heredity by ensuring the orderly development of offspring into a form similar to that of their parents.	Fetal development

Concepts	Related Topics
4. Fertilization produces a zygote, which then begins to grow by mitosis, the first stage of life of the embryo.	
5. Mature cells group together in distinct patterns to form tissues. Tissues unite to form organs, and organs unite to form the lifesystems of the body.	
B. Life processes based on metabolism	Energy transfer mechanisms in living cells
1. All human cells must utilize oxygen through respiration, receive nutrition through digestive processes, eliminate wastes, and grow to their potential stage of maturity.	ATP cycle Aerobic and anaerobic respiration
2. These life processes involve chemical changes (called *metabolism*) that are controlled by enzymes.	Oxidation of carbohydrates Photosynthesis
3. The energy needed for life processes in humans comes from food: proteins, carbohydrates, and fats. Energy from food is used to make adenosine triphosphate (ATP), which is used as a universally available source of energy in all cells of the body.	Protein and lipid synthesis Classification systems for living organisms
4. The cell constantly interacts with its environment through the processes of osmosis and diffusion.	
5. All cellular functions depend on specific types of proteins, especially enzymes. By controlling the manufacture of specific proteins, DNA (with the help of RNA) is able to control all cellular functions.	
6. The maintenance of internal balance (called *homeostasis*) is a major part of metabolism. Internal conditions, such as concentrations of substances in cells or body fluids, pH, and temperature, are kept within narrow ranges by constant regulation. These regulatory activities always require a major expenditure of energy by the organism. Much of homeostasis is done to satisfy the requirements of enzymes, which are always sensitive to physical conditions.	

Concepts	Related Topics
C. Life processes conducted through bodily systems.	Gills, lungs, and tracheae
1. The function of the respiratory system is to transport oxygen to the blood and eliminate carbon dioxide from the blood.	Oxygen and carbon dioxide exchange
a) The quantity of available oxygen determines the effectiveness of respiration.	Positive and negative pressure; breathing; basal metabolic rates
b) Oxygen consumption is directly proportional to the rate of bodily activity and energy use.	Energy production from metabolic processes
c) Metabolic processes of the body are directly affected by oxygen supply.	Factors affecting metabolic rate
d) Changes in oxygen consumption caused by an increase or decrease in activity temporarily affect the concentration of oxygen in the blood, which is then restored to normal by an increase or decrease in respiratory rate.	
2. The circulatory system transports nutrients to the cells and wastes from the cells.	Rhythmic beating of heart Structure of arteries and veins
a) The force of the circulatory flow (blood pressure) is created by the pumping of the heart. This force delivers blood to the capillaries, where exchange of materials between the blood and tissues takes place.	Location of major blood vessels
b) The stimulation of the heart comes from within the heart muscle, but the rate of beating is modified by chemicals (hormones) and nerve transmissions from the brain.	Capillary as medium for exchange
c) The rate of blood flow through the vessels is directly proportional to blood pressure and is partially maintained by the closed nature of the cardiovascular circuit.	Electrolytes Acids and bases
d) The volume of blood pumped through the cardiovascular circuit per unit of time is directly proportional to blood pressure.	Hyper- and hypothermia Blood typing—Rh factor
e) Arteries are able to change their internal diameter by constriction or dilation; blood pressure is inversely proportional to the diameter of arteries.	Clotting mechanism

Concepts	Related Topics

f) In capillaries, exchange of materials between the blood and tissues is accomplished by a combination of blood pressure, diffusion, and osmosis.

Body defenses in blood and lymph

g) Blood is returned to the heart through veins by the passive mechanisms of pushing from behind, squeezing of veins by skeletal muscles, and gravity.

Distribution of body fluids

3. The digestive system breaks down foods and delivers the nutrients to the circulatory system.

Solid and liquid components of blood

a) Food must be ingested into the system, mixed with digestive substances, broken down chemically (digestion), and selectively absorbed into the blood stream.

Materials required for plant growth (auxins, vitamins, etc.)

Variations in digestive systems of living organisms

a. Utilization of large quantities of food
b. Utilization of fluids and soft tissues

b) The rate of digestion is directly related to the quantity of food.

c) The lining of the alimentary tube provides mucus to lubricate the passage of food and protect the lining itself from enzymes or acid.

d) Chemical breakdown is the result of enzymes and activators.

Chemical digestion of carbohydrates, proteins, and fats

e) Nutrients are stored in the liver for reserve supply.

Role of vitamins and minerals

Hydrolysis

f) Waste products are eliminated through the colon.

Structure formula and isomerism
a. hydrocarbons
b. halogen derivatives
c. alcohols and phenols
d. aldehydes and phenols
e. amino acids
f. heterocyclics
g. lids
h. organometallics
i. nucleic acid

Concepts	Related Topics

4. The excretory (renal) system removes metabolic wastes and excess substances from the body.

Invertebrate mechanisms for excretion

   a) The kidneys selectively absorb wastes and excess substances from the blood to form urine.

Role of nephron unit in homeostasis

   b) The kidneys selectively reabsorb substances needed by the body and return them to the blood.

Filtration and dialysis

   c) Selective reabsorption conserves water and electrolytes, which balances their concentrations in the blood and tissues.

Artificial kidney
Excretion of wastes through skin

   d) The circulating volume of the blood has a direct affect on kidney activity.

   e) The ureters connect the kidneys to the bladder, a receptacle for holding urine.

   f) Micturition (urination) is a reflex action.

5. The endocrine system regulates body activities.

Interrelationships of endocrine glands

   a) Endocrine glands secrete hormones into the blood and tissues.

Function of insulin, thyroxin, parathyrin

   b) Hormonal secretion is activated by chemical and neural factors.

Role of pituitary gland
Sex hormones

   c) Hormones regulate primary metabolic processes.

Steroids

   d) Hypo- or hyperactivity of endocrine glands results in disorders.

Release of energy by adrenaline

6. The musculoskeletal system generates motion and maintains posture.

Location of bones in the skeleton and functional relationships of bones to one another

   a) The bones and muscles are combined into individual lever systems to produce motion.

Ligaments and joints

   b) In the human body, a lever system consists of a muscle (force), joint (fulcrum), and a bone (lever). The arrangement of a lever system permits movement with a minimal expenditure of energy.

Function of red and yellow marrow

   c) Joints act as points of balance and are also sculptured to regulate the extent or direction of movement.

Smooth and striated muscles

Concepts	Related Topics

d) Change in position is produced by a shift of weight accomplished by muscular force.

Major muscles of the body and functional relationships of muscles to bones

e) The longer the axis of the lever (bone) being moved, the greater the extent of movement.

Principles of energy and work

f) The use of muscular force consumes a large amount of energy and results in waste heat as a byproduct, used to maintain body temperature.

7. The nervous system provides a means of internal bodily communication that controls and coordinates all activities in response to environmental stimuli.

Plant stimulus-response systems

Responses to light, temperature, touch, and other physical conditions

a) Impulses travel along neurons (nerve cells).

Sensory and motor organs

b) Neurons are grouped together to form the central nervous system (brain and spinal cord) and nerves that connect the central nervous system to all parts of the body.

Brain centers

Spinal nerves

c) Stimuli are changes in either the external or internal environment.

Cranial nerves

d) The central nervous system receives stimuli and ensures that a proper response is given to each stimulus.

Autonomic nervous system

e) Responses are initiated through the central nervous system and consist of either a muscular movement or secretion of a substance by a gland.

II. Human potential for adaptation

Ecological balance

A. Interdependent relationships with other living forms

Producers, consumers, decomposers

1. Humans, like other living things, form complex relationships with the environment.

Movement of energy through ecosystems

2. The kinds and amount of life found in different environments is determined by temperature, moisture, sunlight, and soil.

Biomes

3. Humans, like other animals, depend on animal and plant sources of food (food chains).

Climatic effects on life processes

Concepts	Related Topics
4. Only organisms with chlorophylls, such as plants, can make food.	Composition of sea water
	a. sodium chloride
5. Food chains exist because all living things need energy.	b. magnesium
	c. calcium
6. The survival of humankind (and species in general) is influenced by other species in the same environment.	d. sulfur
	e. oxygen
7. Living organisms in the same environment form an interrelated community in which many species, out of the total number, live in close associations with one another (symbiosis). Most of these symbiotic associations constitute mutualism (benefit to both partners), or parasitism (benefit to one partner at the expense of the other).	
B. Conservation of resources	Classification of matter
1. Supplies of natural resources are finite.	a. organic and inorganic
	b. elements, compounds, mixtures
2. Population growth reduces the amount of resources available to individual humans.	Structure of matter
	a. atoms
	b. molecules
3. Supplies of natural resources can be expanded to some extent by new ways of increasing food production, development of new sources of energy, recycling of waste materials, conservation of natural habitats, and soil conservation.	Forms of matter
	a. liquid
	b. gas
	c. solid
4. Ultimately, population control is the only way to ensure adequate amounts of food, energy, and other resources for individual humans.	Changes in form
	a. physical
	b. chemical
III. Human interaction with the environment	Physiology of plants
	Nitrogen cycle
A. Environmental regulation of life processes	Photosynthesis
1. Inorganic matter is synthesized into food for plants; plants provide food for animals.	Vaporization, distillation
	Carbon-oxygen cycle
	Magnetism

Concepts	Related Topics
2. The physiological phenomena (assimilation, respiration, and growth) are controlled by temperature, light, moisture, nutrient supplies, and general atmospheric conditions.	Light, sound, electricity Pollution and pest control Gamma, Beta, Alpha rays Causative organisms of disease
B. Use and modification of the environment 1. Humans must protect themselves from biological, physical, and radiological hazards.	Koch's postulates Natural and acquired immunity Antibiotics and disinfectants Sterilization, pasteurization, refrigeration
2. Humans must discover and develop new ways of using natural resources to minimize or reverse environmental destruction. Conservation, recycling, and avoidance of "disposable" products are central elements in this strategy.	Community characteristics, principle of succession Solar energy, heat production, transfer convection Nuclear fission

SCIENCE GLOSSARY

Items in capitals have a special entry in the glossary.

A

absolute zero   The lowest temperature a gas can attain. This is 460 degrees below zero on the FAHRENHEIT scale and 273 degrees below zero on the CELSIUS scale.

absorption   The movement of water and/or dissolved substances into a cell, tissue, or organism.

acceleration   A change in the speed of an object. If the object speeds up, this is called *positive acceleration*. If the object goes slower, it is called *negative acceleration*.

acid   A compound with a pH less than 7, which means that it releases hydrogen ions when dissolved in water. An acid changes blue litmus paper to red and tastes sour.

acquired immunity   Immunity that is not natural or congenital; obtained after birth.

active immunity   Immunity brought about by activity of certain cells of the body as a result of being exposed to an antigen.

active transport   An energy-requiring process by means of which materials are moved across a cell membrane.

adsorption   The gathering of molecules of a substance on a surface.

aerobe	Any organism living in the presence of and utilizing free, molecular oxygen (that is, oxygen not in chemical combination) in its oxidative processes.
alchemy	The science of transforming less valuable metals into gold or silver, and the philosophy behind this idea. The theories of the alchemists of the Middle Ages were false, but their experiments laid the foundation for modern chemistry.
alkali	A compound with a pH greater than 7. An alkaline substance changes red litmus paper to blue, and it can combine with hydrogen. *See* BASE.
alkaline	A substance having the properties of an ALKALI.
allantois	One of four extraembryonic membranes attached to the body of the embryo or fetus of a land-dwelling vertebrate. In humans it is modified to form part of the placenta and umbilicus.
amino acid	An organic molecule containing an amino group (NH_2) and a carboxyl group (COOH) bonded to the same carbon atom; the "building blocks" of proteins.
amnion	The innermost of four extraembryonic membranes attached to the body of the embryo or fetus of a land-dwelling vertebrate. It forms a fluid-filled sac around the body that provides an aqueous environment and cushions the embryo from shocks.
ampere	A measurement of electric current, abbreviated *amp*. It was named after French scientist ANDRÉ-MARIE AMPÈRE.
Ampère, André-Marie	A French scientist (1775–1836) whose work and theory laid the foundation for the André-Marie science of electrodynamics. His name lives on in the electrical measurement AMPERE.
amphipods	A crustacean group that includes sand fleas.
anaerobe	Any organism not requiring free, molecular oxygen for its cellular oxidative processes. Some anaerobes are *obligate*, and cannot survive in the presence of oxygen; others are *facultative*, and can survive with or without oxygen.
anatomy	The study of the structure of living things. Usually, "anatomy" refers to the structure of the human body.
anemone	A sea animal (a coelenterate) that resembles the flower of the same name.
antibiotic	A substance derived from lower organisms that can be used to prevent growth of certain pathogens, thus combating infection.
antibody	A specific type of protein molecule that is manufactured in the tissues, blood, or lymph in response to the presence of viruses or foreign cells. Each variety of antibody will attach to the surface of only one type of invader, enabling it to be recognized and marked for destruction by the immune system.

antigens   Protein molecules on the surface of viruses or foreign cells that provoke the manufacture of matching antibodies, enabling invaders to be recognized as such so they can be destroyed.

apolipoprotein   (apo E) A gene that codes for a protein that facilitates the transport of cholesterol and influences human longevity.

ATP   (adenosine triphosphate) The energy-transport compound of a cell.

atrium   The anterior chamber(s) of the heart of vertebrates.

attenuated   The state of being weakened, as in the case of pathogens used to induce active immunity.

auricle   The projecting outer portion, or pinna, of the ear.

autotroph   An organism, such as a green plant, capable of manufacturing its food from inorganic environmental materials.

B

bacteria   Unicellular, microscopic, PROKARYOTIC organisms, mostly SAPRO-TROPHIC or PARASITIC.

base   A compound with a pH greater than 7 that can react with an acid to accept a hydrogen ion and form a salt. *See* ALKALI.

biochemistry   The study of the chemical makeup of organisms. This science is a branch of both chemistry and biology.

biology   The study of living things; a major science.

biome   A type of community recognized by certain characteristics of plants and climate, such as the plains of the Midwest.

bond   The force of attraction that holds 2 atoms together in a molecule. There are two major types of chemical bonds: COVALENT BONDS and IONIC BONDS.

botany   The study of plant life. Botany is a branch of BIOLOGY.

Brahe, Tycho   A Danish astronomer (1546–1601) who made a systematic study of the movement of celestial bodies. He is often referred to only as *Tycho*.

C

carbohydrate   A food substance made up of carbon, hydrogen, and oxygen.

carbon   An important chemical element that forms the basic skeleton of all ORGANIC compounds. Atoms of other elements are bonded to the carbon skeleton to form the many different varieties of organic compounds.

carbon dioxide   A compound made up of 1 atom of carbon and 2 atoms of oxygen. It exists in the form of a gas and is one of the principal waste byproducts resulting from CELLULAR RESPIRATION.

carcinogen   A cancer causing substance that may be physical, chemical, or biological.

catalyst   A chemical substance that lowers the energy necessary for a chemical reaction to take place and makes the reaction proceed more rapidly. ENZYMES act as catalysts in living organisms.

celestial   An adjective referring to the sky.

cell   The basic structural and functional unit of organisms.

cellular respiration   The oxidation of glucose into carbon dioxide and water (or into other products, in the case of anaerobic respiration), leading to the release of energy.

Celsius   A system of measurement of temperature, often referred to as *centigrade*. On the Celsius scale the freezing point for water is 0 degrees and the boiling point is 100 degrees.

centriole   A cellular organelle characteristic of animal cells, but not plant cells, that migrates to the poles during mitosis; spindle fibers and astral rays arise from it.

centromere   The portion of the chromosome that holds the chromatids together and to which spindle fibers apparently attach.

chelicerae   The claw-like head appendages on certain arthropods, such as spiders.

chemistry   The science that studies the composition and transformation of matter; a major science.

Chlamydiae   Small intracellular obligate parasites closely related to the *Rickettsiae*.

chlorophylls   The green pigments of plants, produced in the presence of light and essential for photosynthesis.

chromosomes   Small cellular bodies containing tightly bound and packaged DNA that are formed during MITOSIS and MEIOSIS from loosely packaged DNA (chromatin). The hereditary determinants called GENES are carded on chromosomes.

colloid   A type of mixture intermediate between a SOLUTION and a SUSPENSION, consisting of liquid plus particles that are too small to settle out of the mixture and too large to dissolve. Colloids can exist in the form of a gel and pass through membranes either slowly or not at all.

commensalism   A symbiotic relationship in which one member is benefited, and the other member is neither benefited nor harmed.

compound   The combination of two or more elements into a single unit.

condensation   The transition of water vapor to liquid water due to a lowering of temperature.

conduction   The transfer of heat from one object or physical medium to another by direct contact.

conservation of energy   The principle that energy changes its form but cannot be created or destroyed.

conservation of matter	The principle that matter can change its form but cannot be created or destroyed.
constellation	A particular grouping of stars.
copepod	A small aquatic crustacean.
Copernicus, Nicholas	A Polish astronomer (1473–1543) who proposed the theory that the earth moves through space. It was generally believed up to that time that the earth was the immobile center of the universe.
cosmic year	The time it takes the sun to go around its galaxy.
covalent bond	A type of chemical bond created by the sharing of electrons between 2 atoms to achieve the maximum number of electrons in the outer electron orbit of each atom. Covalent bonds are the strongest type of chemical bonds.
crop rotation	An agricultural method by which crops in an area are changed each year, helping to maintain the fertility of the soil.
crustaceans	A group of aquatic animals with a hard outside covering. They are often included with MOLLUSKS in the group of "shellfish."
crystal	A form of solid in which the constituent atoms or molecules are arranged in a very regular, repeating pattern.
cytoplasm	In a prokaryotic cell, the entire contents of the cell contained within the plasma membrane. In a eukaryotic cell, the region of the cell lying within the plasma membrane but exterior to the nucleus.

D

Dalton, John	An English chemist and physicist (1766–1844) who introduced the theory that matter is made up of atoms.
Darwin, Charles	An English naturalist (1809–1883) who developed a theory of EVOLUTION.
deforestation	The process by which land is cleared of forests.
density	Mass per unit volume, often expressed as grams per milliliter.
dictyosome	The *Golgi apparatus* of a cell, which serves as a collecting and packaging center for secretions.
diffusion	The spontaneous movement of dissolved molecules from an area where they are in high concentration to an area where they are in lower concentration. This process requires no energy and, in living organisms, often takes place across semi-permeable membranes.
distillation	The purification of a liquid substance by heating it until it vaporizes and then cooling it to cause it to condense into liquid again.
DNA	Deoxyribonucleic acid; a large, helical, double-stranded molecule in which the chromosomes code hereditary information.
dorso-ventral	An adjective referring to a back-to-front plane.

Down syndrome A genetic disorder of humans caused by the presence of an extra, third copy of chromosome 21. Individuals with Down syndrome are mentally retarded and possess characteristic physical features.

E

eclipse The obscuring of a celestial body that takes place when one celestial object moves in front of another. When the moon comes between the earth and the sun, it casts a shadow, or *umbra*, on part of the earth. This is known as a *solar* eclipse, since during this time the sun cannot be seen on that part of the earth. When the earth comes between the sun and the moon, it casts a shadow on the moon. Since the moon cannot be seen during this time, this is called a *lunar* eclipse.

Einstein, Albert A German physicist (1879–1955) who lived the last years of his life in the United States. His theories changed the field of PHYSICS. He, more than any other scientist, was responsible for nuclear fission.

electron A negatively charged particle in the atom that moves in an orbit around the NUCLEUS of the atom.

electronics The study of the motion or movement of free electrons and ions, and the application of these phenomena to radio and television.

electrophoresis A biochemical technique used to separate organic molecules such as PROTEINS or NUCLEIC ACIDS out of a mixture. In the most commonly used version of the technique, a sample of the mixture is placed at one end of a slab-shaped gel immersed in a buffer solution. An electric current is passed through the chamber containing the gel, and molecules travel through the gel at different distances according to their size and electrical charge. Each type of molecule accumulates in its own distinct zone or band in the gel.

element One of more than 100 known basic substances. These substances and their combinations make up all matter, as far as is known.

embryology The study of the development of organisms from the time of conception.

energy The capacity to do work.

enthalpy The heat content of the reactants and products in a chemical reaction.

entropy The concept that closed systems move to a state of maximum disorder unless energy enters from the surroundings.

enzyme An organic CATALYST; specific types of proteins produced by cells that govern or otherwise affect all biological reactions. *Exoenzymes* act outside the cells that produce them, and *endoenzymes* act within the cells that produce them. Enzymes are sensitive to the pH and temperature of their environment, and deviations from the optimal pH and temperature for an enzyme will lessen its activity. The maintenance of optimal internal environments for enzymes is a major objective of HOMEOSTASIS.

erg A unit of work or energy.

erythrocytes	Red blood cells.
eugenics	A science that deals with the improvement of hereditary qualities of a race or breed.
eukaryote	An organism characterized by cells containing a true or visible nucleus.
evaporation	The process by which liquids change to gases.
evolution, theory of	Usually refers to Darwin's theory that changes occur in populations because natural selection favors the survival of those organisms best fitted for their environment.
exergonic reaction	Downhill reaction, whose products have less energy than the reactant.
experiment	A test to see if an idea is true or false.

F

Fahrenheit	The system of measuring temperature generally used in the United States was developed by Gabriel Fahrenheit (1686–1736), a German scientist. On the Fahrenheit scale, 32 degrees is the freezing point of water, 212 degrees is the boiling point of water, and 98.6 degrees is the average temperature of the human body. Another widely used temperature measurement is the CELSIUS scale.
Faraday, Michael	An English physicist and chemist (1791–1867) who developed the first dynamo and discovered that a magnet could induce an electric current in a conductor such as metal.
fertility	The ability to reproduce. *See* REPRODUCTION.
force	That which stops, creates, or changes the velocity of motion.
friction	The resistance created to the movement of an object when it rubs or collides with other objects.
fungi	A group of organisms, typically SAPROTROPHIC (or *parasitic*), many of which have a MYCELIUM. A few fungi, such as yeasts, do not have a mycelial body. *See* SAPROTROPH.

G

galaxy	A grouping of stars. Our sun is a star in the galaxy called the *Milky Way*.
Galileo	An Italian astronomer and physicist (1564–1642) who made many contributions to science. He discovered that objects of different weights and shapes fall to the ground at the same rate of speed, attracted by GRAVITY. He was a strong believer in COPERNICUS' theory that the earth moved in space, and he was persecuted for this belief.

gene A hereditary determinant consisting of a segment of a DNA molecule that contains the coded information necessary for assembling a specific type of protein molecule. Each gene occupies a fixed locus on a specific CHROMOSOME, enabling the transmission of hereditary determinants from one generation to the next.

genetic code The sequence of NUCLEOTIDE bases in a molecule of DNA or RNA that, when translated by a RIBOSOME, specifies the sequence of AMINO ACIDS in a PROTEIN molecule.

genetic disorder A metabolic disorder caused by inheritance of a damaged gene, a damaged chromosome, or an incorrect number of chromosomes. *See* DOWN SYNDROME, HEMOPHILIA, PHENYLKETONURIA, and SICKLE CELL ANEMIA.

genetics The study of HEREDITY, or the manner in which hereditary traits are passed on from one generation to the next.

genome The genetic makeup of an individual; the genotype.

geology The study of the formation, structure, and history of the earth.

geriatrics The science of the diseases of aged persons.

glycolysis The anaerobic decomposition of a glucose into two molecules of pyruric acid, with the production of 2 net molecules of ATP.

golgi Storage organelle in plant and animal cells.

gravitation The tendency of objects in space to move toward each other.

gravity The force of attraction between two bodies. It is the force that causes objects to fall to earth.

greenhouse effect A warming of the earth caused by blankets of carbon dioxide and other gases that prevent sun rays that strike the surface from radiating back into space.

H

habitat The immediate surroundings or environment in which a particular species may live.

half-life The length of time required for the degradation to another substance of half the molecules in an amount of radioactive substance. The half-lives of radioactive ISOTOPES of elements can be used to date material containing radioactive substances. An example is the carbon-14 dating of living material.

Harvey, William An English physician and anatomist (1578–1657) who discovered how the blood moves through the body.

heat A form of energy.

heat shock proteins A protein that prevents the denaturation of other proteins when the temperature rises to abnormally high levels.

hemoglobin	A type of protein molecule that is bright red in color and binds reversibly to oxygen. It is carried within ERYTHROCYTES, enabling them to transport oxygen.
hemophilia	A GENETIC DISORDER caused by inheritance of a defective gene for one of the proteins that act as blood-clotting factors. The blood of affected persons fails to clot normally if an injury occurs, creating the danger that they might bleed to death from even minor wounds.
heredity	The transmission of traits from generation to generation.
homeostasis	The maintenance of internal balance by a living organism.
hormone	A chemical regulator of many bodily activities. A hormone is produced by an endocrine gland.
hydridoma	Recombinant (mixed) cells produced by the fusion of plasma cells and cancer cells.
hydrogen	The chemical element with the smallest atom. It exists as a gas and is common in nature. Hydrogen is important to living organisms because it is a constituent of water and most organic compounds.
hypha	A mycelial thread; one of the "strands" making up a MYCELIUM, which is a fungus body.
hypothesis	An unproven explanation of something that has happened or might happen.

I

immunity	Resistance to a particular disease or condition. *See* ACTIVE IMMUNITY, ACQUIRED IMMUNITY, NATURAL IMMUNITY, PASSIVE IMMUNITY.
immunization	The process of making one immune, usually by the giving of antigens to induce active immunity via the production of antibodies.
immunoglobulins	Antibodies.
indicator	A substance whose color is sensitive to the hydrogen-ion concentration of the solution to which it is added.
inorganic	An adjective meaning "not organic" and applying to any atom other than carbon, or to a molecule not containing carbon. *See* ORGANIC.
insecticides	Chemical combinations used to destroy or control harmful insects.
interferon	An antiviral agent secreted by cells under attack from viruses.
interstellar	An adjective meaning "between stars."
ion	An atom or radical that has acquired a positive charge by giving up or losing electron(s), or a negative charge by gaining electron(s).
ionic bond	A type of chemical bond created by one atom giving up all electron or electrons to another atom to achieve the maximum number of electrons in the outer orbit of each atom. Ionic compounds will separate in water to yield IONS in a process called *dissociation*.

isotopes   Atoms that belong to the same chemical element but have a different atomic mass.

K

Kepler, Johannes   A German astronomer (1571–1630) who made important discoveries about the orbits of planets.

kinetic energy   Energy that is in motion. The energy of a boulder tumbling down a mountainside is an example of kinetic energy. *See* POTENTIAL ENERGY.

Koch, Robert   A German doctor (1843–1910) who studied bacteria. He and LOUIS PASTEUR are considered the founders of the science of bacteriology.

Krebs cycle   The aerobic breakdown of glucose, forming carbon dioxide and water.

L

Lamarck, Chevalier de   A French naturalist (1744–1829) who developed a theory of evolution. *See* DARWIN.

Lavoisier, Antoine   A French chemist (1743–1794) who made important discoveries concerning combustion, the conservation of matter, and the role of oxygen in respiration.

leukocytes   White corpuscles or blood cells.

lever system   An assemblage of parts for moving weight with the least amount of applied force. A lever system consists of a rigid rod (*lever*) applied to the weight, a point of balance (*fulcrum*) for the lever, and mechanical force applied to the lever. These parts can be arranged in different ways to accommodate different amounts of weight, but a common principle of all lever systems is that the greatest amount of lifting force is achieved when the point at which the force is applied is farthest from the fulcrum.

light year   The distance light travels in one year.

Linnaeus, Carolus   A Swedish botanist (1707–1778) best known for developing a system of nomenclature for animals and plants.

lipopaly-saccharide   A polymer of simple sugars linked with fragments of lipid molecules.

litmus   An indicator used to test for pH, or hydrogen-ion concentration. Litmus is red in acid solutions and blue in basic solutions.

litmus paper   A special paper containing LITMUS, used by chemists to test for acid and alkali.

lunar   An adjective referring to the moon. A lunar eclipse is an eclipse of the moon. *See* SOLAR; ECLIPSE.

lymph   A colorless fluid that has passed from the bloodstream through capillary walls into the intercellular spaces; lymph is collected by lymph ducts and returned to the bloodstream.

lysosomes   Cellular organelles that contain powerful hydrolytic enzymes.

M

mandible	The lower jaw bone of vertebrates; the mouth part of arthropods that resembles a jaw and functions in biting.
marine	An adjective meaning "of or relating to the sea."
mechanics	The study of the effects of force on moving or motionless bodies; a branch of PHYSICS.
meiosis	A type of cellular division that results in gametes (sex cells) or gametic nuclei. It consists of two divisions resulting in four daughter cells, and the number of chromosomes in each daughter is reduced by half (haploid).
membrane	A thin sheet forming a semipermeable boundary, as in (1) a thin layer of soft tissue; (2) the outer boundary of a cell (*see* PLASMA MEMBRANE); or (3) the enclosing boundary of an intracellular structure (for example, the nucleus).
Mendel, Gregor Johann	An Austrian monk and botanist (1822–1884) who made important discoveries concerning HEREDITY.
metabolism	A cellular process by which food is oxidized for the release of energy and utilized for synthesis of cellular materials.
meteorology	A science that studies the weather and the atmosphere.
microscope	An instrument that produces a magnified image of an object. Light microscopes use a set of glass lenses to focus and magnify rays of light that either pass through or bounce off the object. Electron microscopes use magnetic lenses and beams of electrons to produce more sharply focused and highly magnified images than can be produced with a light microscope.
mineral	An INORGANIC substance that occurs naturally in rocks or soil. Minerals such as calcium, sodium, potassium, and zinc are used by living organisms in various metabolic processes.
mitochondrion	The cellular organelle of EUKARYOTES in which cellular oxidation (*cellular respiration*) generates energy.
mitosis	A type of cellular division that results in exact duplicates of the parent cell, as in asexual reproduction or growth. It consists of one division resulting in two daughter cells, and the number of chromosomes in each daughter is the same as in the parent (diploid).
molecule	The smallest unit into which a compound can be divided and still retain its original properties. Molecules are made up of atoms.
mollusks	Animals of the phylum *Mollusca*, characterized by a *mantle*, a *radula*, and a *muscular foot*. Some mollusks are aquatic, like the octopus, clam, and oyster. Others are terrestrial, like the snail and slug.
mutation	A stable and abrupt change in a gene, and thus in the trait the gene determines, that is transmitted from generation to generation.
mutualism	A symbiotic relationship of mutual benefit to its partners.

mycelium A mass of fungal threads or hyphae, composing the fungus body.

N

natural immunity Immunity or resistance to disease with which a person is born.

nebula A cloudy and gaseous mass found in INTERSTELLAR space.

nephron A functional unit of the kidney, consisting of Bowman's capsule with its glomerulus, and the associated ducts and convoluted tubules, with their capillaries.

neutron A small particle that is part of the atom and has no electrical charge. *See* ELECTRON and PROTON.

Newton, Isaac An English mathematician and natural philosopher (1642–1727) who made major discoveries in astronomy and PHYSICS. His most important work was his study of GRAVITATION and OPTICS.

nonpolar compound A substance in which the electromagnetic charge of each molecule is balanced so that there is no positively or negatively charged end to the molecule. Oils and fats are examples. *See* POLAR and SOLUBLE.

norepinephrine A biogenic amine derivative of tyrosine that serves as a neurotransmitter in the central nervous system and the peripheral nervous system.

nuclear An adjective referring to the NUCLEUS of an atom or cell.

nuclear fission The splitting of an atom in order to produce energy.

nuclear fusion The joining together of lightweight atoms resulting in the release of energy.

nucleic acid DNA and RNA; the nucleic acids code and transcribe information about heredity.

nucleolus A separate area within the NUCLEUS in which RNA is synthesized.

nucleotide The "building unit" of NUCLEIC ACIDS, consisting of a sugar (ribose or deoxyribose), a phosphate, and a base (a purine or a pyrimidine).

nucleus The center core of an object, as (1) the center of an atom, containing protons and neutrons; or (2) the regulatory center of a cell of an organism.

O

observatory A specially constructed building containing one or more telescopes for observation of the heavens.

ohm A unit for measuring electric resistance.

oncogen Specific genes that initiate malignancies.

optics The study of light and its effects; a branch of PHYSICS.

orbit The route that an object in space (such as the moon) takes around another body (such as the earth).

organ	A structure consisting of several different types of TISSUE combined into a single unit. A single organ can perform one or more major functions and is usually linked with other organs to form a *system*.
organelle	An intracellular structure that performs a major function for the cell; the cellular equivalent of an organ.
organic	Characteristic of, pertaining to, or derived from organisms; an adjective referring to living things or organisms.
organism	A living thing, such as a human, a plant, or an animal.
osmosis	The movement of water across a semipermeable membrane.
oxidation	Any chemical reaction that results in a molecule losing an electron, losing a hydrogen atom, or gaining an oxygen atom.
oxide	A compound made of oxygen and another element.

P

parasitism	A symbiotic relationship in which one organism (*parasite*) lives on and at the expense of another (*host*).
passive	Immunity (usually temporary) imparted without the person's body acting in its immunity build-up; the immunity is imparted by the administration of foreign antibodies.
Pasteur, Louis	A French chemist (1822–1895) who made major discoveries in chemistry and biology, especially in the control of many diseases. He and ROBERT KOCH were the founders of the science of bacteriology.
pasteurization	The heating of milk, or some other liquid, to a certain temperature for a definite period of time to destroy certain pathogens without changing the flavor or quality of the beverage.
PCR	Polymerase chain reaction is an in vitro technique for the rapid reproduction of many copies of DNA segments.
peptide bond	A chemical bond that joins two amino acids by connecting the carbohl group of one amino acid and the amino group of the other.
peptidoglycan	A substance in bacterial cell walls made of polypeptide-linked carbohydrates.
pH	A symbol used in expression of acidity or alkalinity. It denotes the negative logarithm of the concentration of hydrogen ions in gram atoms per liter.
phagotroph	An organism that feeds on other organisms, usually while they are still alive, by engulfing them to allow digestion and absorption to take place within the body.

phenylketonuria (PKU) A GENETIC DISORDER caused by inheritance of a damaged gene for the enzyme that converts excess molecules of the AMINO ACID phenylalanine to the AMINO ACID tyrosine. High levels of phenylalanine and phenylketones, molecules intermediate between phenylalanine and tyrosine, accumulate in the blood of the affected person unless dietary intake of phenylalanine is severely restricted. Untreated PKU in infants results in severe brain damage and mental retardation.

physics The study of matter and energy and their interactions.

phytogeographic map A map showing plant life.

Planck, Max A German physicist (1858–1947) who did notable work in thermodynamics; the "father of quantum physics."

planet A large body that moves around the sun, for example, the earth.

plankton A group of sea life—both plant and animal—that drifts with tides and currents.

plasma The liquid portion of the blood in which proteins and other substances are dissolved.

plasma membrane The cell membrane; the living covering of the cell.

plasmid Small circular DNA molecules in bacterial cells capable of self-duplication; often different genes are inserted.

plastids Cellular organelles that are found in plant cells and may contain pigments. The types of plastids are (1) *chloroplasts,* which contain the chlorophyll and carotenoid pigments and which are green; (2) *chromoplasts,* which contain carotenoid pigments and range in color from yellow to brown; and (3) *leucoplasts,* which are colorless.

polar compound A substance (for example, water) in which the electromagnetic charge of each molecule is unevenly distributed so that the molecule is positively charged on one end and negatively charged on the other end. *See* NONPOLAR COMPOUND and SOLUBLE.

potential energy Energy that is available for use. The energy of a boulder balanced on a mountainside is an example of potential energy. It becomes *kinetic energy* when the boulder begins to roll.

precipitation The settling out of particles suspended in liquid. Precipitation can be the result of a chemical reaction in which dissolved reactants form an insoluble product. Material that settles out of a suspension is a *precipitate.*

Priestley, Joseph The English chemist (1738–1804) who discovered oxygen, though the element was named, and its importance first recognized, by LAVOISIER.

primeval An adjective meaning "the first" or "early."

prokaryote An organism characterized by cells not containing a true or definite NUCLEUS surrounded by a nuclear membrane.

protein A complex organic compound consisting of AMINO ACIDS.

proton   A positively charged particle found in the nucleus of atoms.

protoplasm   An outdated term for the living substance within a cell. Current terminology divides cellular content into CYTOPLASM and *nucleoplasm* (material within the nuclear membrane).

protoplast   The entire cellular contents, surrounded by and including the cell membrane. The cell wall and/or capsule are not a part of the protoplast.

R

radical   A group of atoms that carries a charge and stays together as a unit during chemical reactions or in solutions, such as the nitrate ion and the sulfate ion.

radio astronomy The study of radio waves received from outer space.

reduction   Any chemical reaction that results in a molecule gaining an electron, gaining a hydrogen atom, or losing an oxygen atom.

regeneration   The ability of an organism to regrow parts of itself after an injury.

replication   The process by which DNA duplicates itself for distribution to daughter nuclei during mitosis and/or meiosis.

reproduction   The process by which organisms create offspring of their own species.

respiration   In cells, the oxidation of food for the release of energy; in aerobes, the intake of oxygen and the release of carbon dioxide.

restriction fragment A piece of DNA produced by breaking a large piece of DNA at specific points with restriction enzymes extracted from bacteria.

retrovirus   An RNA virus that produces new DNA from its RNA, as catalized by the enzyme reverse transcriptase.

RFLP   (restriction fragment length polymorphism) Differences in the lengths of RESTRICTION FRAGMENTS seen when DNA from different individuals is exposed to the same set of restriction enzymes. Using RFLP's to determine the identity of a person with DNA obtained from blood or other bodily materials is often referred to as "DNA fingerprinting." RFLP's can also be used to diagnose the presence of genetic disorders resulting from damaged genes.

ribosome   An intracellular structure consisting of RNA and protein whose function is to provide a site for the TRANSLATION phase of protein synthesis.

RNA   (ribonucleic acid) A large, helical, single-stranded molecule whose different types perform various tasks in the process of protein synthesis.

S

salinity	The degree of SALT present. Usually refers to the amount of salt in a fluid.
salt	A substance formed when an acid is mixed with a base.
saprotroph	An organism feeding on dead organic matter, usually digesting the food externally and absorbing the digested material into its body.
satellite	An object that orbits around a planet, such as a moon. In recent years, the earth has had several man-made satellites.
serotonin	A biogenic amine derivative of tryptophan that serves as a neurotransmitter in the central nervous system.
serum	The fluid portion of blood plasma after clotting.
sickle cell anemia	A GENETIC DISORDER caused by inheritance of a damaged gene for two of the four PROTEIN subunits of the HEMOGLOBIN molecule. The defective hemoglobin molecules stick to one another, forming clusters that distort the shape of the ERYTHROCYTES, reducing their ability to transport oxygen. Defective erythrocytes can also burst or clog capillaries.
slime mold	Large amoeboid protozoans that form spores similar to those of fungi.
solar	An adjective referring to the sun. A solar eclipse is an eclipse of the sun. See LUNAR; ECLIPSE.
solar system	The sun, planets, satellites, and asteroids.
soluble	The ability of a substance to mix completely with a liquid at the molecular level, such that no particles of any kind are visible in the mixture. The substance must be compatible with the liquid; nonpolar substances will not dissolve in polar liquids or the reverse. Dissolved substances will often be able to pass through semipermeable membranes. *See* NONPOLAR COMPOUND, POLAR COMPOUND, SOLUTE, and SOLUTION.
solute	The substance dissolved in a fluid to form a solution. *See* SOLUTION, SOLUBLE, and SOLVENT.
solution	A solution is a type of mixture formed when one substance mixes completely with a liquid at the molecular level. For example, when sugar (POLAR COMPOUND) is mixed with hot water (also a POLAR COMPOUND), the result is a solution. *See* SOLUTE, SOLVENT, and SOLUBLE.
solvent	The fluid in which a solute is dissolved to form a SOLUTION. *See* SOLUBLE.
sonic	An adjective referring to sound.
spawn	Eggs of certain aquatic animals. Also used as a verb meaning "to lay eggs." Both forms are usually used in connection with fish.

stimulus   Any change in the external or internal environment of a living organism. Many stimuli cause a change in the organism's activity (response). For example, if a person has not eaten for some time, the smell of the food might make his mouth water. The stimulus is the sudden presence of food (detected by smell); the response is secretion of saliva.

sublimation   The transformation of a substance from a solid directly to a gaseous state without passing through a liquid state.

substratum   A layer lying beneath the top layer (geology); the surface of a medium on which microorganisms grow (biology); a material or compound on which enzymes act (biology). Also called the *substrate*.

supersonic   An adjective meaning "faster than sound."

suspension   A type of mixture in which large particles are mixed with a liquid and remain mixed only as long as they are agitated. The particles in a suspension will settle out if not continuously agitated. An example is the suspension of blood cells in the plasma of blood. Particles in suspension will not pass through a semipermeable membrane. *See* COLLOID and SOLUTION.

symbiosis   A relationship between two different species living together. The relationship may be PARASITISM, MUTUALISM, or COMMENSALISM.

synergism   A phenomenon in which the total is greater than the sum of the individual parameters.

T

theory   An explanation of natural events based on hypotheses and confirmed by testing.

thermodynamics   The study of heat and energy flow.

tissue   A group of similar CELLS specialized to perform a single task. When different tissues are combined, they are arranged in sequential layers. *See* ORGAN.

transcription   The formation of messenger RNA from the coded DNA.

transduction   The passage of genetic material from one bacterial cell to another by means of viral parasites called *phages*.

transformation   The passage of genetic material from one bacterium to another through the medium in which they are growing.

translation   The formation of proteins from amino acids by the use of the coded information in the messenger RNA.

translocation   The movement of materials throughout a plant.

U

unicellular   An adjective meaning "one-celled." *See* CELL.

universe   All things that exist in space, taken as a whole.

V

valence The number of electrons that can be accepted, given up, or shared by an atom or RADICAL. Positive valence numbers indicate electrons that can be given up to or shared with another atom or radical; negative valence numbers indicate electrons that can be accepted from another atom or radical. The positive and negative valences of reactants must balance for a chemical reaction to occur.

vapor The gaseous phase of a substance that is usually in a liquid state. Vaporization (*evaporation*) of water or another liquid is accomplished by heating the liquid.

vascular tissue Tissue used to transport materials in multicellular organisms. In higher animals, blood is vascular tissue; in higher plants, xylem and phloem are vascular tissues.

vector An organism, usually an arthropod, that carries and transmits pathogens from one animal to another.

velocity The rate of motion of one object relative to another object.

Vesalius, Andreas A Flemish anatomist (1514–1564) who studied the body. His discoveries were so important that he is often referred to as "the father of anatomy." *See* ANATOMY.

virus An obligate intracellular parasite consisting essentially of a nucleic acid surrounded by a protein coat.

vitamin An organic substance other than an ENZYME that is necessary for the proper maintenance of a metabolic process. A vitamin deficiency will cause metabolic dysfunction and an overall decline in health. Animals, including humans, must get their vitamins from the foods they eat.

volt The practical unit of measurement of electric potential and electromotive force.

W

water table The level nearest to the surface of the ground where water is found.

work The result of energy expenditure. Common examples of work are movement, chemical reactions, and changes from one physical state to another.

Y

yeast A unicellular nonmycelial fungus. Some yeasts are of commercial importance in the brewing and baking industries.

Z

zoology The study of animals; a branch of BIOLOGY.

ANSWER SHEET

CHEMISTRY AND PHYSICS

Test 1

1. Ⓐ Ⓑ Ⓒ Ⓓ	14. Ⓐ Ⓑ Ⓒ Ⓓ	27. Ⓐ Ⓑ Ⓒ Ⓓ	40. Ⓐ Ⓑ Ⓒ Ⓓ	53. Ⓐ Ⓑ Ⓒ Ⓓ
2. Ⓐ Ⓑ Ⓒ Ⓓ	15. Ⓐ Ⓑ Ⓒ Ⓓ	28. Ⓐ Ⓑ Ⓒ Ⓓ	41. Ⓐ Ⓑ Ⓒ Ⓓ	54. Ⓐ Ⓑ Ⓒ Ⓓ
3. Ⓐ Ⓑ Ⓒ Ⓓ	16. Ⓐ Ⓑ Ⓒ Ⓓ	29. Ⓐ Ⓑ Ⓒ Ⓓ	42. Ⓐ Ⓑ Ⓒ Ⓓ	55. Ⓐ Ⓑ Ⓒ Ⓓ
4. Ⓐ Ⓑ Ⓒ Ⓓ	17. Ⓐ Ⓑ Ⓒ Ⓓ	30. Ⓐ Ⓑ Ⓒ Ⓓ	43. Ⓐ Ⓑ Ⓒ Ⓓ	56. Ⓐ Ⓑ Ⓒ Ⓓ
5. Ⓐ Ⓑ Ⓒ Ⓓ	18. Ⓐ Ⓑ Ⓒ Ⓓ	31. Ⓐ Ⓑ Ⓒ Ⓓ	44. Ⓐ Ⓑ Ⓒ Ⓓ	57. Ⓐ Ⓑ Ⓒ Ⓓ
6. Ⓐ Ⓑ Ⓒ Ⓓ	19. Ⓐ Ⓑ Ⓒ Ⓓ	32. Ⓐ Ⓑ Ⓒ Ⓓ	45. Ⓐ Ⓑ Ⓒ Ⓓ	58. Ⓐ Ⓑ Ⓒ Ⓓ
7. Ⓐ Ⓑ Ⓒ Ⓓ	20. Ⓐ Ⓑ Ⓒ Ⓓ	33. Ⓐ Ⓑ Ⓒ Ⓓ	46. Ⓐ Ⓑ Ⓒ Ⓓ	59. Ⓐ Ⓑ Ⓒ Ⓓ
8. Ⓐ Ⓑ Ⓒ Ⓓ	21. Ⓐ Ⓑ Ⓒ Ⓓ	34. Ⓐ Ⓑ Ⓒ Ⓓ	47. Ⓐ Ⓑ Ⓒ Ⓓ	60. Ⓐ Ⓑ Ⓒ Ⓓ
9. Ⓐ Ⓑ Ⓒ Ⓓ	22. Ⓐ Ⓑ Ⓒ Ⓓ	35. Ⓐ Ⓑ Ⓒ Ⓓ	48. Ⓐ Ⓑ Ⓒ Ⓓ	61. Ⓐ Ⓑ Ⓒ Ⓓ
10. Ⓐ Ⓑ Ⓒ Ⓓ	23. Ⓐ Ⓑ Ⓒ Ⓓ	36. Ⓐ Ⓑ Ⓒ Ⓓ	49. Ⓐ Ⓑ Ⓒ Ⓓ	62. Ⓐ Ⓑ Ⓒ Ⓓ
11. Ⓐ Ⓑ Ⓒ Ⓓ	24. Ⓐ Ⓑ Ⓒ Ⓓ	37. Ⓐ Ⓑ Ⓒ Ⓓ	50. Ⓐ Ⓑ Ⓒ Ⓓ	63. Ⓐ Ⓑ Ⓒ Ⓓ
12. Ⓐ Ⓑ Ⓒ Ⓓ	25. Ⓐ Ⓑ Ⓒ Ⓓ	38. Ⓐ Ⓑ Ⓒ Ⓓ	51. Ⓐ Ⓑ Ⓒ Ⓓ	64. Ⓐ Ⓑ Ⓒ Ⓓ
13. Ⓐ Ⓑ Ⓒ Ⓓ	26. Ⓐ Ⓑ Ⓒ Ⓓ	39. Ⓐ Ⓑ Ⓒ Ⓓ	52. Ⓐ Ⓑ Ⓒ Ⓓ	65. Ⓐ Ⓑ Ⓒ Ⓓ

Test 2

1. Ⓐ Ⓑ Ⓒ Ⓓ	9. Ⓐ Ⓑ Ⓒ Ⓓ	17. Ⓐ Ⓑ Ⓒ Ⓓ	25. Ⓐ Ⓑ Ⓒ Ⓓ	33. Ⓐ Ⓑ Ⓒ Ⓓ
2. Ⓐ Ⓑ Ⓒ Ⓓ	10. Ⓐ Ⓑ Ⓒ Ⓓ	18. Ⓐ Ⓑ Ⓒ Ⓓ	26. Ⓐ Ⓑ Ⓒ Ⓓ	34. Ⓐ Ⓑ Ⓒ Ⓓ
3. Ⓐ Ⓑ Ⓒ Ⓓ	11. Ⓐ Ⓑ Ⓒ Ⓓ	19. Ⓐ Ⓑ Ⓒ Ⓓ	27. Ⓐ Ⓑ Ⓒ Ⓓ	35. Ⓐ Ⓑ Ⓒ Ⓓ
4. Ⓐ Ⓑ Ⓒ Ⓓ	12. Ⓐ Ⓑ Ⓒ Ⓓ	20. Ⓐ Ⓑ Ⓒ Ⓓ	28. Ⓐ Ⓑ Ⓒ Ⓓ	36. Ⓐ Ⓑ Ⓒ Ⓓ
5. Ⓐ Ⓑ Ⓒ Ⓓ	13. Ⓐ Ⓑ Ⓒ Ⓓ	21. Ⓐ Ⓑ Ⓒ Ⓓ	29. Ⓐ Ⓑ Ⓒ Ⓓ	37. Ⓐ Ⓑ Ⓒ Ⓓ
6. Ⓐ Ⓑ Ⓒ Ⓓ	14. Ⓐ Ⓑ Ⓒ Ⓓ	22. Ⓐ Ⓑ Ⓒ Ⓓ	30. Ⓐ Ⓑ Ⓒ Ⓓ	38. Ⓐ Ⓑ Ⓒ Ⓓ
7. Ⓐ Ⓑ Ⓒ Ⓓ	15. Ⓐ Ⓑ Ⓒ Ⓓ	23. Ⓐ Ⓑ Ⓒ Ⓓ	31. Ⓐ Ⓑ Ⓒ Ⓓ	39. Ⓐ Ⓑ Ⓒ Ⓓ
8. Ⓐ Ⓑ Ⓒ Ⓓ	16. Ⓐ Ⓑ Ⓒ Ⓓ	24. Ⓐ Ⓑ Ⓒ Ⓓ	32. Ⓐ Ⓑ Ⓒ Ⓓ	40. Ⓐ Ⓑ Ⓒ Ⓓ

HUMAN ANATOMY AND PHYSIOLOGY

TEST 3

1. Ⓐ Ⓑ Ⓒ Ⓓ
2. Ⓐ Ⓑ Ⓒ Ⓓ
3. Ⓐ Ⓑ Ⓒ Ⓓ
4. Ⓐ Ⓑ Ⓒ Ⓓ
5. Ⓐ Ⓑ Ⓒ Ⓓ
6. Ⓐ Ⓑ Ⓒ Ⓓ
7. Ⓐ Ⓑ Ⓒ Ⓓ
8. Ⓐ Ⓑ Ⓒ Ⓓ
9. Ⓐ Ⓑ Ⓒ Ⓓ
10. Ⓐ Ⓑ Ⓒ Ⓓ
11. Ⓐ Ⓑ Ⓒ Ⓓ

12. Ⓐ Ⓑ Ⓒ Ⓓ
13. Ⓐ Ⓑ Ⓒ Ⓓ
14. Ⓐ Ⓑ Ⓒ Ⓓ
15. Ⓐ Ⓑ Ⓒ Ⓓ
16. Ⓐ Ⓑ Ⓒ Ⓓ
17. Ⓐ Ⓑ Ⓒ Ⓓ
18. Ⓐ Ⓑ Ⓒ Ⓓ
19. Ⓐ Ⓑ Ⓒ Ⓓ
20. Ⓐ Ⓑ Ⓒ Ⓓ
21. Ⓐ Ⓑ Ⓒ Ⓓ
22. Ⓐ Ⓑ Ⓒ Ⓓ

23. Ⓐ Ⓑ Ⓒ Ⓓ
24. Ⓐ Ⓑ Ⓒ Ⓓ
25. Ⓐ Ⓑ Ⓒ Ⓓ
26. Ⓐ Ⓑ Ⓒ Ⓓ
27. Ⓐ Ⓑ Ⓒ Ⓓ
28. Ⓐ Ⓑ Ⓒ Ⓓ
29. Ⓐ Ⓑ Ⓒ Ⓓ
30. Ⓐ Ⓑ Ⓒ Ⓓ
31. Ⓐ Ⓑ Ⓒ Ⓓ
32. Ⓐ Ⓑ Ⓒ Ⓓ
33. Ⓐ Ⓑ Ⓒ Ⓓ

34. Ⓐ Ⓑ Ⓒ Ⓓ
35. Ⓐ Ⓑ Ⓒ Ⓓ
36. Ⓐ Ⓑ Ⓒ Ⓓ
37. Ⓐ Ⓑ Ⓒ Ⓓ
38. Ⓐ Ⓑ Ⓒ Ⓓ
39. Ⓐ Ⓑ Ⓒ Ⓓ
40. Ⓐ Ⓑ Ⓒ Ⓓ
41. Ⓐ Ⓑ Ⓒ Ⓓ
42. Ⓐ Ⓑ Ⓒ Ⓓ
43. Ⓐ Ⓑ Ⓒ Ⓓ
44. Ⓐ Ⓑ Ⓒ Ⓓ

45. Ⓐ Ⓑ Ⓒ Ⓓ
46. Ⓐ Ⓑ Ⓒ Ⓓ
47. Ⓐ Ⓑ Ⓒ Ⓓ
48. Ⓐ Ⓑ Ⓒ Ⓓ
49. Ⓐ Ⓑ Ⓒ Ⓓ
50. Ⓐ Ⓑ Ⓒ Ⓓ
51. Ⓐ Ⓑ Ⓒ Ⓓ
52. Ⓐ Ⓑ Ⓒ Ⓓ
53. Ⓐ Ⓑ Ⓒ Ⓓ
54. Ⓐ Ⓑ Ⓒ Ⓓ
55. Ⓐ Ⓑ Ⓒ Ⓓ

TEST 4

1. Ⓐ Ⓑ Ⓒ Ⓓ
2. Ⓐ Ⓑ Ⓒ Ⓓ
3. Ⓐ Ⓑ Ⓒ Ⓓ
4. Ⓐ Ⓑ Ⓒ Ⓓ
5. Ⓐ Ⓑ Ⓒ Ⓓ
6. Ⓐ Ⓑ Ⓒ Ⓓ
7. Ⓐ Ⓑ Ⓒ Ⓓ
8. Ⓐ Ⓑ Ⓒ Ⓓ
9. Ⓐ Ⓑ Ⓒ Ⓓ
10. Ⓐ Ⓑ Ⓒ Ⓓ

11. Ⓐ Ⓑ Ⓒ Ⓓ
12. Ⓐ Ⓑ Ⓒ Ⓓ
13. Ⓐ Ⓑ Ⓒ Ⓓ
14. Ⓐ Ⓑ Ⓒ Ⓓ
15. Ⓐ Ⓑ Ⓒ Ⓓ
16. Ⓐ Ⓑ Ⓒ Ⓓ
17. Ⓐ Ⓑ Ⓒ Ⓓ
18. Ⓐ Ⓑ Ⓒ Ⓓ
19. Ⓐ Ⓑ Ⓒ Ⓓ
20. Ⓐ Ⓑ Ⓒ Ⓓ

21. Ⓐ Ⓑ Ⓒ Ⓓ
22. Ⓐ Ⓑ Ⓒ Ⓓ
23. Ⓐ Ⓑ Ⓒ Ⓓ
24. Ⓐ Ⓑ Ⓒ Ⓓ
25. Ⓐ Ⓑ Ⓒ Ⓓ
26. Ⓐ Ⓑ Ⓒ Ⓓ
27. Ⓐ Ⓑ Ⓒ Ⓓ
28. Ⓐ Ⓑ Ⓒ Ⓓ
29. Ⓐ Ⓑ Ⓒ Ⓓ
30. Ⓐ Ⓑ Ⓒ Ⓓ

31. Ⓐ Ⓑ Ⓒ Ⓓ
32. Ⓐ Ⓑ Ⓒ Ⓓ
33. Ⓐ Ⓑ Ⓒ Ⓓ
34. Ⓐ Ⓑ Ⓒ Ⓓ
35. Ⓐ Ⓑ Ⓒ Ⓓ
36. Ⓐ Ⓑ Ⓒ Ⓓ
37. Ⓐ Ⓑ Ⓒ Ⓓ
38. Ⓐ Ⓑ Ⓒ Ⓓ
39. Ⓐ Ⓑ Ⓒ Ⓓ
40. Ⓐ Ⓑ Ⓒ Ⓓ

41. Ⓐ Ⓑ Ⓒ Ⓓ
42. Ⓐ Ⓑ Ⓒ Ⓓ
43. Ⓐ Ⓑ Ⓒ Ⓓ
44. Ⓐ Ⓑ Ⓒ Ⓓ
45. Ⓐ Ⓑ Ⓒ Ⓓ
46. Ⓐ Ⓑ Ⓒ Ⓓ
47. Ⓐ Ⓑ Ⓒ Ⓓ
48. Ⓐ Ⓑ Ⓒ Ⓓ
49. Ⓐ Ⓑ Ⓒ Ⓓ
50. Ⓐ Ⓑ Ⓒ Ⓓ

BIOLOGY

TEST 5

1. Ⓐ Ⓑ Ⓒ Ⓓ
2. Ⓐ Ⓑ Ⓒ Ⓓ
3. Ⓐ Ⓑ Ⓒ Ⓓ
4. Ⓐ Ⓑ Ⓒ Ⓓ
5. Ⓐ Ⓑ Ⓒ Ⓓ
6. Ⓐ Ⓑ Ⓒ Ⓓ
7. Ⓐ Ⓑ Ⓒ Ⓓ
8. Ⓐ Ⓑ Ⓒ Ⓓ
9. Ⓐ Ⓑ Ⓒ Ⓓ
10. Ⓐ Ⓑ Ⓒ Ⓓ
11. Ⓐ Ⓑ Ⓒ Ⓓ
12. Ⓐ Ⓑ Ⓒ Ⓓ
13. Ⓐ Ⓑ Ⓒ Ⓓ
14. Ⓐ Ⓑ Ⓒ Ⓓ
15. Ⓐ Ⓑ Ⓒ Ⓓ

16. Ⓐ Ⓑ Ⓒ Ⓓ
17. Ⓐ Ⓑ Ⓒ Ⓓ
18. Ⓐ Ⓑ Ⓒ Ⓓ
19. Ⓐ Ⓑ Ⓒ Ⓓ
20. Ⓐ Ⓑ Ⓒ Ⓓ
21. Ⓐ Ⓑ Ⓒ Ⓓ
22. Ⓐ Ⓑ Ⓒ Ⓓ
23. Ⓐ Ⓑ Ⓒ Ⓓ
24. Ⓐ Ⓑ Ⓒ Ⓓ
25. Ⓐ Ⓑ Ⓒ Ⓓ
26. Ⓐ Ⓑ Ⓒ Ⓓ
27. Ⓐ Ⓑ Ⓒ Ⓓ
28. Ⓐ Ⓑ Ⓒ Ⓓ
29. Ⓐ Ⓑ Ⓒ Ⓓ

30. Ⓐ Ⓑ Ⓒ Ⓓ
31. Ⓐ Ⓑ Ⓒ Ⓓ
32. Ⓐ Ⓑ Ⓒ Ⓓ
33. Ⓐ Ⓑ Ⓒ Ⓓ
34. Ⓐ Ⓑ Ⓒ Ⓓ
35. Ⓐ Ⓑ Ⓒ Ⓓ
36. Ⓐ Ⓑ Ⓒ Ⓓ
37. Ⓐ Ⓑ Ⓒ Ⓓ
38. Ⓐ Ⓑ Ⓒ Ⓓ
39. Ⓐ Ⓑ Ⓒ Ⓓ
40. Ⓐ Ⓑ Ⓒ Ⓓ
41. Ⓐ Ⓑ Ⓒ Ⓓ
42. Ⓐ Ⓑ Ⓒ Ⓓ
43. Ⓐ Ⓑ Ⓒ Ⓓ

44. Ⓐ Ⓑ Ⓒ Ⓓ
45. Ⓐ Ⓑ Ⓒ Ⓓ
46. Ⓐ Ⓑ Ⓒ Ⓓ
47. Ⓐ Ⓑ Ⓒ Ⓓ
48. Ⓐ Ⓑ Ⓒ Ⓓ
49. Ⓐ Ⓑ Ⓒ Ⓓ
50. Ⓐ Ⓑ Ⓒ Ⓓ
51. Ⓐ Ⓑ Ⓒ Ⓓ
52. Ⓐ Ⓑ Ⓒ Ⓓ
53. Ⓐ Ⓑ Ⓒ Ⓓ
54. Ⓐ Ⓑ Ⓒ Ⓓ
55. Ⓐ Ⓑ Ⓒ Ⓓ
56. Ⓐ Ⓑ Ⓒ Ⓓ
57. Ⓐ Ⓑ Ⓒ Ⓓ

58. Ⓐ Ⓑ Ⓒ Ⓓ
59. Ⓐ Ⓑ Ⓒ Ⓓ
60. Ⓐ Ⓑ Ⓒ Ⓓ
61. Ⓐ Ⓑ Ⓒ Ⓓ
62. Ⓐ Ⓑ Ⓒ Ⓓ
63. Ⓐ Ⓑ Ⓒ Ⓓ
64. Ⓐ Ⓑ Ⓒ Ⓓ
65. Ⓐ Ⓑ Ⓒ Ⓓ
66. Ⓐ Ⓑ Ⓒ Ⓓ
67. Ⓐ Ⓑ Ⓒ Ⓓ
68. Ⓐ Ⓑ Ⓒ Ⓓ
69. Ⓐ Ⓑ Ⓒ Ⓓ
70. Ⓐ Ⓑ Ⓒ Ⓓ
71. Ⓐ Ⓑ Ⓒ Ⓓ

GENERAL SCIENCE

TEST 6

1. Ⓐ Ⓑ Ⓒ Ⓓ
2. Ⓐ Ⓑ Ⓒ Ⓓ
3. Ⓐ Ⓑ Ⓒ Ⓓ
4. Ⓐ Ⓑ Ⓒ Ⓓ
5. Ⓐ Ⓑ Ⓒ Ⓓ
6. Ⓐ Ⓑ Ⓒ Ⓓ
7. Ⓐ Ⓑ Ⓒ Ⓓ
8. Ⓐ Ⓑ Ⓒ Ⓓ
9. Ⓐ Ⓑ Ⓒ Ⓓ
10. Ⓐ Ⓑ Ⓒ Ⓓ
11. Ⓐ Ⓑ Ⓒ Ⓓ
12. Ⓐ Ⓑ Ⓒ Ⓓ
13. Ⓐ Ⓑ Ⓒ Ⓓ
14. Ⓐ Ⓑ Ⓒ Ⓓ

15. Ⓐ Ⓑ Ⓒ Ⓓ
16. Ⓐ Ⓑ Ⓒ Ⓓ
17. Ⓐ Ⓑ Ⓒ Ⓓ
18. Ⓐ Ⓑ Ⓒ Ⓓ
19. Ⓐ Ⓑ Ⓒ Ⓓ
20. Ⓐ Ⓑ Ⓒ Ⓓ
21. Ⓐ Ⓑ Ⓒ Ⓓ
22. Ⓐ Ⓑ Ⓒ Ⓓ
23. Ⓐ Ⓑ Ⓒ Ⓓ
24. Ⓐ Ⓑ Ⓒ Ⓓ
25. Ⓐ Ⓑ Ⓒ Ⓓ
26. Ⓐ Ⓑ Ⓒ Ⓓ
27. Ⓐ Ⓑ Ⓒ Ⓓ
28. Ⓐ Ⓑ Ⓒ Ⓓ

29. Ⓐ Ⓑ Ⓒ Ⓓ
30. Ⓐ Ⓑ Ⓒ Ⓓ
31. Ⓐ Ⓑ Ⓒ Ⓓ
32. Ⓐ Ⓑ Ⓒ Ⓓ
33. Ⓐ Ⓑ Ⓒ Ⓓ
34. Ⓐ Ⓑ Ⓒ Ⓓ
35. Ⓐ Ⓑ Ⓒ Ⓓ
36. Ⓐ Ⓑ Ⓒ Ⓓ
37. Ⓐ Ⓑ Ⓒ Ⓓ
38. Ⓐ Ⓑ Ⓒ Ⓓ
39. Ⓐ Ⓑ Ⓒ Ⓓ
40. Ⓐ Ⓑ Ⓒ Ⓓ
41. Ⓐ Ⓑ Ⓒ Ⓓ
42. Ⓐ Ⓑ Ⓒ Ⓓ

43. Ⓐ Ⓑ Ⓒ Ⓓ
44. Ⓐ Ⓑ Ⓒ Ⓓ
45. Ⓐ Ⓑ Ⓒ Ⓓ
46. Ⓐ Ⓑ Ⓒ Ⓓ
47. Ⓐ Ⓑ Ⓒ Ⓓ
48. Ⓐ Ⓑ Ⓒ Ⓓ
49. Ⓐ Ⓑ Ⓒ Ⓓ
50. Ⓐ Ⓑ Ⓒ Ⓓ
51. Ⓐ Ⓑ Ⓒ Ⓓ
52. Ⓐ Ⓑ Ⓒ Ⓓ
53. Ⓐ Ⓑ Ⓒ Ⓓ
54. Ⓐ Ⓑ Ⓒ Ⓓ
55. Ⓐ Ⓑ Ⓒ Ⓓ

56. Ⓐ Ⓑ Ⓒ Ⓓ
57. Ⓐ Ⓑ Ⓒ Ⓓ
58. Ⓐ Ⓑ Ⓒ Ⓓ
59. Ⓐ Ⓑ Ⓒ Ⓓ
60. Ⓐ Ⓑ Ⓒ Ⓓ
61. Ⓐ Ⓑ Ⓒ Ⓓ
62. Ⓐ Ⓑ Ⓒ Ⓓ
63. Ⓐ Ⓑ Ⓒ Ⓓ
64. Ⓐ Ⓑ Ⓒ Ⓓ
65. Ⓐ Ⓑ Ⓒ Ⓓ
66. Ⓐ Ⓑ Ⓒ Ⓓ
67. Ⓐ Ⓑ Ⓒ Ⓓ
68. Ⓐ Ⓑ Ⓒ Ⓓ

FINAL SCIENCE EXAMINATION

Test 7

1. Ⓐ Ⓑ Ⓒ Ⓓ
2. Ⓐ Ⓑ Ⓒ Ⓓ
3. Ⓐ Ⓑ Ⓒ Ⓓ
4. Ⓐ Ⓑ Ⓒ Ⓓ
5. Ⓐ Ⓑ Ⓒ Ⓓ
6. Ⓐ Ⓑ Ⓒ Ⓓ
7. Ⓐ Ⓑ Ⓒ Ⓓ
8. Ⓐ Ⓑ Ⓒ Ⓓ
9. Ⓐ Ⓑ Ⓒ Ⓓ
10. Ⓐ Ⓑ Ⓒ Ⓓ
11. Ⓐ Ⓑ Ⓒ Ⓓ
12. Ⓐ Ⓑ Ⓒ Ⓓ
13. Ⓐ Ⓑ Ⓒ Ⓓ
14. Ⓐ Ⓑ Ⓒ Ⓓ
15. Ⓐ Ⓑ Ⓒ Ⓓ

16. Ⓐ Ⓑ Ⓒ Ⓓ
17. Ⓐ Ⓑ Ⓒ Ⓓ
18. Ⓐ Ⓑ Ⓒ Ⓓ
19. Ⓐ Ⓑ Ⓒ Ⓓ
20. Ⓐ Ⓑ Ⓒ Ⓓ
21. Ⓐ Ⓑ Ⓒ Ⓓ
22. Ⓐ Ⓑ Ⓒ Ⓓ
23. Ⓐ Ⓑ Ⓒ Ⓓ
24. Ⓐ Ⓑ Ⓒ Ⓓ
25. Ⓐ Ⓑ Ⓒ Ⓓ
26. Ⓐ Ⓑ Ⓒ Ⓓ
27. Ⓐ Ⓑ Ⓒ Ⓓ
28. Ⓐ Ⓑ Ⓒ Ⓓ
29. Ⓐ Ⓑ Ⓒ Ⓓ
30. Ⓐ Ⓑ Ⓒ Ⓓ

31. Ⓐ Ⓑ Ⓒ Ⓓ
32. Ⓐ Ⓑ Ⓒ Ⓓ
33. Ⓐ Ⓑ Ⓒ Ⓓ
34. Ⓐ Ⓑ Ⓒ Ⓓ
35. Ⓐ Ⓑ Ⓒ Ⓓ
36. Ⓐ Ⓑ Ⓒ Ⓓ
37. Ⓐ Ⓑ Ⓒ Ⓓ
38. Ⓐ Ⓑ Ⓒ Ⓓ
39. Ⓐ Ⓑ Ⓒ Ⓓ
40. Ⓐ Ⓑ Ⓒ Ⓓ
41. Ⓐ Ⓑ Ⓒ Ⓓ
42. Ⓐ Ⓑ Ⓒ Ⓓ
43. Ⓐ Ⓑ Ⓒ Ⓓ
44. Ⓐ Ⓑ Ⓒ Ⓓ
45. Ⓐ Ⓑ Ⓒ Ⓓ

46. Ⓐ Ⓑ Ⓒ Ⓓ
47. Ⓐ Ⓑ Ⓒ Ⓓ
48. Ⓐ Ⓑ Ⓒ Ⓓ
49. Ⓐ Ⓑ Ⓒ Ⓓ
50. Ⓐ Ⓑ Ⓒ Ⓓ
51. Ⓐ Ⓑ Ⓒ Ⓓ
52. Ⓐ Ⓑ Ⓒ Ⓓ
53. Ⓐ Ⓑ Ⓒ Ⓓ
54. Ⓐ Ⓑ Ⓒ Ⓓ
55. Ⓐ Ⓑ Ⓒ Ⓓ
56. Ⓐ Ⓑ Ⓒ Ⓓ
57. Ⓐ Ⓑ Ⓒ Ⓓ
58. Ⓐ Ⓑ Ⓒ Ⓓ
59. Ⓐ Ⓑ Ⓒ Ⓓ
60. Ⓐ Ⓑ Ⓒ Ⓓ

61. Ⓐ Ⓑ Ⓒ Ⓓ
62. Ⓐ Ⓑ Ⓒ Ⓓ
63. Ⓐ Ⓑ Ⓒ Ⓓ
64. Ⓐ Ⓑ Ⓒ Ⓓ
65. Ⓐ Ⓑ Ⓒ Ⓓ
66. Ⓐ Ⓑ Ⓒ Ⓓ
67. Ⓐ Ⓑ Ⓒ Ⓓ
68. Ⓐ Ⓑ Ⓒ Ⓓ
69. Ⓐ Ⓑ Ⓒ Ⓓ
70. Ⓐ Ⓑ Ⓒ Ⓓ
71. Ⓐ Ⓑ Ⓒ Ⓓ
72. Ⓐ Ⓑ Ⓒ Ⓓ
73. Ⓐ Ⓑ Ⓒ Ⓓ
74. Ⓐ Ⓑ Ⓒ Ⓓ
75. Ⓐ Ⓑ Ⓒ Ⓓ

CHEMISTRY AND PHYSICS
TEST 1

65 QUESTIONS ▪ TIME—65 MINUTES

Directions: Read each question carefully and consider all possible answers. When you have decided which choice is best, blacken the corresponding space on your answer sheet. There is only one best answer for each question.

1. Oxygen gas can be obtained in appreciable quantities by heating all of the following EXCEPT

    (A) H_2O
    (B) H_2O_2
    (C) HgO
    (D) PbO_2

2. All of the reactions between the following pairs will produce hydrogen EXCEPT

    (A) copper and hydrochloric acid.
    (B) iron and sulfuric acid.
    (C) magnesium and steam.
    (D) sodium and alcohol.

3. When hydrochloric acid is added to sodium sulfite, and the gas that is formed is bubbled through barium hydroxide, the salt formed is

    (A) $BaCl_2$
    (B) $BaSO_3$
    (C) $NaCl$
    (D) $NaOH$

4. If 3,480 calories of heat are required to raise the temperature of 300 grams of a substance from 50°C to 70°C, the substance would be:

    Use the formula: $c = Q/MDT$

    c = specific heat
    Q = number of calories
    M = mass
    T = temperature

Substances	Specific Heat
(A) ethyl alcohol	0.581
(B) aluminum	0.214
(C) liquid ammonia	1.125
(D) water	1.0

5. Ozone is a molecular variety of

    (A) oxygen.
    (B) chlorine.
    (C) hydrogen.
    (D) sulfur.

6. If a eudiometer tube is filled with 26 milliliters of hydrogen and 24 milliliters of oxygen and the mixture exploded, which of the following would remain uncombined?

    (A) 2 milliliters hydrogen
    (B) 14 milliliters hydrogen
    (C) 23 milliliters hydrogen
    (D) 11 milliliters oxygen

7. The gas resulting when hydrochloric acid is added to a mixture of iron filings and sulfur is

    (A) H_2S
    (B) SO_2
    (C) SO_3
    (D) H_2

8. Calculate the time required for 100 milligrams of I^{131} (dissociation constant, $K = 0.086625$) to decay to 50 milligrams. Use the formula

    $$K = \frac{0.693}{t\frac{1}{2}}$$

    (A) 0.5 days
    (B) 0.4 days
    (C) 64 days
    (D) 8 days

GO ON TO THE NEXT PAGE

9. What is the percentage composition of oxygen in a mole of glucose ($C_6H_{12}O_6$)?

(C = 12, H = 1, O = 16)

(A) 53
(B) 35
(C) 6
(D) 20

10. In sulfuric acid the valence number of sulfur is

(A) + 2
(B) − 2
(C) − 4
(D) + 6

11. The boiling points of the following gases are as follows: argon, −185.7°C; helium, −268.9°C; nitrogen, −195.8°C; oxygen, −183°C. In the fractional distillation of liquid air, the gas that boils off last is

(A) argon.
(B) helium.
(C) nitrogen.
(D) oxygen.

12. The chemical reaction: $2Zn + 2HCl = 2ZnCl + H_2$ is an example of

(A) double displacement.
(B) synthesis.
(C) analysis.
(D) single displacement.

13. When carbon dioxide gas is bubbled through water in a test tube, the product is

(A) ozone.
(B) methane.
(C) hydrogen peroxide.
(D) carbonic acid.

14. Bronze is an alloy of copper and

(A) iron.
(B) lead.
(C) zinc.
(D) tin.

15. Which of the following substances will raise the pH of a solution of hydrochloric acid?

(A) NaCl
(B) H_2CO_3
(C) $NaHCO_3$
(D) HNO_3

16. An oxide whose water solution will turn litmus red is

(A) BaO
(B) Na_2O
(C) P_2O_3
(D) CaO

17. A compound that has a high heat for formation is normally

(A) easy to form from its elements and easy to decompose.
(B) easy to form from its elements and difficult to decompose.
(C) difficult to form from its elements and easy to decompose.
(D) difficult to form from its elements and difficult to decompose.

18. A solution of zinc chloride should NOT be stored in a tank made of aluminum because

(A) aluminum will displace the zinc in the zinc chloride solution.
(B) the zinc will become contaminated.
(C) the chloride ion will react with impurities in the solution.
(D) the two metals will react to produce an undesirable compound.

19. The valence number of sulfur in the ion SO_4^{-2} is

(A) −2
(B) +2
(C) +6
(D) +10

20. The chemical name for sulfuric acid is

(A) hydrogen sulfate.
(B) hydrogen sulfite.
(C) sulfur trioxide.
(D) hydrogen sulfide.

21. The number of grams of hydrogen formed by the action of 6 grams of magnesium (atomic weight = 24) on an appropriate quantity of acid is

(A) 0.5
(B) 8
(C) 22.4
(D) 72

22. The symbol for 2 molecules of hydrogen is

(A) H_2
(B) 2H
(C) 2H+
(D) $2H_2$

23. The formula for sodium bisulfate is

(A) $NaBiSO_4$
(B) $NaHSO_4$
(C) NaH_2SO_4
(D) Na_2SO_4

24. The law of multiple proportions was first proposed by

(A) Dalton.
(B) Davy.
(C) Priestley.
(D) Williams.

25. One liter of a certain gas, under standard conditions, weighs 1.16 grams. A possible formula for the gas is

(A) C_2H_2
(B) CO
(C) NH_3
(D) O_2

26. Which of the following compounds would be classified as a salt?

(A) Na_2CO_3
(B) $Ca(OH)_2$
(C) H_2CO_3
(D) CH_3OH

27. Of the following, which is an aromatic compound?

(A) Benzene
(B) Ethyl alcohol
(C) Iodoform
(D) Methane

28. Of the following, which is a monosaccharide?

(A) Dextrose
(B) Glycogen
(C) Lactose
(D) Sucrose

29. Fats belong to the class of organic compounds represented by the general formula, RCOOR', where R and R' represent hydrocarbon groups; therefore, fats are

(A) ethers.
(B) soaps.
(C) esters.
(D) lipases.

30. Oil and water are immiscible (do not mix) because

(A) oil is polar and water is polar.
(B) oil is nonpolar and water is polar.
(C) water is nonpolar and oil is polar.
(D) water is nonpolar and oil is nonpolar.

31. The chemical bond that forms between the carboxyl (RCOOH) group of one amino acid and the amino (RC-NH2) of another is a/an

(A) peptide bond.
(B) coordinate covalent.
(C) ionic bond.
(D) high energy bond.

32. Two atoms have the same atomic number but different atomic weights (masses); therefore, these atoms are

(A) compounds.
(B) isotopes.
(C) neutrons.
(D) different elements.

33. Commercial bleach has the formula

(A) $CaCl_2$
(B) CaOCL
(C) $CaOCl_2$
(D) $Ca(ClO_3)_2$

GO ON TO THE NEXT PAGE

34. In forming an ionic bond with an atom of chlorine, a sodium atom will
    (A) receive 1 electron from the chlorine atom.
    (B) receive 2 electrons from the chlorine atom.
    (C) give up 1 electron to the chlorine atom.
    (D) give up 2 electrons to the chlorine atom.

35. Which of the following is an example of a transition element? (Refer to the periodic table on page 197.)
    (A) Aluminum
    (B) Astatine
    (C) Nickel
    (D) Rubidium

36. A gas lighter than air is
    (A) CH_4
    (B) C_6H_6
    (C) HCl
    (D) N_2O

37. Of the following gases, which is odorless and heavier than air?
    (A) CO
    (B) CO_2
    (C) H_2S
    (D) N_2

38. In a volume of air at a pressure of one atmosphere at sea level, the partial pressure of oxygen is equal to
    (A) 593 mm of mercury.
    (B) 494 mm of mercury.
    (C) 380 mm of mercury.
    (D) 160 mm of mercury.

39. The complete combustion of carbon disulfide would yield carbon dioxide and
    (A) sulfur.
    (B) sulfur dioxide.
    (C) sulfuric acid.
    (D) water.

40. Alcoholic beverages contain
    (A) wood alcohol.
    (B) isopropyl alcohol.
    (C) glyceryl alcohol.
    (D) ethyl alcohol.

41. Of the following compounds, which is more difficult to decompose than lithium fluoride?
    (A) Lithium bromide
    (B) Lithium chloride
    (C) Lithium iodide
    (D) None of the above

42. Which of the following molecules would be classified as a ketone?

    (A)

    (B)

    (C)

    (D)

43. The periodic table (page 197) shows that the atomic number of fluorine is 9; this indicates that the fluoride atom contains
    (A) nine neutrons in its nucleus.
    (B) nine protons in its nucleus and nine electrons in orbit around the nucleus.
    (C) a total of nine protons and neutrons.
    (D) a total of nine protons and electrons.

44. The elements in group Zero of the periodic table (page 197) are considered inert gases because each has how many electrons in its outermost energy level?
    (A) 8
    (B) 7
    (C) 4
    (D) 2

45. Of four copper wires with the following dimensions, which one would have the greatest resistance to electrical current?

    (A) Length of 1 meter and diameter of 4 millimeters
    (B) Length of 2 meters and diameter of 8 millimeters
    (C) Length of 1 meter and diameter of 8 millimeters
    (D) Length of 2 meters and diameter of 2 millimeters

46. The general formula for an organic acid is

    (A) RCOOR
    (B) ROH
    (C) ROR
    (D) RCOOH

47. An example of a strong electrolyte is

    (A) sugar.
    (B) calcium chloride.
    (C) glycerin.
    (D) boric acid.

48. A lead ball, a wooden ball, and a styrofoam ball, all with a mass of 1 kilogram, are thrown at a wall 16 meters away, and all of them hit the wall in 2 seconds. Which ball will strike the wall with the greatest force?

    (A) Lead ball
    (B) Wooden ball
    (C) Styrofoam ball
    (D) All strike with the same force.

49. Identify the 2 atoms with the same number of electrons in their outermost energy level. (Use the periodic table on page 197.)

    (A) Na/K
    (B) K/Ca
    (C) Na/Mg
    (D) Ca/Na

50. When copper oxide is heated with charcoal, the reaction that occurs is an example of

    (A) reduction only.
    (B) oxidation only.
    (C) both oxidation and reduction.
    (D) neither oxidation nor reduction.

51. Nonmetal oxides, when dissolved in water, tend to form

    (A) acids.
    (B) bases.
    (C) salts.
    (D) hydrides.

52. The most important of the greenhouse gases contributing to global warning and altering the marine carbon cycle is

    (A) SO_2
    (B) CO
    (C) NH_3
    (D) CO_2

53. The best reducing agent is

    (A) mercury.
    (B) hydrogen.
    (C) copper.
    (D) carbon dioxide.

54. For a solution of H_2SO_4, the equivalency between molarity and normality would be (H = I, S = 32, O = 16)

    (A) IM = IN
    (B) IM = 2N
    (C) IN = 2M
    (D) IM = 0.5N

55. The test for a nitrate results in

    (A) a precipitate.
    (B) a red flame.
    (C) a brown ring.
    (D) litmus turning blue.

56. A solution that contains all the solute it can normally dissolve at a given temperature must be

    (A) concentrated.
    (B) supersaturated.
    (C) saturated.
    (D) unsaturated.

GO ON TO THE NEXT PAGE

57. The oxides of barium and sulfur combine to form

(A) a salt.
(B) a base.
(C) an acid.
(D) an anhydride.

58. A pencil is dropped into a glass half filled with water. It looks as if the end that is underwater does not match up with the end that is in the air. This optical illusion is the result of

(A) diffraction of light.
(B) convection of light.
(C) diffusion of light.
(D) refraction of light.

59. The reason why concentrated H_2SO_4 is used extensively to prepare other acids is that concentrated sulfuric acid

(A) is highly ionized.
(B) is an excellent dehydrating agent.
(C) has a high specific gravity.
(D) has a high boiling point.

60. In a 0.001 M solution of HCl, the pH is:

(A) 2
(B) −3
(C) 1
(D) 3

61. By use of the periodic table on page 197, it can be determined that the atoms with the greatest affinity would be

(A) Na and Cl
(B) K and F
(C) Na and F
(D) K and Cl

62. Using the periodic table on page 197, determine if the valence of a sodium ion is:

(A) +1
(B) 0
(C) −1
(D) +12

63. The portion of an atom directly involved in the ionic bonding is/are

(A) protons in the nucleus.
(B) neutrons in the nucleus.
(C) electrons in the outer energy level.
(D) electrons in the innermost energy level.

64. If the toxicity of a pesticide or a herbicide is in the range that a few drops could be fatal, the label should read

(A) Warning.
(B) Caution.
(C) Avoid.
(D) Danger.

65. A tornado passed over a house and destroyed it, primarily because

(A) the air pressure over the roof was lower than the pressure in the attic.
(B) the air pressure over the roof was equal to the pressure in the attic.
(C) the air pressure over the roof was higher than the pressure in the attic.
(D) None of the above

STOP   If you finish before time is called, you may check your work on this section only. Do not turn to any other section in the test.

TEST 2

40 QUESTIONS ▪▫ TIME—40 MINUTES

Directions: Read each question carefully and consider all possible answers. When you have decided which choice is best, fill in the corresponding space on your answer sheet. There is only one best answer for each question.

1. Which of the following properties is considered a physical property?

   (A) Flammability
   (B) Boiling point
   (C) Reactivity
   (D) Osmolarity

2. Which one of the following substances is a chemical compound?

   (A) Blood
   (B) Water
   (C) Oxygen
   (D) Air

3. What are the differentiating factors for potential and kinetic energy?

   (A) Properties—physical or chemical
   (B) State—solid or liquid
   (C) Temperature—high or low
   (D) Activity—in motion or in storage

4. How many calories are required to change the temperature of 2,000 grams of H_2O from 20°C to 38°C?

   (A) 36 calories
   (B) 24 calories
   (C) 18 calories
   (D) 12 calories

5. The oxidation of 1 gram of CHO produces 4 calories. How much CHO must be oxidized in the body to produce 36 calories? (CHO is a carbohydrate.)

   (A) 4 grams
   (B) 7 grams
   (C) 9 grams
   (D) 12 grams

6. What is the atomic weight of the element in the figure below?

   (A) 2
   (B) 3
   (C) 4
   (D) 7

7. Which of the following kinds of radiation is most penetrating?

   (A) Alpha
   (B) Beta
   (C) Gamma
   (D) X rays

8. I^{131} has a half-life of eight days. A 100-milligram sample of this radioactive element would decay to what amount after eight days?

   (A) 50 milligrams
   (B) 40 milligrams
   (C) 30 milligrams
   (D) 20 milligrams

9. A direct physiological effect of radiation on human tissues is

   (A) impairment of cellular metabolism.
   (B) proliferation of white blood cells.
   (C) formation of scar tissue.
   (D) reduction of body fluids.

GO ON TO THE NEXT PAGE

10. What is the gram molecular weight of $C_6H_{12}O_6$? (C = 12, H = 1, O = 16)

    (A) 29 grams
    (B) 174 grams
    (C) 180 grams
    (D) 696 grams

11. Which one of the following equations is balanced?

    (A) $H_2O \rightarrow H_2 \uparrow + O_2 \uparrow$
    (B) $Al + H_2SO_4 \rightarrow Al_2(SO_4)_3 + H_2 \uparrow$
    (C) $S + O_2 \rightarrow SO_3$
    (D) $2HgO \rightarrow 2Hg + O_2 \uparrow$

12. A person with a fever would be expected to have

    (A) an increase in pulse rate.
    (B) a decrease in pulse rate.
    (C) no change in pulse rate.
    (D) All of the above

13. Which of the following bodily substances is a catalyst?

    (A) Bile
    (B) Hemoglobin
    (C) Enzyme
    (D) Mucus

14. In order to increase the temperature of a gas in a closed unit, it would be necessary to

    (A) increase the pressure.
    (B) decrease the density.
    (C) decrease the volume.
    (D) increase the space.

15. Which of the following equations represents an oxidation-reduction reaction?

    (A) $2Na + Cl_2 \rightarrow NaCl$
    (B) $CO_2 + H_2O \rightarrow H_2CO_3$
    (C) $HNO_3 + KOH \rightarrow KNO_3 + H_2O$
    (D) $CaO + H_2O \rightarrow Ca(OH)_2$

16. Which one of the following equations represents neutralization?

    (A) $2Na + Cl_2 \rightarrow 2NaCl$
    (B) $CO_2 + H_2O \rightarrow H_2CO_3$
    (C) $HNO_3 + KOH \rightarrow KNO_3 + H_2O$
    (D) $CaO + H_2O \rightarrow Ca(OH)_2$

17. What happens when a small amount of soap is added to hard water?

    (A) Copious suds are formed.
    (B) A scum is formed.
    (C) All sediments filter out.
    (D) Sediments diffuse equally throughout the solution.

18. A 10-percent solution of glucose will contain

    (A) 1 gram of glucose per 1,000 milliliters of solution.
    (B) 1 gram of glucose per 100 milliliters of solution.
    (C) 1 gram of glucose per 10 microliters of solution.
    (D) 10 grams of glucose per 100 milliliters of solution.

Questions 19–22 refer to the diagrams below.

Each diagram represents one solution: One gram molecular weight of NaOH, one of KOH, and one of HCl, each dissolved in enough H_2O to make 1 liter.

19. What is the molecular weight of NaOH? (Atomic weights: Na = 23; O = 16; H = 1)

    (A) 40×1
    (B) 40×10
    (C) 40×100
    (D) $40 \times 1,000$

20. These are molar quantities because

    (A) their molecular weights are equal to each other.
    (B) the volume for each solution is the same.
    (C) each solution contains 1 gram molecular weight.
    (D) the percentage of solute to solvent is equal in each solution.

21. Identify the products of the chemical reaction between 1 cubic centimeter of KOH and 1 cubic centimeter of HCl.

(A) $K^+ + Cl_2 + 2H + OH$

(B) $KCl + H_2 + O_2$

(C) $K + Cl + HOH$

(D) $KCl + H_2O$

22. CA^{++} (atomic weight 40) is bivalent; hence, 1 gram equivalent weighs

(A) 40 grams.

(B) 30 grams.

(C) 20 grams.

(D) 10 grams.

23. A covalent bond between 2 amino acid molecules can be created by

(A) inserting a water molecule between them.

(B) removing a water molecule from them.

(C) inserting a carbon atom between them.

(D) removing a carbon atom from one of them.

24. Identify those elements in the periodic table that are inert gases (refer to columns).

(A) IA

(B) Zero

(C) IIIB–VIIB

(D) VIII

25. The basic inorganic raw materials for photosynthesis are

(A) water and oxygen.

(B) water and carbon dioxide.

(C) oxygen and carbon dioxide.

(D) sugar and carbon dioxide.

26. Production of Salk vaccine against polio depended upon discovery of a method for

(A) growing the polio virus outside the human body.

(B) killing the polio virus.

(C) observing the polio virus in the human body.

(D) producing a polio antitoxin.

27. Ringworm is caused by a(n)

(A) alga.

(B) bacterium.

(C) fungus.

(D) protozoan.

28. The process responsible for the continuous removal of carbon dioxide from the atmosphere is

(A) respiration.

(B) metabolism.

(C) oxidation.

(D) photosynthesis.

Periodic Table

IA																VIIA	Zero
H 1	IIA											IIIA	IVA	VA	VIA	H 1	He 2
Li 3	Be 4											B 5	C 6	N 7	O 8	F 9	Ne 10
Na 11	Mg 12	IIIB	IVB	VB	VIB	VIIB		VIII		IB	IIB	Al 13	Si 14	P 15	S 16	Cl 17	Ar 18
K 19	Ca 20	Sc 21	Ti 22	V 23	Cr 24	Mn 25	Fe 26	Co 27	Ni 28	Cu 29	Zn 30	Ga 31	Ge 32	As 33	Se 34	Br 35	Kr 36
Rb 37	Sr 38	Y 39	Zr 40	Nb 41	Mo 42	Tc 43	Ru 44	Rh 45	Pd 46	Ag 47	Cd 48	In 49	Sn 50	Sb 51	Te 52	I 53	Xe 54
Cs 55	Ba 56	*La 57	Hf 72	Ta 73	W 74	Re 75	Os 76	Ir 77	Pt 78	Au 79	Hg 80	Tl 81	Pb 82	Bi 83	Po 84	At 85	Rn 86
Fr 87	Ra 88	**Ac 89															

*LANTHANIDE SERIES	Ce 58	Pr 59	Nd 60	Pm 61	Sm 62	Eu 63	Gd 64	Tb 65	Dy 66	Ho 67	Fr 68	Tm 69	Yb 70	Lu 71
**ACTINIDE SERIES	Th 90	Pa 91	U 92	Np 93	Pu 94	Am 95	Cm 96	Bk 97	Cf 98	Es 99	Fm 100	Md 101	No 102	Lr 103

GO ON TO THE NEXT PAGE

29. All of the following concepts in genetics were first clearly stated by Gregor Mendel EXCEPT

    (A) dominance.
    (B) independent assortment.
    (C) segregation.
    (D) hybrid vigor.

30. The relation between termites and their intestinal protozoa is an example of

    (A) trophism.
    (B) parasitism.
    (C) mutualism.
    (D) commensalism.

31. When completed, the number of DNA base pairs comprising the human genome is expected to be approximately

    (A) 10 thousand.
    (B) 10 million.
    (C) 3 billion.
    (D) 3 trillion.

32. A completed human genomic map identifies the nucleotide sequences on the following chromosomal pairs:

    (A) 22 autosomes + 1 sex chromosome
    (B) 48 autosomes + 1 sex chromosome
    (C) 23 autosomes + 1 sex chromosome
    (D) 92 autosomes + 2 sex chromosomes

33. A technique (in which a catheter is inserted into the uterus to retrieve tissue samples) for the prenatal diagnosis of genetic diseases is called

    (A) amniocentesis.
    (B) positional cloning.
    (C) chorionic villus sampling (CVS).
    (D) None of the above

34. Identify the correct statement about DNA fingerprinting analysis of human tissues.

    (A) It is effective with small samples (e.g., less than 100 microliters of blood).
    (B) It produces identical bond patterns from all tissues in an individual.
    (C) It is effective on tissues more than 1,000 years old.
    (D) All of the above

35. In a DNA fingerprinting analysis of blood samples from a mother (M), a child (C), and an alleged father (F), the banding pattern in the child's blood was 50 percent (F), 27.3 percent (M), and 22.3 percent (FM). The statistical probability that the accused man is the child's father is

    (A) 50 percent.
    (B) greater than 50 percent.
    (C) less than 50 percent.
    (D) zero.

36. Glycogenesis occurs primarily in the

    (A) blood cells and spleen.
    (B) pancreas and gallbladder.
    (C) small intestines and stomach.
    (D) liver and muscles.

37. The end products of the Krebs cycle are

    (A) carbon dioxide and water.
    (B) urea and bile pigments.
    (C) lactic acid and pyruvic acid.
    (D) ketones and acetones.

38. The functional unit (or nephron) of the human kidney consists of

    (A) Bowman's capsule and veins.
    (B) Bowman's capsule, the glomerulus, and renal tubule.
    (C) the ureter and renal tubule.
    (D) the ureter, urethra, and renal tubule.

39. An organ that functions both as an endocrine and an exocrine gland is the

(A) salivary gland.
(B) gall bladder.
(C) thyroid gland.
(D) pancreas.

40. Aerobic oxidation of glucose occurs in two major stages; these are

(A) glycolysis and reduction.
(B) synthesis and the Krebs cycle.
(C) glycolysis and the Krebs cycle.
(D) degradation and hydrolysis.

STOP   If you finish before time is called, you may check your work on this section only. Do not turn to any other section in the test.

HUMAN ANATOMY AND PHYSIOLOGY
TEST 3

55 QUESTIONS ▪◻ TIME—55 MINUTES

Directions: Read each question carefully and consider all possible answers. When you have decided which choice is best, fill in the corresponding space on your answer sheet. There is only one best answer for each question.

Cells and Tissues

1. Cholesterol, in spite of its bad reputation, is an essential component of
   - (A) microtubules.
   - (B) the cell membrane.
   - (C) ribosomes.
   - (D) cytosol.

2. Synthesis of phospholipids, steroid hormones, and glycogen occurs within
   - (A) rough endoplasmic reticulum.
   - (B) mitochondria.
   - (C) smooth endoplasmic reticulum.
   - (D) golgi apparatus.

3. Following synthesis at the rough endoplasmic reticulum, new proteins are stored and "packaged" by
   - (A) smooth endoplasmic reticulum.
   - (B) the cell membrane.
   - (C) golgi apparatus.
   - (D) lysosomes.

4. Cell membranes control the movement of substances into and out of the cell and are best described as
   - (A) selectively permeable.
   - (B) freely permeable.
   - (C) impermeable.
   - (D) totally permeable.

5. Mammalian cells suspended within a hypertonic solution will
   - (A) swell and possibly rupture.
   - (B) lose water by osmosis.
   - (C) take on water by osmosis.
   - (D) remain unchanged since intracellular fluid is also hypertonic.

6. Glucose, a primary energy source for skeletal muscle, is insoluble in lipids and is too large to pass through membrane channels. Movement of glucose into skeletal muscle cells occurs via
   - (A) active transport.
   - (B) exocytosis.
   - (C) diffusion.
   - (D) facilitated diffusion.

7. The _____ are the control centers of cellular operations and usually contain nucleoli.
   - (A) nuclei
   - (B) mitochondria
   - (C) ribosomes
   - (D) lysosomes

8. _____, a multifunctional tissue, is comprised of layers of cells that cover both internal and external structures, including all exposed body surfaces. Although avascular, it is characterized by a high level of regeneration.
   - (A) Muscle
   - (B) Nerve
   - (C) Epithelial
   - (D) Connective

9. Connection of skeletal muscle to bones is made by tendons, which consist primarily of _____ fibers.

    (A) collagen
    (B) elastic
    (C) reticular
    (D) nerve

10. Joint cavities are found at articulations, are fluid-filled, and are lined by _____ membranes.

    (A) mucous
    (B) serous
    (C) cutaneous
    (D) synovial

Integumentary System

11. Protection of the skin from the harmful effects of ultraviolet light is provided by the pigment _____, which is produced by specialized cells within the stratum germanitivum.

    (A) carotene
    (B) melanin
    (C) keratin
    (D) hemoglobin

12. Lines of cleavage result from the parallel arrangements of _____ within the skin. They are significant in that incisions made parallel to a cleavage line tend to remain closed whereas incisions crossing lines of cleavage tend to pull open.

    (A) sebaceous glands
    (B) smooth muscle
    (C) blood vessels
    (D) collagen

13. The ear canal is protected against the invasion of foreign particles by a material produced by _____ glands.

    (A) ceruminous
    (B) sebaceous
    (C) apocrine
    (D) merocrine

14. _____ sweat glands become functional at puberty. Its product supports bacterial growth, which intensifies its odor.

    (A) Merocrine
    (B) Apocrine
    (C) Sebaceous
    (D) Ceruminous

15. Merkel discs and Meisnner corpuscles in the skin are functionally involved in

    (A) sweat production.
    (B) transport of blood.
    (C) sensation.
    (D) oil production.

Skeletal System

16. New bone matrix accompanied by increased strength and mass is the result of activity of

    (A) osteoblasts.
    (B) osteoclasts.
    (C) osteocytes.
    (D) lacuna.

17. Blood cell formation in adults is a function of red bone marrow primarily located within

    (A) periosteum.
    (B) endosteum.
    (C) compact bone.
    (D) spongy bone.

18. When blood calcium levels fall to below normal levels, osteoclast activity is stimulated and calcium excretion is decreased under the influence of elevated levels of

    (A) calcitonin.
    (B) parathyroid hormone.
    (C) calcitriol.
    (D) thyroxine.

19. The fetal skeleton begins as a model formed by cartilage. Replacement of cartilage by bone is the process of

    (A) intramembranous ossification.
    (B) endochondral ossification.
    (C) osteoclast activation.
    (D) osteoblast inhibition.

GO ON TO THE NEXT PAGE

20. Freely moveable joints, such as those found at the elbow and ankle, are functionally categorized as

    (A) synarthrosis.
    (B) amphiarthrosis.
    (C) diarthrosis.
    (D) arthritis.

21. Movement at a joint that takes a body part away from the long axis of the body is

    (A) flexion.
    (B) extension.
    (C) abduction.
    (D) adduction.

Muscle

22. Following release of transmitter substance at the neuromuscular junction, the action of that transmitter is terminated by

    (A) acetylcholine.
    (B) acetylcholinesterase.
    (C) epinephrine.
    (D) monoamine oxidase.

23. Following production of an action potential at the end plate, that electrical activity is conducted to the interior of the cell via the

    (A) motor neuron.
    (B) muscle capillaries.
    (C) epimysium.
    (D) transverse tubules.

24. Skeletal muscle contraction, resulting from the interaction of myosin and actin, is a consequence of the release of calcium ions from the

    (A) motor neuron.
    (B) end plate.
    (C) mitochondria.
    (D) sarcoplasmic reticulum.

25. In a(n) _____ voluntary contraction, muscle length changes, movement occurs, and work is done.

    (A) isometric
    (B) isotonic
    (C) paralytic
    (D) flaccid

26. Relaxed muscles produce more energy than is required for resting metabolism. That energy is stored in the form of

    (A) ATP.
    (B) ADP.
    (C) creatine.
    (D) creatine phosphate.

27. Lifting progressively heavier weight requires the activation of an increased number of motor units, which is

    (A) complete tetanus.
    (B) recruitment.
    (C) muscle tone.
    (D) a twitch.

28. Slow muscle fibers are particularly resistant to fatigue, a property due in part to the presence of _____, a protein that reversibly binds oxygen.

    (A) hemoglobin
    (B) myoglobin
    (C) ATP
    (D) ADP

29. Intercalated discs form connections between adjacent _____ muscle cells and play a major role in the function of that type of muscle.

    (A) striated
    (B) voluntary
    (C) cardiac
    (D) smooth

30. Individual muscle fibers and motor units either produce maximal tension in response to a stimulus or develop no tension at all. This is referred to as the _____ principle.

    (A) muscle tone
    (B) tetanus
    (C) twitch
    (D) all-or-none

Nervous System

31. _____ are glial cells within the central nervous system that play a role in maintaining the blood-brain barrier.

    (A) Ependymal cells
    (B) Microglia
    (C) Astrocytes
    (D) Oligodendrocytes

32. Following an action potential, sodium is returned to the extracellular space through the process of

    (A) diffusion.
    (B) filtration.
    (C) osmosis.
    (D) active transport.

33. An increase in potassium permeability at the postsynaptic membrane will result in a(n)

    (A) depolarization.
    (B) action potential.
    (C) excitatory postsynaptic potential.
    (D) inhibitory postsynaptic potential.

34. Spinal cord transection will result in a loss of respiration if the trauma is at upper _____ levels interrupting outflow of the phrenic nerve.

    (A) cervical
    (B) thoracic
    (C) lumbar
    (D) sacral

35. Sensitivity of muscle spindles is controlled by the central nervous system through its ability to activate

    (A) alpha motor neurons.
    (B) gamma motor neurons.
    (C) large diameter afferent axons.
    (D) the neuromuscular junction.

36. Damage to the _____ lobe of the cerebral cortex may result in deficits in conscious perception of auditory stimuli.

    (A) frontal
    (B) parietal
    (C) occipital
    (D) temporal

37. Sensory and motor innervation of the face is the domain of the ophthalmic, maxillary, and mandibular branches of the _____ nerve.

    (A) trochlear
    (B) trigeminal
    (C) facial
    (D) vestibulocochlear

38. Information regarding fine touch to the body surface ascends the spinal cord within the

    (A) spinothalamic tracts.
    (B) lateral corticospinal tracts.
    (C) posterior (dorsal) columns.
    (D) spinocerebellar tracts.

39. Active dreaming and autonomic alterations of blood pressure along with EEG tracings resembling the awake state are characteristic of

    (A) slow wave sleep.
    (B) rapid eye movement (REM) sleep.
    (C) coma.
    (D) arousal.

40. Parasympathetic autonomic outflow to the heart, lungs, and digestive system is a primary function of cranial nerve number

    (A) I
    (B) II
    (C) X
    (D) XII

Endocrinology and Reproduction

41. Release of thyroid hormones is triggered by _____ from the anterior pituitary gland.

    (A) thyrotropin releasing hormone
    (B) thyrotropin
    (C) thyroxine
    (D) iodide

42. In response to the release of _____ by the adenohypophysis, levels of glucocorticoids are elevated.

    (A) corticotropin releasing hormone
    (B) cortisol
    (C) aldosterone
    (D) adrenocorticotropic hormone

GO ON TO THE NEXT PAGE

43. _____ stimulates the smooth muscle of the uterine wall during the labor and delivery process. After delivery, it promotes the ejection of milk.

   (A) Oxytocin
   (B) Vasopressin
   (C) Somatotropin
   (D) Prolactin

44. In females, _____ promotes estrogen secretion from cells within the ovaries, while in males, it stimulates sperm production within the testes.

   (A) testosterone
   (B) melanotropin
   (C) follicle stimulating hormone
   (D) luteinizing hormone

45. Pancreatic beta cells produce the hormone _____, which lowers blood glucose levels by promoting glucose uptake and utilization.

   (A) glucagon
   (B) insulin
   (C) epinephrine
   (D) renin

46. An individual with an abnormally high basal metabolic rate accompanied by weight loss and unusual temperature sensitivity is probably suffering from

   (A) high levels of growth hormone.
   (B) low levels of growth hormone.
   (C) high levels of thyroid hormones.
   (D) low levels of thyroid hormones.

47. Insulin is released by the beta cells of the pancreas in response to

   (A) low blood glucose levels.
   (B) high blood glucose levels.
   (C) high prolactin levels.
   (D) high growth hormone levels.

48. The mineralocorticoid _____ is a product of the adrenal cortex.

   (A) epinephrine
   (B) norepinephrine
   (C) ACTH
   (D) aldosterone

49. Abnormally low levels of parathyroid hormone could result in

   (A) convulsions.
   (B) hyperglycemia.
   (C) hypoglycemia.
   (D) excess water loss via the kidneys.

50. Type I diabetes mellitus is characterized by

   (A) high insulin levels.
   (B) ineffective insulin receptors.
   (C) low blood glucose levels.
   (D) decreased insulin production.

51. Glycogenesis occurs primarily in the

   (A) blood cells and spleen.
   (B) pancreas and gallbladder.
   (C) small intestines and stomach.
   (D) liver and muscles.

52. The end products of the Krebs cycle are

   (A) carbon dioxide and water.
   (B) urea and bile pigments.
   (C) lactic acid and pyruvic acid.
   (D) ketones and acetones.

53. The functional unit (or nephron) of the human kidney consists of

   (A) Bowman's capsule and veins.
   (B) Bowman's capsule, the glomerulus, and renal tubule.
   (C) the ureter and renal tubule.
   (D) the ureter, urethra, and renal tubule.

54. An organ that functions both as an endocrine and an exocrine gland is the

(A) salivary gland.
(B) gallbladder.
(C) thyroid gland.
(D) pancreas.

55. Aerobic oxidation of glucose occurs in two major stages; these are

(A) glycolysis and reduction.
(B) synthesis and the Krebs cycle.
(C) glycolysis and the Krebs cycle.
(D) degradation and hydrolysis.

S T O P   If you finish before time is called, you may check your work on this section only. Do not turn to any other section in the test.

TEST 4

50 QUESTIONS ▪ TIME—50 MINUTES

Directions: Read each question carefully and consider all possible answers. When you have decided which choice is best, fill in the corresponding space on your answer sheet. There is only one best answer for each question.

Blood

1. Maintenance of the osmotic pressure of plasma is a major role of

    (A) albumin.
    (B) globulins.
    (C) fibrinogen.
    (D) platelets.

2. Anemia is a condition resulting from abnormally low levels of

    (A) platelets.
    (B) plasma proteins.
    (C) leukocytes.
    (D) erythrocytes or hemoglobin.

3. Production of red blood cells is stimulated by the release of _____ from specialized cells of the kidneys in response to hypoxia (low oxygen levels).

    (A) platelets
    (B) erythrocytes
    (C) erythropoietin
    (D) leukocytes

4. Blood typing is a classification determined by the identification of

    (A) erythrocyte surface antigens.
    (B) erythrocyte surface antibodies.
    (C) plasma antigens.
    (D) plasma antibodies.

5. Rh-positive blood indicates the presence of

    (A) the Rh antigen in plasma.
    (B) the Rh antigen on the surfaces of erythrocytes.
    (C) the Rh antibody on erythrocyte surfaces.
    (D) the Rh antibody in plasma.

6. Transfusion of blood from a Type A donor to a Type B recipient will result in

    (A) agglutination.
    (B) blood vessel spasm.
    (C) platelet plug formation.
    (D) slowly progressive anemia.

7. The most numerous leukocytes are _____. They are granulocytes and represent one of the earliest defenses against infection.

    (A) lymphocytes
    (B) monocytes
    (C) basophils
    (D) neutrophils

8. T cells, B cells, and NK cells are classes of _____, agranulocytes involved in immunity processes.

    (A) monocytes
    (B) lymphocytes
    (C) neutrophils
    (D) eosinophils

9. Release of ADP, thromboxane A_2, and serotonin are events associated with the _____ phase of hemostasis.

    (A) vascular
    (B) platelet
    (C) coagulation
    (D) inflammation

10. The last step in the final common pathway of coagulation involves the production of insoluble strands of the protein

    (A) prothrombin.
    (B) thrombin.
    (C) fibrinogen.
    (D) fibrin.

Cardiovascular

11. Action potentials in cardiac cells are longer in duration than those in skeletal muscle. The long plateau seen in cardiac action potentials is primarily due to

  (A) calcium entry into the cell.
  (B) calcium exit from the cell.
  (C) sodium entry into the cell.
  (D) sodium exit from the cell.

12. Conducting cells of the heart do not maintain a stable resting membrane potential. The rate of spontaneous depolarizations is greatest within

  (A) the A-V node.
  (B) the S-A node.
  (C) bundle branch fibers.
  (D) purkinje fibers.

13. Depolarization of the ventricles is reflected in the _____ of the electrocardiogram.

  (A) P wave
  (B) QRS complex
  (C) T wave
  (D) P-R segment

14. The maximum ventricular volume within a cardiac cycle is expressed as the

  (A) stroke volume.
  (B) ejection fraction.
  (C) end-systolic volume.
  (D) end-diastolic volume.

15. The amount of tension the ventricles must produce in order to open semilunar valves and eject blood is the

  (A) preload.
  (B) afterload.
  (C) cardiac output.
  (D) stroke volume.

16. Norepinephrine acts at _____ receptors of the heart, resulting in an increase in heart rate.

  (A) alpha 1
  (B) alpha 2
  (C) beta 1
  (D) beta 2

17. Exchange of materials from the vascular system to surrounding interstitial fluids is a property of

  (A) arteries.
  (B) arterioles.
  (C) capillaries.
  (D) veins.

18. Pressure in veins is low and significantly influenced by the force of gravity. In the extremities, unidirectional blood flow is maintained by

  (A) venous valves.
  (B) venous smooth muscle.
  (C) precapillary sphincters.
  (D) semilunar valves.

19. Pulse pressure, the difference between systolic and diastolic pressure, is greatest within

  (A) arteries.
  (B) arterioles.
  (C) capillaries.
  (D) veins.

20. The primary responsibility for rapid correction of blood pressure alterations involves

  (A) angiotensin.
  (B) antidiuretic hormone.
  (C) chemoreceptors.
  (D) baroreceptor reflexes.

Respiration

21. During the act of swallowing, entry of liquids and solid materials into the respiratory tract is prevented by the

  (A) glottis.
  (B) epiglottis.
  (C) pharynx.
  (D) hard palate.

GO ON TO THE NEXT PAGE

22. Septal (Type II) cells in the lung produce _____, which reduces the surface tension within alveoli. Infant respiratory distress syndrome results in individuals producing an inadequate amount of the substance.

    (A) serous fluid
    (B) pleural fluid
    (C) surfactant
    (D) mucous

23. _____ is the volume of air moved into or out of the respiratory system during a single respiratory cycle.

    (A) Tidal volume
    (B) Minute volume
    (C) Residual volume
    (D) Inspiratory reserve volume

24. The volume of air in the respiratory conduction passages that does NOT participate in gas exchange is the

    (A) vital capacity.
    (B) expiratory reserve volume.
    (C) anatomical dead space.
    (D) total lung capacity.

25. Movement of respiratory gases is primarily dependent upon the presence of a(n) _____ gradient.

    (A) concentration
    (B) osmotic
    (C) partial pressure
    (D) temperature

26. Contraction of the diaphragm results in inspiration as a result of

    (A) increased thoracic cavity volume.
    (B) decreased thoracic cavity volume.
    (C) increased abdominal cavity volume.
    (D) decreased abdominal cavity volume.

27. Oxygen unloading at the tissue level is accelerated by

    (A) elevated blood pressure.
    (B) lowered blood pressure.
    (C) elevated pH.
    (D) decreased pH.

28. Although most carbon dioxide is transported as bicarbonate, and some is dissolved in plasma, about 20% is carried

    (A) by leukocytes.
    (B) by plasma proteins.
    (C) as carbaminohemoglobin.
    (D) on the surface of erythrocytes.

29. The reaction of carbon dioxide and water leading to the formation of carbonic acid is catalyzed by

    (A) antigens on the surface of erythrocytes.
    (B) antibodies within plasma.
    (C) enzymes in plasma.
    (D) carbonic anhydrase within erythrocytes.

30. Length of inspiration is shortened by inhibitory impulses originating within the

    (A) apneustic center.
    (B) pneumotaxic center.
    (C) inspiratory center.
    (D) precentral gyrus.

Renal

31. Decline in systemic blood pressure leads to the release of renin, which results in the production of

    (A) angiotensinogen.
    (B) angiotensin I.
    (C) angiotensin II.
    (D) carbonic anhydrase.

32. Angiotensin II has multiple direct and indirect effects, including

    (A) vasoconstriction.
    (B) vasodilation.
    (C) inhibition of aldosterone release.
    (D) increased urine output.

33. _____ are examples of substances that are NOT significantly reabsorbed by the kidneys and are therefore excreted.

    (A) Amino acids
    (B) Vitamins
    (C) Nitrogenous products of protein catabolism
    (D) Water and electrolytes

34. Glucose and most other nutrients, such as amino acids and vitamins, are reabsorbed within the _____ of the nephron.

(A) collecting duct
(B) proximal convoluted tubule
(C) loop of Henle
(D) distal convoluted tubule

35. The movement of urine from the kidneys to the bladder is driven by

(A) gravity alone.
(B) peristalsis.
(C) bladder pressure.
(D) blood pressure.

36. Urinary continence is maintained by contraction of the external urethral sphincter, which is innervated by the

(A) sympathetic division of the ANS.
(B) parasympathetic division of the ANS.
(C) phrenic nerve.
(D) pudendal nerve.

37. The cation in the highest concentration within extracellular fluid that plays a major role in water distribution is

(A) sodium.
(B) potassium.
(C) calcium.
(D) magnesium.

38. The hormone most responsible for the renal regulation of sodium is

(A) thyroxine.
(B) insulin.
(C) glucagon.
(D) aldosterone.

39. Acid-base regulation is most powerful and most complete by

(A) buffers.
(B) respiratory mechanisms.
(C) renal mechanisms.
(D) urinary bladder activity.

40. Uncontrolled diabetes mellitus results in

(A) respiratory acidosis.
(B) respiratory alkalosis.
(C) metabolic acidosis.
(D) metabolic alkalosis.

Digestion

41. Absorption of vitamin B_{12} (required for erythrocyte production) is promoted by intrinsic factor—a product of cells found within the

(A) small intestine.
(B) stomach.
(C) pancreas.
(D) large intestine.

42. Bile that is NOT immediately needed for digestion is stored and concentrated within the

(A) liver.
(B) gallbladder.
(C) pancreas.
(D) ileum.

43. Secretion of pancreatic juice is stimulated by _____, released in response to proteins and fats within the small intestine.

(A) secretin
(B) cholecystokinin
(C) insulin
(D) aldosterone

44. Diarrhea and constipation result primarily from altered motility of the

(A) stomach.
(B) small intestine.
(C) liver.
(D) large intestine.

45. In order to be absorbed, carbohydrates must be reduced to the form of

(A) monosaccharides.
(B) disaccharides.
(C) polysaccharides.
(D) oligosaccharides.

GO ON TO THE NEXT PAGE

46. Protein digestion begins in the stomach by a group of proteolytic enzymes referred to as

    (A) lipase.
    (B) sucrase.
    (C) pepsin.
    (D) amylase.

47. Vitamin _____ is water-soluble and readily absorbed from the intestine by diffusion.

    (A) A
    (B) D
    (C) E
    (D) C

48. Gastric ulcers occur when the protective inner layer of the stomach is damaged and the _____ layer, with its blood vessels and nerve cells, is exposed to acid.

    (A) serosal
    (B) mucosal
    (C) submucosal
    (D) muscular

49. Saliva contains mucus, water, and _____, which partially digests polysaccharides.

    (A) lipase
    (B) amylase
    (C) pepsin
    (D) insulin

50. Smooth muscle activity of the digestive system is stimulated by increased levels of _____ activity.

    (A) parasympathetic autonomic
    (B) sympathetic autonomic
    (C) thyroid gland
    (D) aldosterone

STOP   If you finish before time is called, you may check your work on this section only. Do not turn to any other section in the test.

BIOLOGY
TEST 5

71 QUESTIONS ▪◻ TIME—65 MINUTES

Directions: For each of the following items, select the choice that best answers the question or completes the statement. Fill in the corresponding space on your answer sheet.

1. Passage of water through the membrane of a cell is called
   - (A) assimilation.
   - (B) osmosis.
   - (C) circulation.
   - (D) transpiration.

2. The largest portion of the iron supplied to the body by foods is used by the body for the
   - (A) growth of hard bones and teeth.
   - (B) manufacture of insulin.
   - (C) development of respiratory enzymes.
   - (D) formation of hemoglobin.

3. Phenylketonuria is a genetic disorder that involves an inability of
   - (A) blood to clot properly.
   - (B) one amino acid to be convened to another.
   - (C) blood cells to carry a sufficient load of oxygen.
   - (D) lung alveoli to stay open.

4. A new drug for treatment of tuberculosis was being tested in a hospital. Patients in group A received doses of the new drug; those in group B were given only sugar pills. Group B represents a(n)
   - (A) scientific experiment.
   - (B) scientific method.
   - (C) experimental error.
   - (D) experimental control.

5. Which is most closely associated with the process of transpiration?
   - (A) Spiracles of a grasshopper
   - (B) Root of a geranium
   - (C) Leaf of a maple
   - (D) Gills of a fish

6. Which term includes all the others?
   - (A) Organ
   - (B) Tissue
   - (C) System
   - (D) Organism

7. When several drops of pasteurized milk were placed in a petri dish containing sterilized nutrient agar, many colonies developed. This experiment shows the milk
   - (A) contained some bacteria.
   - (B) contained harmful bacteria.
   - (C) should have been sterilized.
   - (D) was incorrectly stamped "pasteurized."

8. The growth of green plants toward light is related most specifically to the distribution of _____ in the plant.
   - (A) minerals
   - (B) enzymes
   - (C) auxins
   - (D) amino acids

9. In humans, the digestion of carbohydrates begins in the
   - (A) stomach.
   - (B) small intestine.
   - (C) mouth.
   - (D) liver.

GO ON TO THE NEXT PAGE ▶

10. To determine whether an unknown black guinea pig is pure or hybrid black, it should be crossed with

    (A) a white guinea pig.
    (B) a hybrid black guinea pig.
    (C) a pure black guinea pig.
    (D) another unknown.

11. In a series of rock layers arranged one on top of another, fossils found in the lowest layers are

    (A) completely different from fossils found in the upper layers.
    (B) older than the fossils found in the upper layers.
    (C) of organisms simpler than the organisms fossilized in the upper layers.
    (D) of organisms more complex than organisms fossilized in the upper layers.

12. The principal way in which forests help to prevent soil erosion is that the

    (A) trees provide homes for wildlife.
    (B) leaves of the trees manufacture food.
    (C) forest floors absorb water.
    (D) forest shields the soil from the sun's heat.

13. Which factor in the environment of an organism causes it to react?

    (A) A stimulus
    (B) A response
    (C) A reflex
    (D) An impulse

14. A breeder wanted to develop a strain of beef cattle with high-quality meat and the ability to thrive in a hot, dry climate. How can she best accomplish this?

    (A) Continued selection among the members of a prize herd
    (B) Crossbreeding followed by selection
    (C) Inbreeding to bring out desirable hidden traits
    (D) Inbreeding followed by selection

15. The inhaling and the exhaling of air by the human lungs is mainly an application of

    (A) Boyl's Law—the inverse relationship between the pressure and the volume of a gas.
    (B) the volume of a gas at standard temperature and pressure (STP).
    (C) Charles' Law—the direct relationship between the temperature and the volume of a gas.
    (D) the number of O_2 and CO_2 particles per mole.

16. Which plant tissues are mostly concerned with storage?

    (A) Phloem and xylem
    (B) Phloem and cambium
    (C) Palisade cells and epidermis
    (D) Pith and spongy cells

17. The Hubble Telescope is able to produce images of very distant celestial objects more clearly than other telescopes because

    (A) its reflector is able to concentrate more light on the lens.
    (B) its images are enhanced by computer.
    (C) its view is not obstructed by atmosphere.
    (D) it has a larger lens.

18. Which reagent should be used in the urine test for diabetes?

    (A) Iodine
    (B) Nitric acid
    (C) Ammonia
    (D) Benedict's solution

19. The major benefit of buffer systems is that they

    (A) increase pH significantly.
    (B) resist significant changes in pH.
    (C) decrease pH significantly.
    (D) None of the above

20. The Kreb cycle produces

    (A) H_2O and NADH.
    (B) CO_2 and H_2.
    (C) pyruvic acid and lactic acid.
    (D) amino acids.

21. The removal for microscopic examination of a small bit of living tissue from a patient is called
    (A) biopsy.
    (B) surgery.
    (C) dissection.
    (D) therapy.

22. The presence of which substance is most important for all cell activity?
    (A) Light
    (B) Carbon dioxide
    (C) Water
    (D) Chlorophyll

23. The end products of digestion that enter the lacteals are
    (A) glucose.
    (B) amino acids.
    (C) minerals.
    (D) fatty acids.

24. A student in the laboratory tossed two pennies from a container 100 times and recorded these results: both heads, 25; one head and one tail, 47; both tails, 28. Which cross between plants would result in approximately the same ratio?
    (A) Aa × AA
    (B) Aa × Aa
    (C) AA × aa
    (D) Aa × aa

25. In the equation below for photosynthesis, the oxygen comes

    $$CO_2 + H_2O \rightarrow C_6H_{12}O_6 + O_2$$

    (A) entirely from CO_2.
    (B) from a simple sugar molecule.
    (C) partially from CO_2 and H_2O.
    (D) entirely from H_2O.

26. Tissue culture has been extensively used as a research method in all of the following fields of biological investigation EXCEPT
    (A) photosynthesis.
    (B) virology.
    (C) development of nerve cells.
    (D) experimental embryology.

27. After each transfer of a culture of bacteria, the wire loop should be
    (A) dipped into alcohol.
    (B) held in a flame.
    (C) dipped into liquid soap.
    (D) washed repeatedly in water.

28. Identify the statement that is NOT true of cellular respiration.
    (A) It is a downhill process.
    (B) It occurs in both plant and animal cells.
    (C) It uses CO_2 and H_2O for reactants.
    (D) It is an exergonic process.

29. In which one of the following ways does combustion differ from cellular respiration?
    (A) More heat is produced.
    (B) More energy is wasted.
    (C) It is less rapid.
    (D) It occurs at a higher temperature.

30. Of the following, an enzyme responsible for the digestion of proteins is
    (A) maltase.
    (B) trypsin.
    (C) ptyalin.
    (D) steapsin.

31. Failure of blood to clot readily when exposed to air may be due to a(n)
    (A) oversupply of erythrocytes.
    (B) deficiency of leucocytes.
    (C) overabundance of fibrin.
    (D) inadequacy of thrombokinase.

32. Cone cells are most closely associated with the function of
    (A) digestion.
    (B) absorption.
    (C) vision.
    (D) secretion.

33. The part of the vertebrate eye that controls the amount of light entering the eye is the
    (A) cornea.
    (B) ciliary body.
    (C) iris.
    (D) conjunctiva.

GO ON TO THE NEXT PAGE

34. Most of the carbon dioxide in the blood is carried in the
    (A) liquid portion.
    (B) leucocytes.
    (C) erythrocytes.
    (D) platelets.

35. Increased blood pressure may be brought about by excess secretion of
    (A) thyroxin.
    (B) insulin.
    (C) ACTH.
    (D) adrenaline.

36. Of the following, the plant hormone concerned with growth is
    (A) auxin.
    (B) estrogen.
    (C) testosterone.
    (D) ATP.

37. Bread mold resembles ferns in that both develop
    (A) mycelia.
    (B) hyphae.
    (C) pinnules.
    (D) spores.

38. Sap rises in woody stems because of root pressure and
    (A) transpiration pull.
    (B) enzyme action.
    (C) molecular adhesion.
    (D) photosynthesis.

39. Vascular tissues present in the body of a flowering plant are xylem and
    (A) cambium.
    (B) phloem.
    (C) meristem.
    (D) lenticels.

40. Stored food for the embryo of a bean seed is found in the
    (A) plumule.
    (B) hypocotyl.
    (C) cotyledons.
    (D) testa.

41. Which of the following is NOT a characteristic of cancer cells?
    (A) High power for self-affinity
    (B) Altered genetic material
    (C) Uncontrolled division
    (D) Loss of normal functions

42. In the structure of a flower, the stigma is most closely positioned to the
    (A) style.
    (B) ovary.
    (C) sepal.
    (D) ovule.

43. The basic structure of cell membranes is a
    (A) protein bilayer.
    (B) protein-impregnated phospholipid bilayer.
    (C) carbohydrate bilayer.
    (D) phospholipid bilayer.

44. When catalyzed by sucrase, sucrose decomposes to yield glucose + fructose. The reaction is
    (A) fermentation.
    (B) hydrolysis.
    (C) denaturation.
    (D) condensation.

45. Continental drift is caused by
    (A) fluctuations in the earth's magnetic field.
    (B) extrusion of molten rock through cracks in sea floors.
    (C) fragmentation of larger land masses into smaller ones.
    (D) Coriolis force generated by the rotation of the earth.

46. Carbohydrates are a combination of carbon, hydrogen, and oxygen in an approximate ratio of
    (A) 2:1:2
    (B) 3:2:1
    (C) 1:2:1
    (D) 1:1:1

47. Rod-shaped bacteria are classified as
    (A) bacilli.
    (B) cocci.
    (C) vibrios.
    (D) spirilla.

48. A stain used in classifying bacteria is
    (A) Gram's.
    (B) Wright's.
    (C) Loeffler's.
    (D) Giemsa.

49. A bacteriophage is a kind of
    (A) enzyme.
    (B) toxin.
    (C) bacterium.
    (D) virus.

50. Of the following, the marsupial native to the United States is the
    (A) raccoon.
    (B) wombat.
    (C) opossum.
    (D) armadillo.

51. The first fully terrestrial vertebrates were the
    (A) amphibians.
    (B) reptiles.
    (C) birds.
    (D) mammals.

52. Enzyme molecules are all of the following EXCEPT
    (A) lipids.
    (B) proteins.
    (C) macromolecules.
    (D) biological catalysts.

53. The size of most eukaryotic cells is
    (A) 0.1–1.0 microns.
    (B) 10–100 microns.
    (C) 1.0–10 microns.
    (D) greater than 100 microns.

54. Sickle cell anemia is a genetic disorder that involves an inability of
    (A) erythrocytes to contain a sufficient amount of hemoglobin.
    (B) bone marrow to produce a sufficient number of erythrocytes.
    (C) bone marrow to produce erythrocytes of normal size.
    (D) erythrocytes to carry a sufficient load of oxygen.

55. Of the following, a crustacean that lives on land is the
    (A) centipede.
    (B) millipede.
    (C) sow bug.
    (D) tick.

56. Where would you find a leucoplast?
    (A) In a liver cell
    (B) In white blood cell
    (C) In a white potato
    (D) In a bacterium

57. Of the following, the hydra is most closely related to
    (A) coral.
    (B) flatworm.
    (C) sponge.
    (D) roundworm.

58. An unforeseen result of the widespread use of DDT is the
    (A) control of mosquitoes.
    (B) development of insects immune to DDT.
    (C) development of fishes immune to DDT.
    (D) destruction of harmful birds.

59. Cytoplasmic structures that contain powerful hydrolysis enzymes, which could lead to cell destruction in the absence of surrounding membranes, are
    (A) lysosomes.
    (B) golgi.
    (C) ribosomes.
    (D) None of the above

60. If the carrying capacity (k-value) represents the maximum number of individuals of a species that a habitat can support, it suggests that the population
    (A) is regulated by density-dependent factors.
    (B) will ultimately become extinct.
    (C) is regulated by density-independent factors.
    (D) can increase at an exponential rate, indefinitely.

GO ON TO THE NEXT PAGE

61. The relation between termites and their intestinal protozoa is an example of
    (A) trophism.
    (B) parasitism.
    (C) mutualism.
    (D) commensalism.

62. When completed, the number of DNA base pairs comprising the human genome is expected to be approximately
    (A) 10 thousand.
    (B) 10 million.
    (C) 3 billion.
    (D) 3 trillion.

63. A completed human genomic map identifies the nucleotide sequences on the following chromosomal pairs:
    (A) 22 autosomes + 1 sex chromosome
    (B) 48 autosomes + 1 sex chromosome
    (C) 23 autosomes + 1 sex chromsome
    (D) 92 autosomes + 2 sex chromosomes

64. A technique (in which a catheter is inserted into the uterus to retrieve tissue samples) for the prenatal diagnosis of genetic diseases is called
    (A) amniocentesis.
    (B) positional cloning.
    (C) chorionic villus sampling (CVS).
    (D) None of the above

65. Identify the correct statement about DNA fingerprinting analysis of human tissues.
    (A) It is effective with small samples (e.g., less than 100 microliters of blood).
    (B) It produces identical bond patterns from all tissues in an individual.
    (C) It is effective on tissues more than 1,000 years old.
    (D) All of the above

66. In a DNA fingerprinting analysis of blood samples from a mother (M), a child (C), and an alleged father (F), the banding pattern in the child's blood was 50 percent (F), 27.3 percent (M), and 22.3 percent (FM). The statistical probability that the accused man is the child's father is
    (A) 50 percent.
    (B) greater than 50 percent.
    (C) less than 50 percent.
    (D) zero.

67. The basic inorganic raw materials for photosynthesis are
    (A) water and oxygen.
    (B) water and carbon dioxide.
    (C) oxygen and carbon dioxide.
    (D) sugar and carbon dioxide.

68. Production of Salk vaccine against polio depended upon the discovery of a method for
    (A) growing the polio virus outside the human body.
    (B) killing the polio virus.
    (C) observing the polio virus in the human body.
    (D) producing a polio antitoxin.

69. Ringworm is caused by a(n)
    (A) alga.
    (B) bacterium.
    (C) fungus.
    (D) protozoan.

70. The process responsible for the continuous removal of carbon dioxide from the atmosphere is

    (A) respiration.

    (B) metabolism.

    (C) oxidation.

    (D) photosynthesis.

71. All of the following concepts in genetics were first clearly stated by Gregor Mendel EXCEPT

    (A) dominance.

    (B) independent assortment.

    (C) segregation.

    (D) hybrid vigor.

STOP If you finish before time is called, you may check your work on this section only. Do not turn to any other section in the test.

GENERAL SCIENCE
TEST 6

68 QUESTIONS ▄ TIME—68 MINUTES

Directions: For each of the following items, select the choice that best answers the question or completes the statement. Fill in the corresponding space on your answer sheet.

1. A tree native to China and NOT to the United States is the

   (A) silvery maple.
   (B) chestnut.
   (C) gingko.
   (D) tulip tree.

2. Mammals are believed to have evolved directly from

   (A) fish.
   (B) amphibians.
   (C) reptiles.
   (D) birds.

3. The biochemical technique that would be used to separate differently sized pieces of DNA created by digesting a sample of DNA with a restriction enzyme is

   (A) diapedesis.
   (B) liquid scintillation.
   (C) electrophoresis.
   (D) kinesthesia.

4. Which of the following groups, in primate phylogeny, includes the primate most closely related to humans?

   (A) Old World monkeys
   (B) Great apes
   (C) New World monkeys
   (D) Lemurs

5. Stanley Miller recently obtained evidence supporting the possibility of spontaneous generation by achieving laboratory synthesis of

   (A) amino acids.
   (B) DNA.
   (C) RNA.
   (D) glucose.

6. The part of a compound light microscope that focuses light before it passes through the specimen is the

   (A) objective.
   (B) micrometer.
   (C) ocular.
   (D) condenser.

7. Choose the correct structural formula for acetylene, C_2H_2.

   (A) $HC = CH$
   (B) $HC - CH$
   (C) $HC \equiv CH$
   (D) $HC \equiv CH$

8. We can see only one side of the moon because the

   (A) earth rotates on its own axis.
   (B) moon makes one rotation as it makes one revolution around the earth.
   (C) moon has no refractive atmosphere.
   (D) sun does not shine on the moon's unseen side.

9. Which of the following is NOT an essential biotic element of all ecosystems?

   (A) Producers
   (B) Water
   (C) Consumers
   (D) Decomposers

10. The deadly property of carbon monoxide, if inhaled, is due to its

    (A) high affinity for O_2.
    (B) low affinity for hemoglobin.
    (C) high affinity for hemoglobin.
    (D) conversion to cyanide gas.

11. Of the following, vitamin B_{12} is most useful in combating

    (A) pernicious anemia.
    (B) night blindness.
    (C) rickets.
    (D) goiter.

12. Choose the correct description, relative to scolar and vector quantities.

    (A) Vectors = magnitude and direction
    (B) Scolar = direction
    (C) Vector = magnitude
    (D) Scolar = magnitude and direction

13. An emission device in modern cars that uses platinum beads to oxidize carbon monoxide and hydrocarbons to carbon dioxide and water is the

    (A) carburetor.
    (B) catalytic converter.
    (C) PCV valve.
    (D) air filter.

14. Of the following electrical devices found in the home, the one that develops the highest voltage is the

    (A) electric broiler.
    (B) radio tube.
    (C) television picture tube.
    (D) electric steam-iron.

15. Most soluble food substances enter the blood stream through the

    (A) small intestine.
    (B) duodenum.
    (C) capillaries in the stomach.
    (D) hepatic vein.

16. Air-polluting sulfa dioxide (SO_2) results primarily from

    (A) natural gas furnaces.
    (B) leaded gasoline.
    (C) paper waste.
    (D) coal burning power plants.

17. The "dark" side of the moon refers to the

    (A) craters, into which no sunlight has ever reached.
    (B) south pole of the moon's axis.
    (C) hemisphere that has never reflected the sun's rays on the earth.
    (D) moon itself in the early phases of the month.

18. Of the following, the one NOT characteristic of poison ivy is

    (A) milky juice.
    (B) shiny leaves.
    (C) three-leaflet clusters.
    (D) white berries.

19. Glucose is a reducing sugar, which if boiled in Benedict's reagent, produces an orange to brick-red color. Choose the chemical species it reduces.

    (A) OH^-
    (B) $C\Phi^{++}$
    (C) $C\Phi$
    (D) $C\Phi^{--}$

20. A patient whose total body complement of physiological reactions has reached equilibrium is best described as

    (A) dead.
    (B) stable.
    (C) moribund.
    (D) healthy.

GO ON TO THE NEXT PAGE

21. Of the following, the one present in greatest amounts in dry air is
    (A) carbon dioxide.
    (B) oxygen.
    (C) water vapor.
    (D) nitrogen.

22. Which is NOT a characteristic of enzymes?
    (A) They are proteins.
    (B) They catalize metabolics reactions.
    (C) They act on substances.
    (D) They are phospholipids.

23. Nerve cells transmit impulses by varying the permeability of their membranes primarily to
    (A) Na^+ and K^+
    (B) Cl^- and K^+
    (C) Na^+ and Cl^-
    (D) K^+ and Mg^{++}

24. Identify the statement which is NOT characteristic of exergonic reactions.
    (A) They are downhill reactions.
    (B) They have a negative energy change ($-H$).
    (C) They are uphill reactions.
    (D) The products have less energy than the reactants.

25. As electrons from aerobic respiration are moved through the electron transport system (ETS), the final electron acceptor is
    (A) hydrogen.
    (B) carbon dioxide.
    (C) oxygen.
    (D) water.

26. The normal height of a mercury barometer at sea level is
    (A) 15 inches.
    (B) 30 inches.
    (C) 32 feet.
    (D) 34 feet.

27. One of the necessary parameters for supporting the theory of evolution by natural selection is the age of the earth, which is, by geographical indices, approximately (in years)
    (A) 1 billion.
    (B) 400 million.
    (C) 4 billion.
    (D) 100 million.

28. Of the following, the statement that best describes a "high" on a weather map is that the air
    (A) extends farther up than normal.
    (B) pressure is greater than normal.
    (C) temperature is higher than normal.
    (D) moves faster than normal.

29. The nerve endings for the sense of sight are located in the part of the eye called the
    (A) cornea.
    (B) sclera.
    (C) iris.
    (D) retina.

30. Malaria is caused by
    (A) bacteria.
    (B) mosquitoes.
    (C) protistans.
    (D) bad air.

31. A 1,000-ton ship must displace a weight of water equal to
    (A) 500 tons.
    (B) 1,000 tons.
    (C) 1,500 tons.
    (D) 2,000 tons.

32. Of the following instruments, the one that can convert light into an electric current is the
    (A) radiometer.
    (B) dry cell.
    (C) electrolysis apparatus.
    (D) photoelectric cell.

33. On the film in a camera, the lens forms an image that by comparison with the original subject, is

    (A) right side up and reversed from left to right.
    (B) upside down and reversed from left to right.
    (C) right side up and not reversed from left to right.
    (D) upside down and not reversed from left to right.

34. The development of insecticide resistant insects is based on

    (A) inheritance of acquired characteristics.
    (B) gradualism.
    (C) natural selection.
    (D) sexual selection.

35. Which of the following insects belongs to the order of insects containing the largest number of species?

    (A) Housefly
    (B) Flour beetle
    (C) Grasshopper
    (D) Cockroach

36. Which of the following could react chemically with ammonia?

    $$H:N:H$$
    $$H$$

    (A) H
    (B) Cl^-
    (C) Na
    (D) H^+

37. Photosynthesis is a cellular process, which

    (A) is an exergonic reaction.
    (B) produces simple sugar and O_2.
    (C) is initiated by chemical energy.
    (D) produces CO_2 and H_2O.

38. One-celled eukaryotes belong to the group of living things known as

    (A) protistans.
    (B) poriferans.
    (C) annelids.
    (D) arthropods.

39. Spiders can be distinguished from insects because spiders have

    (A) hard outer coverings.
    (B) large abdomens.
    (C) four pairs of legs.
    (D) biting mouth parts.

40. The greenhouse effect, allegedly the cause of global warming, is believed to be due, primarily, to

    (A) pesticide accumulation in soil.
    (B) carbon dioxide increase in the atmosphere.
    (C) oxygen increase in the atmosphere.
    (D) pesticide increase in the water.

41. The lightest element known on earth is

    (A) hydrogen.
    (B) helium.
    (C) oxygen.
    (D) air.

42. Of the following gases in the air, the most plentiful is

    (A) argon.
    (B) nitrogen.
    (C) oxygen.
    (D) carbon dioxide.

43. The time it takes for light from the sun to reach the earth is approximately

    (A) four years.
    (B) four months.
    (C) 8 minutes.
    (D) sixteen years.

GO ON TO THE NEXT PAGE

44. The composition of edible sodium chloride (NaCl) from an explosive metal (Na) and a poisonous gas (Cl) illustrates which characteristic of matter?

    (A) Impenetrability
    (B) Malleability
    (C) Density
    (D) Emergent properties

45. The time it takes for the earth to rotate 45 degrees is

    (A) 1 hour.
    (B) 3 hours.
    (C) 4 hours.
    (D) 10 hours.

46. Of the following glands, the one that regulates the metabolic rate is the

    (A) adrenal.
    (B) salivary.
    (C) thyroid.
    (D) thymus.

47. In the small intestine, a digestive enzyme can break the peptide bond between two amino acids in a protein molecule by

    (A) removing a water molecule from them.
    (B) inserting a water molecule between them.
    (C) removing a carbon atom from one of them.
    (D) inserting a carbon atom between them.

48. The major cause for seasonal changes in temperature and light on earth is

    (A) distance of earth from the sun.
    (B) a 23.5 inclination of the earth on its axis.
    (C) alignment between earth, sun, and moon.
    (D) rotation of earth on its axis.

49. Passive immunity to diphtheria may be achieved by taking an injection of a(n)

    (A) vaccine.
    (B) toxin.
    (C) toxoid.
    (D) antitoxin.

50. Of the following, the only safe blood transfusion would be

    (A) group A blood into a group O person.
    (B) group B blood into a group A person.
    (C) group O blood into a group AB person.
    (D) group AB blood into a group B person.

51. If the effect of two or more factors is greater than the sum of the individual effects (e.g., $2 + 2 > 4$), the phenomenon is called

    (A) synergism.
    (B) coopeativity.
    (C) antagonism.
    (D) None of the above

52. The water-conducting tissue in an angiosperm is

    (A) phloem.
    (B) xylem.
    (C) pith.
    (D) cambium.

Questions 53 and 54 refer to the diagram below.

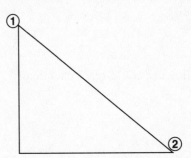

The boulder at the top of an inclined plane has potential energy, $E_p = mgh$, and if it rolls down the plane the energy becomes kinetic, $E_k = \frac{1}{2} mV^2$. Therefore, $mgh = \frac{1}{2} mV^2$.

53. Choose the correct formula for calculating the boulder's velocity when it reaches position 2.

    (A) $V = \sqrt{2gh}$
    (B) $V = 2gh$
    (C) $V = mgh^2$
    (D) $V = \sqrt{mg^2h}$

54. The above expression mgh $= \frac{1}{2}mV^2$ represents

(A) conservation of momentum.
(B) constancy of velocity.
(C) variability of acceleration.
(D) conservation of energy.

55. Completion of the human genome project gave further proof that genes are

(A) nucleic acid.
(B) phospholipids.
(C) protein.
(D) protein and nucleic acid.

56. Of the following, the process that will result in water most nearly chemically pure is

(A) aeration.
(B) chlorination.
(C) distillation.
(D) filtration.

57. The number of degrees on the Fahrenheit thermometer between the freezing point and the boiling point of water is

(A) 100 degrees.
(B) 180 degrees.
(C) 212 degrees.
(D) 273 degrees.

58. One is most likely to feel the effects of static electricity on a

(A) cold, damp day.
(B) cold, dry day.
(C) warm, humid day.
(D) warm, dry day.

59. Of the following planets, the one that has the largest number of satellites is

(A) Jupiter.
(B) Mercury.
(C) Neptune.
(D) Pluto.

60. The deserts of the earth generally occur on the _____ side of the continents.

(A) west
(B) north
(C) east
(D) south

61. Atmospheric moisture (H_2O) combines with oxides of carbon, nitrogen, and sulfur (CO_2, NO_3, and SO_2) to produce

(A) alkaline precipitation.
(B) acid rain.
(C) alcohol.
(D) None of the above

62. As water is warmed, its solubility of oxygen (O_2)

(A) increases.
(B) decreases.
(C) remains constant.
(D) fluctuates randomly.

63. The chlorinated hydrocarbon pesticide, DDT, was banned from use in the United States during the 1970s because it

(A) has high affinity for milk and adipose tissues.
(B) is deliterious to eggs of several species of birds.
(C) is a biological concentration in ecosystem food chains.
(D) All of the above

64. Of the 92 naturally occurring elements, the number found in the human body is closer to

(A) 50
(B) 10
(C) 25
(D) 75

65. Inasmuch as the molecular formula for glucose is $C_6H_{12}O_6$ and the molecular formula for fructose is $C_6H_{12}O_6$, the two substances are

(A) hextomers.
(B) isomers.
(C) heteromers.
(D) anomers.

66. Which of the following elements is the most abundant in the human body?

(A) Carbon
(B) Potassium
(C) Nitrogen
(D) Oxygen

GO ON TO THE NEXT PAGE

67. The density of gold (Au) is 19.3g/cm^3 and that of iron (Fe) is 7.9g/com^3. A comparison of the volumes (V) of 50 gram samples of each metal would show that

(A) $V_{Au} = V_{Fe}$

(B) $V_{Au} < V_{Fe}$

(C) $V_{Au} > V_{Fe}$

(D) There is no predictable relationship between volumes.

68. The genomic diversity between *E. coli*, fruit flies, and humans results from

(A) different types of chemical bases.

(B) different types of amino acids.

(C) same number of bases with different sequences.

(D) different numbers and different sequences of bases.

STOP   If you finish before time is called, you may check your work on this section only. Do not turn to any other section in the test.

FINAL SCIENCE EXAMINATION
TEST 7

75 QUESTIONS ▬ **TIME—75 MINUTES**

Directions: After carefully reading each test item, select the best answer. Fill in the corresponding space on your answer sheet.

1. Of the following human traits, the one under both genetic and hormonal control is
   - (A) hemophilia.
   - (B) color blindness.
   - (C) baldness.
   - (D) blood type.

2. If a sexually reproducing animal has a diploid number of 12, how many chromosomes would a mature sperm have?
   - (A) 3
   - (B) 24
   - (C) 4
   - (D) 6

3. The tissue to which gland cells belong is
   - (A) connective.
   - (B) epithelial.
   - (C) secretory.
   - (D) nerve.

4. Of the following, which is closest to the speed of sound in air at sea level?
   - (A) $\frac{1}{5}$ mile per second
   - (B) $\frac{1}{2}$ mile per second
   - (C) 1 mile per second
   - (D) 5 miles per second

5. The general formula for the acetylene series of hydrocarbons is
   - (A) $C_nH_2n + 2$
   - (B) C_nH_2n
   - (C) $C_nH_2n - 2$
   - (D) None of the above

6. How many molecules of ATP are required to activate a molecule of glucose in glycolysis?
   - (A) 2
   - (B) 6
   - (C) 3
   - (D) None

7. The vitamin that helps clotting of the blood is
   - (A) C
   - (B) D
   - (C) E
   - (D) K

8. Each nucleotide in a DNA molecule contains
   - (A) a sugar.
   - (B) a nitrogen base.
   - (C) a phosphate group.
   - (D) All of the above

9. The wavelength (nM) of the visible portion of the electromagnetic spectrum is in the range of
   - (A) 350–700
   - (B) 800–1,000
   - (C) 200–350
   - (D) 550–900

10. A person is more buoyant when swimming in salt water than in fresh water because
    - (A) the person keeps his or her head out of salt water.
    - (B) salt water has greater tensile strength.
    - (C) salt coats the person's body with a floating membrane.
    - (D) salt water is denser than an equal volume of fresh water.

GO ON TO THE NEXT PAGE

11. Two parameters (e.g., the volume and the temperature of a gas) are directly proportional if a constant value can be calculated from their

    (A) product.
    (B) ratio.
    (C) sum.
    (D) difference.

12. Cellular proteins are synthesized in

    (A) ribosomes.
    (B) mitochondria.
    (C) lysosomes.
    (D) golgi.

13. All of the following mechanisms affect the amount of glucose in the blood EXCEPT

    (A) adrenaline secretion.
    (B) insulin secretion.
    (C) level of oxygen intake.
    (D) level of physical activity.

14. The most active mixing of many digestive juices occurs in the

    (A) stomach.
    (B) duodenum.
    (C) ileum.
    (D) jejunum.

15. A *cold-blooded* animal is one that

    (A) has a body temperature colder than that of other types of animals.
    (B) uses heat from its blood to warm other tissues of the body, lowering the blood temperature.
    (C) depends on external heat sources to regulate its body temperature.
    (D) is incapable of regulating its body temperature.

16. The basic mechanism of hereditary transmission is

    (A) sexual reproduction.
    (B) polyploidy.
    (C) separation of chromosomes.
    (D) the mitotic mechanism.

17. If the electrical voice waves produced by a whistle are formed in 1 second, what is the wave frequency demonstrated in the following figure?

    (A) 4 hertz
    (B) 8 hertz
    (C) 12 hertz
    (D) 16 hertz

18. Of the following, the highest bactericidal activity of light occurs at a wavelength in angstrom units of

    (A) 2,536
    (B) 3,256
    (C) 5,236
    (D) 6,532

19. In the diagram below, the refraction of the light rays indicates that the lens is

    (A) thicker in the center than the edges.
    (B) thinner at the center than the edges.
    (C) uniform in thickness.
    (D) consistent in dimensions.

20. Which of the following compounds is an ether?

    (A) CH_2CHO
    (B) CH_3-O-CH_3
    (C) CH_3-COOH
    (D) CH_3-CH_2OH

21. Which of the following statements about wavelengths is true?

    (A) Visible wavelengths vary in lengths.
    (B) The wavelength of green is the longest.
    (C) Radio waves are electromagnetic waves shorter than infrared.
    (D) Infrared rays are shorter than red light rays.

22. An object appears white, or colorless, when it

    (A) absorbs the light reaching it.
    (B) transmits only blue light.
    (C) rejects all colors.
    (D) reflects all colors at the same time.

23. Another name for animal starch is

    (A) cellulose.
    (B) lecithin.
    (C) glycogen.
    (D) chitin.

24. Of the following, a human blood disease that has been definitely shown to be due to a hereditary factor or factors is

    (A) pernicious anemia.
    (B) sickle cell anemia.
    (C) polycythemia.
    (D) leukemia.

25. All of the following elements are major constituents of a cell EXCEPT

    (A) carbon.
    (B) potassium.
    (C) hydrogen.
    (D) phosphorus.

26. If a machine listed for 1,800 watts is plugged into a 110-volt system, approximately how many amps will it use?

    (A) 6.6
    (B) 13.0
    (C) 16.0
    (D) 19.8

27. The selection of algae as a possible additional food for humans is based primarily on their ability to carry on

    (A) fermentation.
    (B) digestion.
    (C) photosynthesis.
    (D) oxidation.

28. A nurse administered a medication at 10^{-4} molar concentrated to a patient. The doctor instructed that the dosage be reduced by one-half strength, which was

    (A) $10^{-2}M$
    (B) $5 \times 10^{-5}M$
    (C) $10^{-8}M$
    (D) $10^{-3}M$

29. In eukaryotic cells, the phase of division that produces two daughter cells is

    (A) G.
    (B) mitosis.
    (C) G_2.
    (D) cytokinesis.

30. Efficiency (mechanical and biological) is a relationship between input, output, and total available energy for work. The correct formula for efficiency is

    (A) $E = \dfrac{Input}{Output} \times 100$

    (B) $E = \dfrac{Input \times Output}{100}$

    (C) $E = \dfrac{Output - Input}{100}$

    (D) $E = \dfrac{Output}{Input} \times 100$

31. When a molecule of glucose in humans is degraded, the percent of its energy capable of generating ATP is nearest to

    (A) 100
    (B) 50
    (C) 25
    (D) 80

GO ON TO THE NEXT PAGE

32. Velocity, defined as the rate of displacement of an object, is

    (A) scalar.
    (B) inertia.
    (C) vector.
    (D) centripetal.

33. The fundamental principle expressed by the Einstein Equation ($E = mc^2$) on mass-energy equivalency is that

    (A) small mass = much energy.
    (B) small mass = little energy.
    (C) little energy = great mass.
    (D) All of the above

34. Exophthalmic goiter is caused by

    (A) hypoactivity of the thyroid.
    (B) hyperactivity of the thyroid.
    (C) deficiency of vitamin A.
    (D) radioactive iodine.

35. If other factors are compatible, a person who can most safely receive blood from any donor belongs to the basic blood group

    (A) 0
    (B) A
    (C) B
    (D) AB

36. The Schick test indicates whether or not a person is probably immune to

    (A) tuberculosis.
    (B) diptheria.
    (C) poliomyelitis.
    (D) scarlet fever.

37. Evaporation of water is likely to be greatest on days of

    (A) high humidity.
    (B) low humidity.
    (C) little or no wind.
    (D) low pressure.

38. The generic formula for alkane, aliphatic hydrocarbons is $C_NH_{2N}+2$, from which the formula for propane is derived, is

    (A) C_2H_e
    (B) C_3H_8
    (C) NaNO
    (D) C_3H_4

39. The percentage of oxygen by weight in $Al_2(SO_4)_3$ (atomic weights: Al = 27, S = 32, O = 16) is approximately

    (A) 19
    (B) 21
    (C) 56
    (D) 92

40. In backcrossing, a hybrid is always mated with

    (A) its own parent.
    (B) another hybrid.
    (C) a pure dominant.
    (D) a pure recessive.

41. The diameter of a light microscope on low power is 2 mm. The number of 50Φ wide paramecia (side-by-side) that stretches across the entire field is

    (A) 400
    (B) 500
    (C) 40
    (D) 4

42. Of the following, a structure found in mammals but NOT in reptiles is the

    (A) lung.
    (B) brain.
    (C) diaphragm.
    (D) ventricle.

43. If the osmotic pressure of human blood is determined by the number of dissolved particles, and a 0.315 molar glucose solution is isotonic to blood, the concentration of isotonic sodium chloride (NaCl) would be

    (A) 0.630M
    (B) 0.3M
    (C) 0.157M
    (D) 0.2M

44. The resistance of matter to changes in motion is
    (A) elasticity.
    (B) inertia.
    (C) momentum.
    (D) inflexible.

45. Some substances are transported across cell membranes by proteins known as
    (A) ligases.
    (B) permeases.
    (C) hydrolases.
    (D) monomers.

46. Which sequence correctly illustrates a food chain?
    (A) algae-insect larvae-fish-human
    (B) algae-fish-insect larvae-human
    (C) insect larvae-algae-fish-human
    (D) fish-insect larvae-algae-human

47. Grasses are usually pollinated by
    (A) wind.
    (B) water.
    (C) birds.
    (D) insects.

48. Among vertebrates the embryonic ectoderm gives rise to which of the following?
    (A) Nervous system
    (B) Digestive system
    (C) Skeletal system
    (D) Respiratory system

49. Generally, life depends directly or indirectly for food, energy, and oxygen upon
    (A) parasitic organisms.
    (B) green plants.
    (C) fungi.
    (D) animals.

50. Pathogenic bacteria responsible for food poisoning are becoming resistant to the antibiotic, Cipro. This phenomenon illustrates that the populations are
    (A) photosynthesizing nutrients.
    (B) encapsulating practices.
    (C) evolving.
    (D) dominating amino acids.

51. The weight in grams of 22.4 liters of nitrogen (atomic weight = 14) is
    (A) 3
    (B) 7
    (C) 14
    (D) 28

52. In the production of sounds, the greater the number of vibrations per second, the
    (A) greater the volume.
    (B) higher the tone.
    (C) lower the volume.
    (D) lower the tone.

53. A segment of a DNA molecule transcribes a base sequence, AGAUAU, on an mRNA codon. The compatible sequence on the tRNA anticodon is
    (A) UUAGCG
    (B) UCUAUA
    (C) AAUAUA
    (D) CGCAAA

54. Which of the following species will combine with a chloride ion to produce ammonium chloride?
    (A) NH_3
    (B) K^+
    (C) NH_4^+
    (D) Al^{+++}

55. The most promising agent as a vaccine for a human cancer would control the HPV-16 virus of the
    (A) cervix.
    (B) lungs.
    (C) colon.
    (D) breasts.

GO ON TO THE NEXT PAGE

56. Which one of the following graphs represents Boyle's Law?

(A)

(B)

(C)

(D)

57. Which of the following minerals is restored to the soil by plants of the pea and bean family?

    (A) Sulfates
    (B) Nitrates
    (C) Carbonates
    (D) Phosphates

58. In humans, any hereditary defect caused by a gene on the Y chromosome would occur

    (A) only in males.
    (B) only in females.
    (C) only if the gene were recessive.
    (D) about equally in males and females.

59. There is no oxidation-reduction in a reaction that involves

    (A) single replacement.
    (B) double replacement.
    (C) simple decomposition.
    (D) direct combination of elements.

60. A cross between two black guinea pigs yields 3 black and 1 white offspring. The white allele in the parents was

    (A) dominant.
    (B) recessive.
    (C) sex-linked.
    (D) absent.

61. The cellular organelle where respiratory reactions for the release of energy occurs is a

    (A) centrosome.
    (B) chromosome.
    (C) chromoplast.
    (D) mitochondrion.

62. Members of a population that are reproductively isolated from other populations form a

    (A) race.
    (B) species.
    (C) community.
    (D) genus.

63. The most efficient cellular respiratory process, in terms of energy-yield per molecule of glucose, is

    (A) aerobic respiration.
    (B) anaerobic respiration.
    (C) fermentation.
    (D) phosphorylation.

64. Which of the following is/are not a requirement for photosynthesis?

    (A) Oxygen
    (B) Carbon dioxide and water
    (C) Sunlight
    (D) Chlorophyll

65. A cellular organelle found in typical plant cells but not in typical animal cells is the

    (A) chloroplast.
    (B) ribosome.
    (C) mitochondrion.
    (D) centrosome.

66. In the absence of oxygen, plants and microbes convert pyruvic acid into

    (A) alcohol and CO_2.
    (B) lactic acid.
    (C) CO_2 and H_2O.
    (D) amino acids.

67. Every cell contains

    (A) a cell membrane and cytoplasm.
    (B) a cell wall and cytoplasm.
    (C) a nucleus and cell wall.
    (D) plastids and pigments.

68. Digestion in humans is

(A) extracellular.

(B) intracellular.

(C) vacuolar.

(D) intercellular.

69. An example of an obligate intracellular parasitic microorganism is a

(A) tapeworm.

(B) virus.

(C) bacterium.

(D) spirochaete.

Questions 70–72 refer to the following graph and equation.

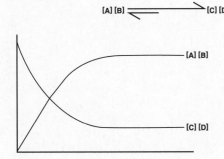

70. At time zero, the percentage of substance that is [A] [B] is approximately

(A) 100

(B) 0

(C) 50

(D) 25

71. The comparative affinity of the reactants and products is

(A) [C] [D] > [A] [B]

(B) [A] [B] = [C] [D]

(C) [A] [B] > [C] [D]

(D) None of the above

72. Choose the incorrect statement, relative to the reaction at equilibrium.

(A) Concentration of reactants and products remains constant.

(B) Reaction is shifted to the right.

(C) Forward and reverse reactions occur at equal rates.

(D) Reaction is shifted to the left.

73. The second law of thermodynamics (entropy) states that systems (ranging from a single organism to the entire universe) become increasingly disordered or random with time. Early scientists erroneously believed that the human body, by maintaining its structural and functional integrity violated this law.

It is currently understood that the human body conforms to the second law of thermodynamics because it is a(an)

(A) closed system.

(B) assembly of organic molecules.

(C) open system.

(D) composite of inorganic and organic molecules.

74. Data from the human genome project have shown that the total number of genes in humans is close to

(A) 30

(B) 1,000,000

(C) 3,000

(D) 30,000

75. The smallest chromosome in the human genome is

(A) 1

(B) 51

(C) 21

(D) Y

S T O P If you finish before time is called, you may check your work on this section only. Do not turn to any other section in the test.

ANSWER KEY

CHEMISTRY AND PHYSICS

TEST 1

1. A	14. D	27. A	40. D	53. B
2. A	15. C	28. A	41. D	54. B
3. B	16. C	29. C	42. C	55. C
4. A	17. B	30. B	43. B	56. C
5. A	18. A	31. A	44. A	57. A
6. D	19. C	32. B	45. D	58. D
7. D	20. A	33. C	46. D	59. D
8. D	21. A	34. C	47. B	60. B
9. A	22. D	35. C	48. D	61. B
10. D	23. B	36. A	49. A	62. A
11. D	24. A	37. B	50. C	63. C
12. D	25. A	38. D	51. A	64. D
13. D	26. A	39. B	52. D	65. A

TEST 2

1. B	9. A	17. B	25. B	33. C
2. B	10. C	18. D	26. A	34. D
3. D	11. D	19. A	27. C	35. B
4. A	12. A	20. C	28. D	36. D
5. C	13. C	21. D	29. D	37. A
6. D	14. A	22. C	30. C	38. B
7. C	15. A	23. B	31. C	39. D
8. A	16. C	24. B	32. A	40. C

HUMAN ANATOMY AND PHYSIOLOGY

Test 3

1. **B**	12. **D**	23. **D**	34. **A**	45. **B**
2. **C**	13. **A**	24. **D**	35. **B**	46. **C**
3. **C**	14. **B**	25. **B**	36. **D**	47. **B**
4. **A**	15. **C**	26. **D**	37. **B**	48. **D**
5. **B**	16. **A**	27. **B**	38. **C**	49. **A**
6. **D**	17. **D**	28. **B**	39. **B**	50. **D**
7. **A**	18. **B**	29. **C**	40. **C**	51. **D**
8. **C**	19. **B**	30. **D**	41. **B**	52. **A**
9. **A**	20. **C**	31. **C**	42. **D**	53. **B**
10. **D**	21. **C**	32. **D**	43. **A**	54. **D**
11. **B**	22. **B**	33. **D**	44. **C**	55. **C**

Test 4

1. **A**	11. **A**	21. **B**	31. **B**	41. **B**
2. **D**	12. **B**	22. **C**	32. **A**	42. **B**
3. **C**	13. **B**	23. **A**	33. **C**	43. **B**
4. **A**	14. **D**	24. **C**	34. **B**	44. **D**
5. **B**	15. **B**	25. **C**	35. **B**	45. **A**
6. **A**	16. **C**	26. **A**	36. **D**	46. **C**
7. **D**	17. **C**	27. **D**	37. **A**	47. **D**
8. **B**	18. **A**	28. **C**	38. **D**	48. **C**
9. **B**	19. **A**	29. **D**	39. **C**	49. **B**
10. **D**	20. **D**	30. **B**	40. **C**	50. **A**

BIOLOGY

TEST 5

1. D	16. D	30. B	44. B	58. B
2. D	17. C	31. D	45. B	59. A
3. B	18. D	32. C	46. C	60. A
4. D	19. B	33. C	47. A	61. C
5. C	20. B	34. A	48. A	62. C
6. D	21. A	35. D	49. D	63. A
7. A	22. C	36. A	50. C	64. C
8. C	23. D	37. D	51. B	65. D
9. A	24. B	38. A	52. A	66. B
10. A	25. D	39. B	53. B	67. B
11. B	26. A	40. C	54. D	68. A
12. C	27. B	41. A	55. C	69. C
13. A	28. C	42. A	56. C	70. D
14. B	29. D	43. B	57. A	71. D
15. A				

GENERAL SCIENCE

TEST 6

1. C	15. A	29. D	43. C	56. C
2. C	16. D	30. C	44. D	57. B
3. C	17. C	31. B	45. B	58. B
4. B	18. A	32. D	46. C	59. A
5. A	19. B	33. B	47. B	60. A
6. D	20. A	34. C	48. B	61. B
7. C	21. D	35. B	49. D	62. B
8. B	22. D	36. D	50. C	63. D
9. B	23. A	37. B	51. A	64. C
10. C	24. C	38. A	52. B	65. B
11. A	25. C	39. C	53. A	66. D
12. A	26. B	40. B	54. D	67. B
13. B	27. C	41. A	55. A	68. D
14. C	28. B	42. B		

FINAL SCIENCE EXAMINATION

Test 7

1. C	16. C	31. B	46. A	61. D
2. D	17. A	32. C	47. A	62. B
3. B	18. A	33. A	48. A	63. A
4. A	19. B	34. B	49. B	64. C
5. C	20. B	35. D	50. C	65. A
6. A	21. A	36. B	51. D	66. A
7. D	22. D	37. B	52. B	67. A
8. D	23. C	38. B	53. A	68. A
9. A	24. B	39. C	54. C	69. B
10. D	25. B	40. D	55. A	70. A
11. B	26. C	41. C	56. B	71. D
12. A	27. C	42. C	57. B	72. D
13. C	28. B	43. C	58. A	73. C
14. B	29. D	44. B	59. B	74. D
15. C	30. D	45. B	60. B	75. C

EXPLANATORY ANSWERS

CHEMISTRY AND PHYSICS

TEST 1

1. **The correct answer is (A).** Heating water to a very high temperature (about 2,000°C) will cause only about 2 percent of the water to dissociate into hydrogen and oxygen—not a very economical or efficient way of obtaining oxygen. Electrolysis will decompose water at a much lower temperature. Hydrogen peroxide and many oxides or metals can be decomposed more easily by heating alone.

2. **The correct answer is (A).** All acids contain hydrogen, which may be displaced by certain metals. However, copper ranks below hydrogen in the *electromotive* or *activity series. Activity* refers to the activity of a metal in displacing hydrogen in acids and in water. Metals ranked below hydrogen in the series do not displace hydrogen from acids.

3. **The correct answer is (B).** Hydrochloric acid can react with sodium hydrogen sulfite to produce sodium chloride, water, and sulfur dioxide. Sulfur dioxide can react with barium hydroxide to form barium sulfite and water.

4. **The correct answer is (A).** The problem can be solved by using the formula: $c = Q/MDT$. Inasmuch as Q, M, D, and T are given, no algebraic rearrangement is necessary to solve for c (specific heat).

5. **The correct answer is (A).** Ozone is a molecule variety of oxygen in which 3 oxygen atoms bond to make 1 molecule of O_3. Ozone is easily formed by the action of electricity or ultraviolet radiation on the normal diatomic form (O_2) of oxygen.

6. **The correct answer is (D).** Since there is twice as much hydrogen as there is oxygen in a molecule of water (H_2O), the 26 milliliters of hydrogen could combine with only 13 milliliters of oxygen. This would leave 11 of the 24 milliliters of oxygen uncombined.

7. **The correct answer is (D).** Hydrochloric acid reacts with active metals, forming the chloride of that metal and releasing hydrogen.

8. **The correct answer is (D).** Inasmuch as 100 milligrams will decay to 50.0 milligrams, the formula: $K = \dfrac{0.693}{t\frac{1}{2}}$ should be algebraically rearranged to solve for $t\frac{1}{2}$ (half-life). To do this, multiple both sides by $t\frac{1}{2}$ and divide both sides by K.

9. **The correct answer is (A).** The percentage composition of oxygen in 1 mole of glucose (180 grams) is calculated as follows

Atomic Mass	No. of Atoms
Carbon $12 \times 6 =$	72
Hydrogen $1 \times 12 =$	12
Oxygen $16 \times 6 =$	96
	180

$$\% \text{ Comp. } O_2 = \frac{96}{180} \times 100$$

10. **The correct answer is (D).** Sulfuric acid (H_2SO_4) contains 4 oxygens, each with a valence of -2; the total negative valence is 8. Each of the 2 hydrogens has a valence of $+1$; the total hydrogen valence equals $+2$. Therefore, sulfur would need a valence of $+6$ to equalize the positive and negative valences in the molecule.

11. **The correct answer is (D).** Fractional distillation can be used to separate the components of a mixture; the mixture is heated to boiling and the temperature is constantly raised. The component with the lowest boiling point vaporizes first; the component with the highest boiling point will vaporize last. Liquid oxygen has a boiling point of $-183°C$, which is higher than the boiling point of the other components; therefore, oxygen will boil off last.

12. **The correct answer is (D).** Only one substance (HCl) is dissociated; therefore, the reaction is a single displacement.

13. **The correct answer is (D).** Free carbon dioxide and water will combine to produce carbonic acid (H_2CO_3). Different reactants would be needed to produce ozone (O_3), methane (CH_4), or hydrogen peroxide (H_2O_2).

14. **The correct answer is (D).** Bronze is an alloy of copper and tin. An alloy is made by mixing two or more metals while in molten condition and then allowing the mixture to cool and solidify. The metals remain completely dissolved in one another after solidification, forming a homogenous substance with properties different from any of the constituent metals in their pure forms. For example, bronze is both harder and more resistant to corrosion than pure copper.

15. **The correct answer is (C).** $NaHCO_3$ will combine with HCl (hydrochloric acid) to form NaCl and H_2CO_3. H_2CO_3 is a weaker acid than HCl; therefore, the net effect of replacing HCl molecules with H_2CO_3 molecules is to raise the pH of the solution. In causing this reaction, $NaHCO_3$ is acting as a *buffer*. NaCl is a salt that will have no effect on the pH of an HCl solution. The other two compounds are acids that would lower the pH of the solution further if added.

16. **The correct answer is (C).** Litmus turns red in acid solution. When phosphorus trioxide dissolves in water, phosphorus acid is formed. The other compounds named form alkaline solutions.

17. **The correct answer is (B).** The amount of heat absorbed or lost in a chemical reaction is the heat of reaction. It equals the heat content of the product(s) minus the heat content of the reactants. Heat is absorbed if more energy is stored in the products than in the reactants, and released if more energy is stored in the reactants than in the product(s). In the formation of a compound, the heat of reaction is called the heat of formation for that compound. A compound with more energy stored in it than in the reactants (a compound with a high heat of formation) can be formed, but it is difficult to decompose.

18. **The correct answer is (A).** Zinc is ranked above the others but below aluminum in the activity series of metals. The higher the metal is ranked, the more energetic it is in its displacement ability. Therefore, aluminum could displace zinc in the zinc chloride solution, forming aluminum chloride. For this reason, zinc chloride should not be stored in a tank made of aluminum because aluminum will displace the zinc in the zinc chloride.

19. **The correct answer is (C).** The 4 oxygen ions would have a total *valence* of -8 (each oxygen, -2); if the valence of the SO_4 ion is -2, the remaining valence of 6 would be matched to a positive valence. Therefore, sulfur must have a valence of $+6$.

20. **The correct answer is (A).** Sulfuric acid is composed of 2 hydrogen ions and 1 sulfate ion. The chemical formula is H_2SO_4; thus, its chemical name is hydrogen sulfate.

21. **The correct answer is (A).** Magnesium has an atomic weight of 24; hydrogen's atomic weight is approximately 1. As is true with many metals, magnesium can react with an acid, such as hydrochloric acid, to produce hydrogen ($Mg + 2HCl \rightarrow MgCl_2 + H_2$). The amount of hydrogen produced can be calculated by using the following equation:

$$\frac{\text{amount Mg}}{\text{atomic weight}} = \frac{\text{amount } H_2O}{\text{atomic weight}}$$

Substituting in the equation, we get the following:

$$\frac{6 \text{ grams}}{24} = \frac{x \text{ grams}}{2} = 0.5 \text{ grams}$$

In working out problems in which one must determine the amount of a substance derived from a given reaction, the chemical equation must be balanced and molecular weight must be used. Thus, for diatomic gases, use twice the atomic weight.

22. **The correct answer is (D).** Hydrogen in molecular form is composed of 2 atoms; the formula for 1 molecule of hydrogen is H_2. Therefore, 2 molecules of hydrogen is $2H_2$.

23. **The correct answer is (B).** Sodium bisulfate differs from sodium sulfate in having hydrogen as a part of the molecule. Since the sulfate ion has a valence of -2, and hydrogen and sodium each have a valence of $+1$, then one sodium and one hydrogen must be in combination with the sulfate ion ($NaHSO_4$).

24. **The correct answer is (A).** John Dalton discovered the facts concerning chemical combinations and suggested that materials are composed of atoms. He first proposed the law of multiple proportions in 1804. The law states that in a series of compounds formed by the same two or more elements, given a definite weight for one element, the different weights of the second element are in the ratio of small whole numbers to the weight of the first. For example, in sulfur dioxide (SO_2), the weight of oxygen is 32 (atomic weight = 16); in sulfur trioxide (SO_3), the weight of oxygen is 48. Therefore, the ratio is 2:3.

25. **The correct answer is (A).** One mole (*gram molecular weight*) of a gas occupies 22.4 liters under standard conditions. Since 1 liter of the gas in question is $\frac{1}{22.4}$ of one mole, it is $\frac{1}{22.4}$ of its gram molecular weight. Knowing this, the molecular weight of the gas can be determined. We can set up the equation as follows:

$$\frac{x \text{ unknown gram mol. wt.}}{22.4 \text{ liters}} = \frac{1.16 \text{ grams}}{1 \text{ liters}}$$

Solving the equation, we get 26 as 1 gram molecular weight. C_2H_2 (ethane) fits this weight (C = 12 × 2, H = 1 × 2).

26. **The correct answer is (A).** A salt is an ionic compound that yields ions other than hydrogen ions (H^+) or hydroxide ions ($OH-$) when it dissociates. Na_2CO_3 will yield neither when it dissociates into $2 Na^+ + CO_3^{2-}$. $Ca(OH)_2$ will yield hydroxide ions when it dissociates, and H_2CO_3 will yield hydrogen ions. CH_3OH is a covalent compound and will not dissociate.

27. **The correct answer is (A).** *Aromatic* compounds are so named because of their odors; they occur in ring structure (molecular structure) and include such compounds as benzene, tolulene, and xylene.

28. **The correct answer is (A).** Dextrose is a *monosaccharide,* in that its molecule is composed of one "sugar unit" and cannot be hydrolyzed into simpler sugars. Lactose and sucrose are *disaccharides,* each yielding two monosaccharides by hydrolysis. Glycogen is a *polysaccharide* composed of a large number of monosaccharide units.

29. **The correct answer is (C).** Fats are glyceryl esters that, when hydrolized, yield glycerol and fatty acids. The cleavage of the ester linkage upon hydrolysis can be achieved by saponification, acids, superheated steam, or lipase, which is an enzyme that hydrolyzes fats. This may be represented as follows:

$$RCOOR' + H_2O \rightarrow RCOOH + R'OH$$

30. **The correct answer is (B).** As a rule, polar liquids dissolve in polar liquids and nonpolar liquids dissolve in nonpolar liquids. Water is polar and oil is nonpolar. Therefore, oil and water are immiscible.

31. **The correct answer is (A).** The bond formed between the carboxy (RCOOH) and the amino ($R - (NH_2)$) of two amino acids is a peptide bond, and the resulting compound is a depeptide.

32. **The correct answer is (B).** The *atomic number* represents the number of protons within the nucleus of an atom; since an atom is electrically neutral, the atomic number also equals the number of electrons of the atom. The atomic weight (*mass number*) represents the total number of nuclear particles (protons plus neutrons). All atoms of the same element have the same number of protons and, thus, the same atomic number. If the number of neutrons differ, the mass number is different; these atoms, then, are *isotopes.*

33. **The correct answer is (C).** Calcium hypochlorite ($CaOCl_2$) is effective as a bleach due to the oxidizing activity of hypochlorous acid ($HClO$), which is produced from calcium hypochloride, and from which chlorine gas can also be liberated.

34. **The correct answer is (C).** An ionic bond will form between 2 atoms if the loss of electrons from one to the other will result in both atoms having a completely filled outer electron orbit. A sodium atom has 11 electrons, 2 in its first electron orbit, 8 in its second electron orbit, and 1 in its outer electron orbit. The loss of 1 electron from the sodium atom will eliminate its outer electron orbit, making the next orbit in toward the nucleus the new outer orbit with a full complement of 8 electrons. A chlorine atom has 17 electrons, 2 in its first electron orbit, 8 in its second, and 7 in its outer electron orbit. The acceptance of 1 electron by the chlorine atom will fill its outer electron orbit with the full complement of 8 electrons.

35. **The correct answer is (C).** Transition elements are characterized by atoms in which the two highest energy levels are incompletely filled. Consulting the periodic table indicates that of those listed, only nickel is a transition element (see the periodic table on page 197).

36. **The correct answer is (A).** Air is a mixture of gases; the gases present in greatest quantity are nitrogen and oxygen. The quantity of nitrogen in the air is almost four times that of oxygen. Of the compounds listed, methane (CH_4), with a molecular weight of 16, is lighter than air.

37. **The correct answer is (B).** Carbon dioxide is an odorless gas that is heavier than air. It is colorless, soluble in water, and about one and one-half times as heavy as air. It is a component of air, but comprises less than 0.05 percent of it.

38. **The correct answer is (D).** The pressure of a gas is measured by the distance in millimeters that it will lift a column of mercury in a barometer. The pressure of air is 760 mm of mercury at sea level. Air is a mixture of gases, and the pressure of each gas in such a mixture, referred to as its *partial pressure,* is equal to its concentration in the mixture. Oxygen constitutes 21% of air; therefore, its partial pressure at sea level would be 21% of 760 mm of mercury of pressure, or 160 mm of mercury.

39. **The correct answer is (B).** Carbon disulfide is highly inflammable; its complete combustion yields carbon dioxide and sulfur dioxide.

$$CS_2 + 3O_2 \rightarrow CO_2 + 2SO_2$$

40. **The correct answer is (D).** The ethyl alcohol of alcoholic beverages is produced by fermentation of monosaccharides; usually yeast is used to supply the enzymes needed, and the fermentation process supplies the energy needed by the yeast.

$$C_6H_{12}O_6 \rightarrow 2C_2H_5OH + 2CO_2$$

41. **The correct answer is (D).** Because fluorine is extremely active, it does not occur freely in nature but combines naturally with all elements except the inert gases, forming very stable compounds. Because it is a vigorous oxidizing agent, it cannot be oxidized by other oxidizing agents. For these reasons, fluorides are more difficult to decompose than are compounds of the other halogens.

42. **The correct answer is (C).** A *ketone* is an organic molecule that contains a carbon atom double-bonded to an oxygen atom located between 2 other carbon atoms $\overset{-C-C-C-}{\underset{O}{\parallel}}$. The compound shown in choice (**A**) is an aldehyde because it contains a terminal CHO $\underset{C=O}{\overset{H}{|}}$ group. The compound shown in choice (**B**) is an alcohol because it contains an OH group bonded to a carbon. The compound shown in choice (**D**) is both an alcohol and an aldehyde.

43. **The correct answer is (B).** The atomic number indicates the number of *protons* (positively charged particles) within the nucleus of an atom. Since an atom is electrically neutral, the number of protons is equal to the number of *electrons* (negatively charged particles) of the atom. Thus, the atomic number can indicate the number of electrons as well as the number of protons.

44. **The correct answer is (A).** The atoms of each element in group Zero have 8 electrons in the outermost energy level. The elements have atoms with complete octets of electrons, producing stable energy levels.

45. **The correct answer is (D).** The resistance of a metal wire is directly proportional to its length and inversely proportional to its cross-sectional area. The longest wire with the smallest diameter will therefore have the greatest resistance.

46. **The correct answer is (D).** An *organic* acid is characterized by the presence of a carboxyl group (—COOH), or $-\overset{O}{\underset{OH}{C}}$. R represents a hydrocarbon group or a radical derived from a hydrocarbon.

47. **The correct answer is (B).** An *electrolyte* is a substance that forms an electrically conducting solution when dissolved in water. This is caused by the dissociation of the compound into ions, or *ionization*. The greater the ionization, the stronger the electrolyte. Calcium chloride ionizes to a much greater degree than the others and is a strong electrolyte.

48. **The correct answer is (D).** Force is a function of mass, distance, and acceleration. Since all of these factors are equal in this example, all of the balls strike the wall with the same force. The force is calculated as $1 \text{ kg} \times 16 \text{ m}/(2 \text{ sec})^2 = 4$ newtons.

49. **The correct answer is (A).** Sodium (Na) and potassium (K) are both in group IA, with 1 electron in the outer energy level. Sodium and potassium have three and four energy levels, respectively.

50. **The correct answer is (C).** Charcoal is an amorphous form of carbon, and carbon can react with oxides of many metals and other substances to form CO, CO_2, and the carbides of the metals. Thus, the oxides would be reduced by the removal of oxygen, and carbon would be oxidized to carbon monoxide or carbon dioxide; therefore, oxidation and reduction would occur.

51. **The correct answer is (A).** Nonmetal oxides, such as oxides of sulfur, carbon, and nitrogen, can react with water to form acids. The equations below are examples:

$$CO_2 + H_2O \rightarrow H_2CO_3$$
$$SO_2 + H_2O \rightarrow H_2SO_3$$

52. **The correct answer is (D).** Carbon dioxide (CO_2) comprises only approximately 0.04 percent of the earth's atmospheric gases. When this percentage increases, it prevents sun rays that strike the earth from radiating back into space. This produces warming of the atmosphere and the earth's surface, causing the greenhouse effect.

53. **The correct answer is (B).** Although hydrogen is relatively inert at ordinary temperatures, it can combine with free oxygen, with oxygen that is in chemical combination, with some metallic elements, and with many nonmetallic elements. The addition of hydrogen reduces a substance.

54. **The correct answer is (B).** A 1.0 molar solution of a substance is prepared by dissolving 1 gram-molecular weight of solution in enough solvent to equal 1 liter of solution. A 1 normal solution is prepared by dissolving an amount of solute (gram-molecular weight/total positive valence) in enough solvent to equal 1 liter of solution. (Atomic weights H = 1.0; S = 32; O = 16). mol. wt. = 98, $\frac{98g}{L} = 1M$ $\frac{98}{2} = \frac{49g}{L} = 1N$.

55. **The correct answer is (C).** The nitrate test involves the use of a sulfate, such as iron sulfate, and sulfuric acid. The nitrate and sulfate ions react, forming nitric oxide. Nitric oxide then combines with the ferrous ion to form a ferrous-nitrogen-oxygen complex, which produces a brown color.

56. **The correct answer is (C).** A *saturated* solution is one that is in equilibrium; a condition of equilibrium exists between the solvent and the solute, and no more of the solute can dissolve.

57. **The correct answer is (A).** Oxides of barium and sulfur can combine to produce barium sulfate, a salt.

$$BaO + SO_3 \rightarrow BaSO_4$$

58. **The correct answer is (D).** The optical illusion described is the result of refraction, the abrupt bending of a ray of light when it passes at an angle from a medium of one density to a medium of a different density. Air and water have very different densities, resulting in the refraction of light. Diffraction is the separation of light into bands of different wavelengths, as in a rainbow. Diffusion is the scattering of light, such as the effect produced when light passes through frosted glass. Convection does not apply to light; it is the transfer of heat by circulation of air or water.

59. **The correct answer is (D).** Sulfuric acid has a high boiling point: 317°C. Because of this, it is not very volatile and can be used to prepare more volatile acids, such as hydrochloric and nitric acids.

$$NaCl + H_2SO_4 \rightarrow NaHSO_4 + HCl$$

60. **The correct answer is (B).** The pH of a solution is a measure of the negative logarithm of the hydrogen ion concentration (e.g., pH = $-\log[H^+]$). The H+ in question is 1×10^{-3}. Therefore, the pH = $^+3$.

61. **The correct answer is (B).** Reactivity of elements in group IA increases from top to bottom because valence electrons are progressively further from the positive charges in the nucleus of atoms. Reactivity of elements in group VIIA increases from bottom to top because valence electrons are progressively closer to the positive charges of the nucleus.

62. **The correct answer is (A).** Sodium (Na) is a metal in group IA, with 1.0 electron in its outermost shell. Its most stable configuration is achieved by donating 1.0 electron, resulting in a +1 valence.

63. **The correct answer is (C).** The electrons in the outer energy level comprise the portion of an atom directly involved in ionic bonding. The outer energy level will either gain or lose electrons in order to achieve a complete octet (8 electrons).

64. **The correct answer is (D).** The Federal Government requires that all pesticides have a label with a signal word. The pesticide will read DANGER (highly toxic) if only a few drops could be fatal.

65. **The correct answer is (A).** The circular winds that form a tornado create an area of extremely low pressure in the center. When rotating areas of low pressure move over most structures that have areas of higher air pressure, the structure explodes outward, as air is forced down a pressure gradient.

TEST 2

1. **The correct answer is (B).** Physical properties are those that do not involve any change in the nature or chemical composition of the substance. Heating a substance to the temperature at which it boils (its *boiling point*) will change its physical state but will not alter its chemical state.

2. **The correct answer is (B).** Water is a compound formed by oxygen and hydrogen in chemical combination. Blood and air are mixtures, and oxygen is an element.

3. **The correct answer is (D).** *Potential energy* is, in effect, energy in storage that can be released when conditions are conducive. *Kinetic energy* is energy of activity; it is released as the activity occurs.

4. **The correct answer is (A).** One calorie (kilocalorie) will raise 1 kilogram (1,000 grams) of water 1 degree Celsius. It would take 18 calories to raise 1,000 grams of water 18 degrees ($38° - 20°$), or 36 calories to raise 2,000 grams of water 18 degrees Celsius.

5. **The correct answer is (C).** If 1 gram of carbohydrate produces 4 calories, 9 grams are required to produce 36 calories. 36 calories ÷ 4 calories/gram = 9 grams.

6. **The correct answer is (D).** The atomic weight (or mass number of an atom) equals the total of the number of protons and neutrons in the nucleus of the atom, or the total number of particles in the nucleus.

7. **The correct answer is (C).** Nearly every unstable nucleus of an atom gives off one or more of the three kinds of radiation: alpha, beta, and gamma. *Alpha* and *beta* radiation are particle emission; *gamma rays* are shortwave energy rays similar to X rays, but stronger and more penetrating. Both gamma rays and X rays are more penetrating than alpha and beta radiation.

8. **The correct answer is (A).** The *half-life period* can be defined as the time needed for half of a given amount of a substance to undergo spontaneous decomposition. This varies with different radioactive elements. There would be 50 milligrams left of a 100 milligram sample of material with a half-life of eight days after the eight days pass.

9. **The correct answer is (A).** Radiation can cause *mutations*, or genetic change. Any change in the genetic code would alter or destroy the trait associated with that particular gene. This could involve changes in enzymes produced and other factors associated with cellular metabolism.

10. **The correct answer is (C).** Gram molecular weight may be defined as the weight of the molecule expressed in grams. The molecular weight of glucose ($C_6H_{12}O_6$) is 180, as the following indicates: The weight of the six atoms of carbon equals 72 (6×12); twelve hydrogens weigh 12 (12×1); the weight of the six oxygens equals 96 (6×16). The total is 180; thus, the gram molecular weight of glucose is 180 grams.

11. **The correct answer is (D).** Equation (D) is balanced, because the amount of each substance is equal on both sides of the equation. There are two mercury atoms and two oxygen atoms on each side.

12. **The correct answer is (A).** A person with a fever has a higher temperature than normal. This reflects an increase in metabolic activities, since heat is given off as a waste product when energy in the form of ATP is used for metabolic purposes. Consequently, the pulse rate of a person with a fever is higher than normal because the heart is pumping blood at a greater rate so that the transport of materials like oxygen and glucose in the blood can accommodate this increased metabolic activity. Also, the circulatory system has to work harder to carry the greater amount of heat generated away from the tissues to be radiated from the surface of the body.

13. **The correct answer is (C).** Enzymes are called *organic catalysts*, in that they are produced by the organisms and catalyze reactions that occur within that organism. The other substances named do not function as catalysts.

14. **The correct answer is (A).** Gases are affected by temperature and pressure. If the gas is in a closed system, it cannot change its volume if temperature or pressure changes. Therefore, in a closed system, increasing the pressure would increase the temperature.

15. **The correct answer is (A).** For every oxidation, there must be a reduction. Oxidation can involve the removal of electrons, the removal of hydrogen, or the addition of oxygen; reduction, the opposite. In equation (**A**) metallic sodium loses an electron to become a positively charged ion; chlorine gains an electron to become a negatively charged chloride ion. Thus, sodium is oxidized and chlorine is reduced.

16. **The correct answer is (C).** Nitric acid reacts with the base potassium hydroxide to form potassium nitrate and water. For each hydrogen ion of the acid, there is a hydroxyl ion of the base to combine with it to form water. Therefore, neutralization occurs.

17. **The correct answer is (B).** Hard water contains calcium sulfate, calcium bicarbonate, or magnesium compounds. Soap is a mixture of sodium salts of organic acids that will react with these dissolved minerals. The insoluble calcium salt of the organic acid is precipitated out. This is the *scum,* or insoluble curdy material, that forms first. If enough soap is added, the soap acts as a cleansing agent after the first portion has precipitated the calcium ion.

18. **The correct answer is (D).** The concentration of a solution, on a percentage basis, contains a specific amount of solute in grams per 100 milliliters of solution. Thus, a 10-percent solution would have 10 grams of solute per 100 milliliters of solution.

19. **The correct answer is (A).** The molecular weight of sodium hydroxide (NaOH) is 40×1 or 40. This can be calculated by adding the atomic weights of the atoms composing the molecule.

20. **The correct answer is (C).** A molar solution contains one gram molecular weight (the molecular weight of the molecule expressed in grams), or one mole per liter of solution. Therefore, each is a one-molar solution.

21. **The correct answer is (D).** Potassium hydroxide (KOH) and hydrochloric acid (HCl) react to form potassium chloride (KCl) and water. This is a double displacement.

$$KOH + HCl \rightarrow K^+ Cl^- + H_2O$$

22. **The correct answer is (C).** An *equivalent weight* of an element is that weight of the element that combines with or displaces one atomic weight of hydrogen. Since calcium has a valence of $+2$ while hydrogen has a valence of $+1$, one half of the atomic weight of calcium will displace one atomic weight of hydrogen. Calcium has an atomic weight of 40; therefore, its equivalent weight is 20, or, expressed as grams, 20 grams. The following equation can apply:

equivalent weight = [atomic weight/valence]

23. **The correct answer is (B).** Two amino acid molecules can be bonded together by removing a hydrogen atom from the amino group (NH_2) of one amino acid molecule and removing a hydroxyl ion (OH^-) from the carboxyl group (COOH) of the other. The result is a molecule of water removed from the two amino acids and a covalent bond between the nitrogen atom in the amino group of one amino acid and the carbon atom in the carboxyl group of the other. This type of reaction is called *dehydration synthesis* and results in the production of water within cells that is called *metabolic water*. Creation of a bond between two amino acids can be illustrated as follows (R represents any of the 20 different side chains that can be included in amino acids):

Removing this water molecule will create a bond between the nitrogen and carbon.

24. **The correct answer is (B).** The periodic table places elements according to similarities in properties due to the number and arrangement of electrons in the atom. Group Zero is the inert gases. Metals and nonmetals are included in the remaining groups.

25. **The correct answer is (B).** Carbon dioxide and water, in the presence of light and the chlorophylls, yield glucose and oxygen. The water is absorbed by the root system of green plants and translocated through xylem to the leaves and other parts, which are the photosynthetic organs. Carbon dioxide enters the plants through epidermal stomates.

26. **The correct answer is (A).** Salk vaccine is prepared from inactivated polio virus. Viruses are obligate intracellular parasites; therefore, a method for growing viruses outside the human body had to be discovered and refined. Viruses typically are cultured in chick embryos.

27. **The correct answer is (C).** Ringworm is caused by fungi known as dermatophytes. These are sometimes known as the *Tineas*.

28. **The correct answer is (D).** *Photosynthesis* is the process characteristic of green plants by which carbon dioxide and water react to produce glucose and oxygen. The carbon dioxide used in the process enters the tissue from the air, passing in through stomata of the epidermis; oxygen produced by the reaction passes through the stomata into the air. This process occurs only in the presence of light, and therefore, continuous carbon dioxide removal occurs only in the presence of light.

29. **The correct answer is (D).** Mendel's Laws clearly stated the concepts of dominance and segregation (first law—Law of Segregation) and of independent assortment (second law—Law of Independent Assortment), but did not deal with the concept of hybrid vigor.

30. **The correct answer is (C).** Any relationship between two individual species is *symbiosis*. The word *symbiosis* means "life together." There are several kinds of symbiotic relationships, including commensalism, parasitism, and mutualism. A *mutualistic* relationship is one in which strong bonds exist between the two species, and each member benefits from the relationship. This kind of symbiotic relationship exists between termites and the protozoans (flagellates) of their intestinal tract. There is evidence that some bacteria in the termite's intestinal tract also play a role in the relationship. The flagellates and bacteria digest the cellulose that the termites consume.

31. **The correct answer is (C).** The Human Genome Project, which is funded by the National Institutes of Health and the Department of Energy, was initiated in 1990 and is expected to be completed (identify about 3 billion base pairs) by the beginning of the next millennium.

32. **The correct answer is (A).** The human genomic contains 22 pairs of autosomes and 1 pair of sex chromosomes in each somatic cell.

33. **The correct answer is (C).** Chorionic villus sampling (CVS) involves inserting a catheter into the uterus to take samples of the fetal chorion.

34. **The correct answer is (D).** DNA fingerprinting analyses produce identical band patterns from all tissues of an individual and can be done with less than 100 microliters of tissue. These techniques have been done on samples from Egyptian mummies over 2,000 years old.

35. **The correct answer is (B).** All bands in the child's blood were inherited from either the father or the mother. Inasmuch as the father, in this case, produced half of the bands and contributed to an additional one quarter of them, paternity can be assigned with high statistical confidence.

36. **The correct answer is (D).** *Glycogenesis* is the formation of glycogen from glucose; glycogen is the form in which carbohydrates are stored in animals. Glycogen is stored in larger quantities and more permanently in the liver; some is produced and stored temporarily in muscle.

37. **The correct answer is (A).** Carbon dioxide and water are the end products of the Krebs cycle, which is the second phase of aerobic cellular oxidation of glucose for the release of energy.

38. **The correct answer is (B).** The kidney has the function of filtering wastes from the blood. Each nephron performs this function; thus, it is the functional unit. Wastes and water are filtered out from the blood in the glomerulus, a mass of capillaries lying in Bowman's capsule; the water and wastes pass through the capsule wall into the renal tubule. Much of the water is reabsorbed into the bloodstream through the walls of the capillaries surrounding the loop of Henle of the renal tubule. The remaining liquid, or urine, passes into the renal pelvis, to the ureter and bladder, and is eventually eliminated through the urethra.

39. **The correct answer is (D).** An endocrine (or ductless) gland secretes hormone(s) directly into the bloodstream. The hormone is transported by the blood and will affect only the target tissue. An exocrine gland passes its secretion through a duct to a specific site. The pancreatic islet cells secrete the hormone insulin; other cells of the pancreas secrete pancreatic juice, containing enzymes, through the pancreatic duct into the duodenum.

40. **The correct answer is (C).** In the first stage of aerobic oxidation, glucose is oxidized to pyruvic acid; this is known as glycolysis. The two pyruvates resulting from glycolysis of a molecule of glucose enter into the Krebs cycle (Citric Acid cycle) and are oxidized to carbon dioxide and water.

HUMAN ANATOMY AND PHYSIOLOGY

Test 3

1. **The correct answer is (B).** Cholesterol is an essential component of cell membranes. Microtubules are comprised of proteins arranged in very small diameter tubes. Ribosomes contain proteins and RNA. Cytosol is the fluid component of cytoplasm.

2. **The correct answer is (C).** The function of smooth endoplasmic reticulum is lipid and carbohydrate synthesis. Rough endoplasmic reticulum is involved in the production of proteins. Mitochondria are devoted to energy (ATP) production and golgi apparatus function in the storage and packaging of cellular secretory products.

3. **The correct answer is (C).** Golgi apparatus function on the storage and packaging of secretory products and lysosomal enzymes. The function of smooth endoplasmic reticulum is lipid and carbohydrate synthesis. Control of the entry and exit of materials is the primary function of the cell's membrane and lysosomes are responsible for the removal of unwanted intracellular items.

4. **The correct answer is (A).** Cell membranes are selective permeable, which determines which substances may cross and which may not. Freely permeable and totally permeable membranes would allow any substances to pass through, and an impermeable membrane is one through which nothing can pass.

5. **The correct answer is (B).** The cell will lose water by osmosis down water's concentration gradient, which is lower in a hypertonic solution. Cells will swell when placed in a hypotonic solution. Osmosis cannot move water from an area of low concentration (the hypertonic solution) into the cell interior with its higher water concentration. Intracellular fluid is not hypertonic.

6. **The correct answer is (D).** Glucose enters skeletal muscle cells by facilitated diffusion via a carrier protein, which must be activated by insulin. Active transport is not involved in glucose movement into muscle cells. Exocytosis is a process of removing substances from the cell's interior. Glucose cannot enter these cells by simple diffusion because of its lipophobic properties and its size.

7. **The correct answer is (A).** The nucleus stores information to control protein synthesis and determines the structure and function of the cell. Mitochondria are sites of energy production. Ribosomes manufacture proteins intracellularly and lysosomes are intracellular vesicles containing enzymes.

8. **The correct answer is (C).** Epithelia line all body surfaces and provide a multiplicity of functions, including protection and control of permeability. Muscle is primarily characterized by the ability to contract, and neural tissue provides for the rapid conduction of action potentials. Connective tissues are found throughout the body, but they are never exposed to the external environment.

9. **The correct answer is (A).** Tendons consist primarily of collagen fibers, which are characterized by extreme flexibility and strength. Elastic fibers return to their original length after stretching. Reticular fibers provide the structural framework of organs, such as the spleen and liver. Nerve tissue is not connective in function.

10. **The correct answer is (D).** Synovial membranes surround the joint cavities, which are filled with synovial fluid. Mucous membranes line cavities that communicate with the external environment, while serous membranes line the components of the ventral body cavity and do not communicate with the external environment. The cutaneous membrane is skin.

11. **The correct answer is (B).** Melanin is the brown/black protective pigment produced by melanocytes within the deepest layer of the epidermis. Carotene is an orange-yellow pigment most commonly found in the stratum corneum of light-skinned individuals. Keratin is a protective protein that begins to appear in the middle layers of the epidermis. Hemoglobin is the oxygen-carrying substance found within red blood cells.

12. **The correct answer is (D).** Collagen and elastic fibers in the skin are arranged in parallel bundles orientated to resist applied forces. Smooth muscle within the skin does not have a directional orientation. Sebaceous glands, or oil glands, produce sebum. Blood vessels within the skin do not alter the opening properties of an incision and do not have a parallel pattern of organization.

13. **The correct answer is (A).** Ceruminous glands produce cerumen (ear wax). Sebaceous glands produce sebum, which protects and conditions hair shafts and skin. Apocrine and merocrine glands are forms of sweat glands.

14. **The correct answer is (B).** Apocrine glands do not become functional until puberty when sex hormone levels rise; merocrine gland activity is lifelong. Sebaceous glands produce sebum and ceruminous glands produce cerumen (ear wax).

15. **The correct answer is (C).** Merkel discs and Meisnner corpuscles are sensory receptors found within cutaneous tissue. Sweat production is provided by sudoriferous glands and oil production is provided by sebaceous glands. Blood transport is provided by components of the vascular system.

16. **The correct answer is (A).** Osteoblasts produce and release the components of bone matrix, leading to increased bone mass and strength. Osteoclasts remove bone matrix, causing bone to weaken. Osteocytes are mature bone cells, which maintain and monitor protein and mineral content of bone. Lacunae are fluid-filled pockets within which osteocytes are found.

17. **The correct answer is (D).** Red bone marrow, found within the trabecular network of spongy bone, is a major site of blood cell formation in adults. Periosteum is the membrane covering the outer surface of bone and endosteum is the membranous lining of the medullary cavity. Compact bone comprises the shafts of long bones and does not contain blood-forming functions.

18. **The correct answer is (B).** Parathyroid hormone levels increase in response to hypocalcemia to promote bone resorption and reduce renal elimination of calcium. Calcitonin lowers blood calcium by inhibiting osteoclast activity. Calcitriol acts within the digestive tract to promote calcium absorption. Thyroxine stimulates osteoblast activity and lowers blood calcium levels.

19. **The correct answer is (B).** Endochondral ossification is the process of replacing hyaline cartilage with bone. Intramembranous ossification is the formation of bone on or within loose fibrous connective tissue. Osteoclast activation and osteoblast inhibition would both slow the rate of bone formation.

20. **The correct answer is (C).** Diarthrosis refers to freely movable (synovial) joints. Synarthroses refers to immovable joints such as the sutures of the skull. Amphiarthroses are slightly movable joints exemplified by the symphysis at the junction of the left and right pubic bones of the pelvis. Arthritis refers to a group of pathologies of the joints.

21. **The correct answer is (C).** Abduction is movement away from the axis and away from the anatomical position. Flexion is movement of the anterior-posterior plane resulting in a decreased angle of the joint. Extension increases the angle at a joint and returns the body to the anatomical position. Adduction is movement toward the longitudinal axis and restoration of the anatomical position.

22. **The correct answer is (B).** Acetylcholinesterase breaks down the transmitter substance, acetylcholine, into acetate and choline, which are inactive at the neuromuscular junction. Epinephrine is not involved with the neuromuscular junction, and monoamine oxidase is an enzyme that regulates levels of available catechol amines.

23. **The correct answer is (D).** Electrical activity initiated on the muscle surface sweeps across the membrane and descends each transverse tubule into the muscle interior. Motor neurons deliver action potential activity to the neuromuscular junction. Blood vessels are not involved in electrical activity propagation. Epimysium is the connective tissue covering of an entire muscle.

24. **The correct answer is (D).** Sarcoplasmic reticulum stores calcium ions released upon the arrival of action potential activity via the transverse tubules. The motor neuron delivers action potentials to the end plate on the surface of the muscle. Mitochondria are involved in energy production and are not calcium storage sites.

25. **The correct answer is (B).** Isotonic contractions are characterized by muscle shortening accompanied by constant muscle tone throughout the contraction. During isometric contractions, muscle tone increases but muscle length remains unchanged and no movement results. Paralytic implies the absence of voluntary motor activity and flaccid refers to a loss of muscle tone.

26. **The correct answer is (D).** Muscles at rest transfer high energy phosphate groups from ATP to creatine, forming creatine phosphate and ADP. When needed, that energy is transferred back to ADP, resulting in production of ATP.

27. **The correct answer is (B).** Recruitment is the process of activating additional motor units to meet the demand for increased contraction force. Complete tetanus refers to muscle contraction in which there is no relaxation phase. Muscle tone is the partial contracture of resting muscle. A twitch is a single stimulus-contraction-relaxation sequence.

28. **The correct answer is (B).** Myoglobin is a red pigment that reversibly binds oxygen in muscle. It is structurally related to hemoglobin, the oxygen-carrying pigment found in blood. ATP and ADP are involved in phosphate energy group utilization.

29. **The correct answer is (C).** Cardiac muscle cells influence the electrical activity of adjacent cells through intercalated discs. "Striated" and "voluntary" are synonymous with skeletal muscle, which does not have intercalated discs. Smooth muscle cells communicate through dense bodies.

30. **The correct answer is (D).** The all-or-none principle states that a muscle fiber (or motor unit) is either maximally contracted or not contracted at all. Muscle tone is the partial contracture present in a resting muscle. Tetanus occurs when stimuli are produced so rapidly that there is no muscle relaxation. A twitch is a single stimulus-contraction-relaxation sequence.

31. **The correct answer is (C).** Astrocytes interface neurons and blood vessels, regulating movement of substances between those compartments. Ependymal cells are involved in the production and circulation of cerebrospinal fluid. Microglia function to remove unwanted materials from the brain and oligodendrocytes myelinate CNS axons.

32. **The correct answer is (D).** Following action potential activity, sodium and potassium are returned to their respective starting compartments by the active transport of the sodium-potassium pump. Since these movements are against concentration gradients, diffusion would be ineffective. Filtration is a process of capillaries, and osmosis refers to the movement of water.

33. **The correct answer is (D).** Increasing postsynaptic permeability to potassium will permit potassium to exit the cell, resulting in a more negative intracellular space. Depolarization, action potentials, and excitatory postsynaptic potentials require an increase in sodium permeability; all would be opposed by increased potassium permeability.

34. **The correct answer is (A).** The phrenic nerve, which supplies the diaphragm, exits the spinal cord at upper cervical levels. While the outflow of lower spinal levels may influence respiration, they are unable to sustain adequate ventilation.

35. **The correct answer is (B).** Gamma motor neurons (efferents), when activated, render the muscle spindles more sensitive to stretch. Alpha motor neurons and large diameter afferents are axons going away from muscle to the CNS. The neuromuscular junction does not normally influence reflex activity.

36. **The correct answer is (D).** The temporal lobe functions in the conscious perception of auditory and olfactory stimuli. The frontal lobe contains centers for voluntary control of skeletal muscle and plays a role in emotion. Parietal lobe function includes conscious perception of skin sensations such as touch, pain, and temperature. The occipital lobe is involved in the conscious perception of visual stimuli.

37. **The correct answer is (B).** The trigeminal nerve is the major component of sensory and motor innervation to the face. Trochlear function involves control of eye movements. The facial nerve subserves taste receptors from the anterior $\frac{2}{3}$ of the tongue, and the vestibulocochlear nerve functions in auditory and vestibular activities.

38. **The correct answer is (C).** The posterior columns contain the ascending pathways for fine touch and pressure to the body surface. Spinothalamic tract axons carry information about pain, temperature, and crude touch. The lateral corticospinal tract is part of the motor system (descending), and the spinocerebellar tracts subserve proprioception.

39. **The correct answer is (B).** REM sleep is characterized by active, often visual dreaming, accompanied by changes in autonomic activity; the EEG shows a high frequency and resembles the awake EEG. The EEG in slow wave (non-REM) sleep shows a characteristic low frequency wave. Arousal is the awakening from sleep and dreaming is not a component of coma.

40. **The correct answer is (C).** The tenth (vagus) nerve contains the primary autonomic outflow to the organs of the thoracic and abdominopelvic cavities. The first (olfactory) cranial nerve functions in the sense of smell (olfaction). The second (optic) cranial nerve subserves the sense of vision, while the twelfth (hypoglossal) nerve controls the musculature of the tongue.

41. **The correct answer is (B).** Thyrotropin from the anterior pituitary regulates the growth and development of the thyroid gland and controls its release of thyroid hormones. Thyrotropin releasing hormone, from the hypothalamus, promotes the release of thyrotropin. Thyroxine is one of the hormones released by the thyroid gland. Iodide is a constituent of thyroid hormones.

42. **The correct answer is (D).** Adrenocorticotropic hormone (ACTH) from the adenohypophysis (anterior pituitary) stimulates the release of glucocorticoids, including cortisol, from the adrenal cortex. Corticotropin releasing hormone (CRH) is produced by the hypothalamus and promotes the release of ACTH. Aldosterone is a mineralocorticoid produced by the adrenal cortex.

43. **The correct answer is (A).** Oxytocin promotes labor and delivery by inducing uterine smooth muscle contraction. Vasopressin (antidiuretic hormone—ADH) promotes water reabsorption by the kidneys. Somatotropin (growth hormone) stimulates cell growth by accelerating protein synthesis. Prolactin participates in the stimulation of mammary gland development and promotes milk production.

44. **The correct answer is (C).** Follicle stimulating hormone (FSH), a gonadotropin from the anterior pituitary, promotes follicle development and estrogen secretion in females, whereas in males it promotes sperm cell production. Testosterone is an androgen with most of its effects seen in males. Melanotropin activates melanocytes within the skin. Luteinizing hormone is responsible for initiating ovulation.

45. **The correct answer is (B).** Insulin is the hormone that lowers blood glucose levels through a number of mechanisms including activating receptors involved in the facilitated diffusion of glucose into muscle. Glucagon is the pancreatic hormone responsible for elevating blood glucose levels; epinephrine also elevates blood glucose. Renin, a hormone from the kidneys, initiates the renin-angiotensin system, which is involved in blood pressure control.

46. **The correct answer is (C).** These symptoms suggest high levels of thyroid hormones (hyperthyroidism); opposite symptoms (i.e., low basal metabolic rate, weight gain, and sensitivity to cold) would be symptomatic of hypothyroidism. Neither high nor low levels of growth hormone would produce these symptoms.

47. **The correct answer is (B).** Insulin is released by beta cells when blood glucose exceeds normal levels (70–110 mg/dL). Low blood glucose triggers the release of glucagon from the pancreas. Prolactin is not involved in the control of blood glucose. Elevated growth hormone levels cause elevations of blood glucose.

48. **The correct answer is (D).** Aldosterone is the hormone from the adrenal cortex that participates in the regulation of sodium and potassium levels. Epinephrine and norepinephrine are products of the adrenal medulla. ACTH is produced by the anterior pituitary.

49. **The correct answer is (A).** Low parathyroid hormone levels would lead to hypocalcemia, which in turn could cause convulsions. Parathyroid hormone is not involved in the regulation of blood glucose levels, nor does it influence water retention/loss mechanisms in the kidneys.

50. **The correct answer is (D).** Type I diabetes mellitus results from inadequate insulin production by the beta cells of the pancreas; high insulin levels would reflect just the opposite. Ineffective insulin receptors are associated with Type II diabetes. Both Type I and Type II diabetic patients display high blood glucose levels.

51. **The correct answer is (D).** *Glycogenesis* is the formation of glycogen from glucose; glycogen is the form in which carbohydrates are stored in animals. Glycogen is stored in larger quantities and more permanently in the liver; some is produced and stored temporarily in muscle.

52. **The correct answer is (A).** Carbon dioxide and water are the end products of the Krebs cycle, which is the second phase of aerobic cellular oxidation of glucose for the release of energy.

53. **The correct answer is (B).** The kidney has the function of filtering wastes from the blood. Each nephron performs this function; thus, it is the functional unit. Wastes and water are filtered out from the blood in the glomerulus, a mass of capillaries lying in Bowman's capsule; the water and wastes pass through the capsule wall into the renal tubule. Much of the water is reabsorbed into the bloodstream through the walls of the capillaries surrounding the loop of Henle of the renal tubule. The remaining liquid, or urine, passes into the renal pelvis, to the ureter and bladder, and is eventually eliminated through the urethra.

54. **The correct answer is (D).** An endocrine (or ductless) gland secretes hormone(s) directly into the bloodstream. The hormone is transported by the blood and will affect only the target tissue. An exocrine gland passes its secretion through a duct to a specific site. The pancreatic islet cells secrete the hormone insulin; other cells of the pancreas secrete pancreatic juice, containing enzymes, through the pancreatic duct into the duodenum.

55. **The correct answer is (C).** In the first stage of aerobic oxidation, glucose is oxidized to pyruvic acid; this is known as glycolysis. The two pyruvates resulting from glycolysis of a molecule of glucose enter into the Krebs cycle (Citric Acid cycle) and are oxidized to carbon dioxide and water.

TEST 4

1. **The correct answer is (A).** Albumin is the major plasma protein and is responsible for maintaining osmotic pressure and plasma volume. Globulins function in the transport of materials and have immune functions. Fibrinogen is a clotting factor. Platelets do not significantly alter plasma osmotic pressure.

2. **The correct answer is (D).** Anemia, a decrease in oxygen delivery, results from deficiencies in erythrocytes or hemoglobin within erythrocytes. Platelets, plasma proteins, and leukocytes do not participate in oxygen transport.

3. **The correct answer is (C).** Erythropoietin is released by cells in the kidneys when they are faced with low oxygen levels; erythropoietin promotes erythropoiesis, red blood cell formation. Neither platelets nor leukocytes are involved in oxygen delivery. Erythrocytes are red blood cells.

4. **The correct answer is (A).** Blood typing is based on the identification of antigens (agglutinogens) located on the surfaces of erythrocytes. Antibodies relevant to blood typing (agglutinins) are found in plasma, but blood type is based on red blood cell surface antigens.

5. **The correct answer is (B).** Rh+ indicates the presence of the Rh (D) antigen on the surfaces of erythrocytes; Rh- indicates the absence of that antigen. Rh antigens are not found in plasma, nor are Rh antigens. Rh antibodies are found in plasma.

6. **The correct answer is (A).** The anti-A antibodies from the plasma of the Type B blood will attack the A-antigens of the Type A blood, leading to agglutination, the clumping and breakdown of erythrocytes. Blood vessel spasm and platelet plug formation are processes involved in hemostasis. The onset of decreased oxygen delivery would be very rapid.

7. **The correct answer is (D).** Neutrophils are granulocytes and are usually the first white blood cells to arrive at an injury site or infection. Lymphocytes and monocytes are agranulocytes. Basophils, accounting for less than 1% of the circulating leukocyte population, produce histamine and heparin.

8. **The correct answer is (B).** T cells, B cells, and NK cells are classes of lymphocytes (indistinguishable under the light microscope), which are involved in immune processes. Neutrophils and eosinophils are granulocytes and are not involved in immunity.

9. **The correct answer is (B).** During the platelet phase of hemostasis, platelets stick to damaged endothelium and become activated, releasing ADP, thromboxane A_2, and serotonin, substances that participate in the hemostasis process. The vascular phase is characterized by contraction of the smooth muscle of the blood vessel wall. Coagulation refers to blood clotting. There is no inflammation phase of hemostasis.

10. **The correct answer is (D).** The last step in the final common pathway produces insoluble strands of fibrin that form the matrix of the blood clot. The conversion of prothrombin to thrombin is the initial step in the final common pathway. Fibrinogen, a plasma protein, is the precursor to fibrin.

11. **The correct answer is (A).** Calcium entry into cardiac cells results in a plateau of about 175 m/sec. Calcium exit from the cell would shorten the action potential. Sodium entry into the cell leads to the rapid initial depolarization, and sodium exit occurs after the action potential is completed.

12. **The correct answer is (B).** Spontaneous depolarizations occur most rapidly within the S-A node and it is therefore the normal pacemaker of the heart. The A-V node, bundle branch fibers, and purkinje fibers also depolarize spontaneously but at a slower rate than the S-A cells.

13. **The correct answer is (B).** The QRS complex results from ventricular depolarization. The P wave reflects atrial depolarization and the T wave relates to ventricular repolarization. The P-R segment reflects the time between atrial and ventricular depolarization.

14. **The correct answer is (D).** End-diastolic volume is the quantity of blood in the ventricles just before the initiation of ventricular contraction (systole). Stroke volume is the quantity of blood ejected during ventricular contraction. Ejection fraction evaluates the efficiency of ventricular emptying during systole. End-diastolic volume is the quantity of blood remaining within the ventricles after ventricular contraction.

15. **The correct answer is (B).** Afterload reflects the forces that the ventricles must overcome in order to eject blood. Preload is the degree of stretching during ventricular diastole and is directly proportional to the end-diastolic volume. Cardiac output measures the volume of blood pumped by the ventricles in one minute. Stroke volume is the quantity of blood ejected during ventricular contraction.

16. **The correct answer is (C).** Beta 1 receptor activation by norepinephrine results in increased heart rate and increased force of contraction. Alpha 1 receptor activation leads to vasoconstriction. Alpha 2 receptors in the CNS cause vasodilation. Beta 2 receptors primarily influence bronchioles, producing bronchodilation.

17. **The correct answer is (C).** Capillaries are the only blood vessels involved in exchange of materials. Arteries carry blood from the heart under high pressure. Arterioles control the flow of blood into capillary beds. Veins return blood to the heart.

18. **The correct answer is (A).** Venous valves prohibit backflow of blood toward the capillaries. Smooth muscle in veins alters vessel diameter but does not impede backflow. Precapillary sphincters control blood flow into capillary beds. Semilunar valves are found within the heart.

19. **The correct answer is (A).** Pulse pressure is much greater in arteries. Arterioles have a small pulse pressure, while blood flow through capillaries and veins is not pulsatile.

20. **The correct answer is (D).** Baroreceptor reflexes are responsible for rapid adjustments of blood pressure. Chemoreceptors are primarily concerned with control of respiration. Angiotensin II and antidiuretic hormone are involved in long-term regulation of blood pressure.

21. **The correct answer is (B).** During swallowing, material is kept out of the respiratory tract by the folding of the epiglottis over the glottis. The pharynx is the chamber shared by the digestive and respiratory systems. The hard palate forms the anterior roof of the mouth.

22. **The correct answer is (C).** Surfactant reduces surface tension within alveoli and prevents alveolar collapse. Serous fluid is produced by serous membranes that line surfaces not accessing the external environment. Pleural fluid increases the surface tension within the pleural space (between the visceral and parietal pleura). Mucus increases surface tension.

23. **The correct answer is (A).** Tidal volume is the volume of a single breath. Minute volume is the volume of air moved within 1 minute. Residual volume is the amount of air remaining in the lungs after a maximal expiration. Inspiratory reserve volume is the amount of air that can be inhaled in excess of a tidal inspiration.

24. **The correct answer is (C).** Anatomical dead space never goes further than the conducting passages and is not involved in gas exchange. Vital capacity is the maximal amount of air that an individual can move into or out of the lungs in a single respiratory cycle. Total lung capacity is the total volume of the lungs.

25. **The correct answer is (C).** Gases diffuse down a partial pressure gradient, not a concentration gradient. Osmotic pressures and gradients refer to properties of fluids. Within normal limits, temperature plays a minimal role in gas movement.

26. **The correct answer is (A).** Increasing thoracic volume leads to decreased intrathoracic pressure and inspiration. Decreasing thoracic volume increases intrathoracic pressure, leading to expiration. Changes in abdominal volumes do not directly affect respiration except through their influences on thoracic volumes.

27. **The correct answer is (D).** Declining blood pH weakens the hemoglobin-oxygen bond (the Bohr Effect) and promotes oxygen release to tissues. Conversely, elevated pH will strengthen the bond. Changes in blood pressure do not appreciably affect oxygen unloading.

28. **The correct answer is (C).** A significant portion of carbon dioxide is transported within erythrocytes as carbaminohemoglobin. Blood gases are not transported by plasma proteins or leukocytes, nor are they transported on the surface of red blood cells.

29. **The correct answer is (D).** Carbonic anhydrase within erythrocytes reversibly catalyzes the reaction of carbon dioxide and water, a reaction which is very slow in the absence of the enzyme. Antigens, antibodies, and plasma enzymes do not influence the reaction.

30. **The correct answer is (B).** The pneumotaxic center of the pons sends inhibitory signals to the inspiratory center, resulting in shortened duration of inspiration.

31. **The correct answer is (B).** Angiotensin I is the result of the action of renin on angiotensinogen. Angiotensin II is subsequently formed from angiotensin I. Carbonic anhydrase is the enzyme that catalyzes the reaction of carbon dioxide and water.

32. **The correct answer is (A).** Angiotensin II is a potent vasoconstrictor and an important component in reversing a hypotensive condition; it is not a vasodilator. Angiotensin II promotes aldosterone release and acts to conserve water rather than eliminate water.

33. **The correct answer is (C).** Nitrogenous byproducts of protein catabolism (including uric acid, creatinine, and urea) are not significantly reabsorbed and therefore appear in urine. Amino acids, vitamins, water, and electrolytes are all reabsorbed within the nephron.

34. **The correct answer is (B).** Nutrients are reabsorbed from the proximal convoluted tubule. The other segments of the nephron are primarily involved in the regulation of the blood levels of electrolytes and of water.

35. **The correct answer is (B).** Peristaltic waves of the smooth muscle of the ureters propel urine from the kidneys to the bladder; gravity does not play a significant role. Bladder pressure would not promote flow toward the bladder and blood pressure is not a factor in ureters action.

36. **The correct answer is (D).** The somatic motor fibers of the pudendal nerve regulate the contracture of the external sphincter. As a skeletal muscle structure, the external sphincter is not innervated by the autonomic nervous system. The phrenic nerve innervates the diaphragm.

37. **The correct answer is (A).** Sodium is the major positive-charged ion within extracellular fluid and is a primary controller of water distribution. Potassium and magnesium are more concentrated within intracellular fluid. Calcium does not play a major role in water distribution.

38. **The correct answer is (D).** Aldosterone promotes the reabsorption of sodium within the kidneys. Thyroxine is a thyroid hormone and is not involved with sodium levels. Insulin and glucagon are involved in the control of blood glucose levels.

39. **The correct answer is (C).** Although generally slower, the kidneys are the most powerful and complete correctors of pH imbalance. Buffers are the most rapid but the weakest mechanisms. Although more powerful than buffers, respiratory mechanisms rarely complete a correction of pH imbalance. The bladder is not involved in acid-base balance.

40. **The correct answer is (C).** Lack of insulin leads to the utilization of fats for energy. Byproducts include ketone bodies, which are acidic and responsible for the acidosis seen in these patients. Diabetic patients are not alkalotic, and diabetes does not result in acid production through actions on the respiratory system.

41. **The correct answer is (B).** Intrinsic factor is produced by cells of the stomach and promotes the absorption of vitamin B_{12}. The small intestine is the site of action of intrinsic factor but not the source. The pancreas and large intestine do not participate in vitamin B_{12} absorption.

42. **The correct answer is (B).** The gallbladder stores bile and concentrates it up to tenfold. Bile is manufactured in the liver but not stored there. Neither the pancreas nor the ileum are involved in bile storage.

43. **The correct answer is (B).** Cholecystokinin (CCK) is released from the intestine in response to the presence of proteins or fats. Secretin is released in response to the presence of acid from the stomach. Neither insulin nor aldosterone are released from intestinal tissues.

44. **The correct answer is (D).** Because of its role in water reabsorption, excess motility of the large intestine may lead to diarrhea, while decreased motility may lead to constipation. The stomach, liver, and small intestine are not controllers of water reabsorption.

45. **The correct answer is (A).** Carbohydrates must be reduced to monosaccharides in order for intestinal absorption to occur. Disaccharides are enzymatically broken down in the small intestine, as are polysaccharides (glycogen and starch), which are broken down into oligosaccharides.

46. **The correct answer is (C).** Pepsin results in the breakdown of proteins into polypeptides. Lipase participates in fat digestion. Sucrase breaks sucrose down into monosaccharides. Amylase initiates the digestion of starch.

47. **The correct answer is (D).** Vitamin C is a water-soluble vitamin. Vitamins A, D, E and K are fat-soluble.

48. **The correct answer is (C).** Pain and bleeding associated with gastric ulcers result from erosion of the mucosal layer, which exposes the vascular and highly innervated submucosal layer. The muscular layer and the outer (serosal) layer generally are not involved in ulcer production.

49. **The correct answer is (B).** Amylase is an enzyme found in saliva, which begins the breakdown of starch. Lipase is involved in fat digestion; pepsin begins the digestion of proteins; and insulin is involved in glucose processes.

50. **The correct answer is (A).** Digestive smooth muscle is activated by the parasympathetic division of the autonomic nervous system. The sympathetic division inhibits digestive activity. Neither the thyroid gland nor aldosterone are involved in control of gastrointestinal smooth muscle.

BIOLOGY

TEST 5

1. **The correct answer is (D).** Although other mechanisms may be involved in passage of materials through a cell membrane, the passage of some materials, especially water, occurs by diffusion; *diffusion* occurs from regions of higher concentration of the substance to regions of lower concentration. Diffusion through a membrane, such as the cell membrane, is known as *osmosis*.

2. **The correct answer is (D).** Iron is a part of the hemoglobin molecule, and, as such, is essential for its formation. Hemoglobin is the oxygen-carrying pigment found in red corpuscles.

3. **The correct answer is (B).** *Phenylketonuria (PKU)* is a genetic disorder characterized by the inability of the affected person to convert excess molecules of the amino acid phenylalanine to molecules of the amino acid tyrosine. It is caused by inheriting a defect in the gene for the enzyme that catalyzes the conversion.

4. **The correct answer is (D).** A *control* is used with experiments for comparison. The control is treated in the same manner as is the experimental group except for one variable. In this case, the variable would be the administering of the drug or sugar pills. Thus, any differences between the groups in experimental results could be attributed to this one variable.

5. **The correct answer is (C).** *Transpiration* is the loss of water in a gaseous state, through epidermal stomata, from the aerial parts of a plant. Most transpiration occurs through the leaf epidermis. Stomata are not found in root epidermis.

6. **The correct answer is (D).** An organism is a living thing or individual. An organism consists of "systems," which are made up of organs. Organs consist of tissues, especially in the case of higher organisms. This statement would not apply to lower organisms that have not reached the system level of phylogenetic development.

7. **The correct answer is (A).** Milk is not sterile; it contains numerous bacteria. Pasteurization does not sterilize milk, but does destroy certain harmful bacteria that can be carried in milk.

8. **The correct answer is (C).** *Auxins* are growth hormones found in plants; in stems, auxins stimulate growth. If a plant is unevenly illuminated, auxins are more concentrated on the side of the stem that is more poorly illuminated, stimulating growth on that side. This will cause the stem to bend toward the light.

9. **The correct answer is (A).** In humans, carbohydrate digestion begins in the mouth with the enzyme ptyalin, produced by the salivary glands.

10. **The correct answer is (A).** Black is dominant over white in this case; therefore, the white guinea pig carries only white genes and is *homozygous* or pure recessive. When such a test backcross is made, the offspring will indicate the genotype of the black guinea pig. If the black guinea pig is hybrid or *heterozygous* black (carrying one white gene), black and white offspring will result in a theoretical ratio of 1:1; if the black guinea pig is pure or homozygous black, all offspring will be black because of dominance, although all of the offspring will be hybrid because they carry a white gene.

11. **The correct answer is (B).** Fossils found in the lowest rock layers are the oldest because these layers were deposited before the ones above. Fossils in upper layers are not always different from the lower layers. Some species have very long histories and leave fossils in more than one layer. Conversely, fossils in upper layers are never completely the same as fossils in lower layers. At least some species of organisms whose fossils lie in lower layers would have become extinct and been replaced by fossils of different organisms by the time upper layers were deposited. Older organisms were not always simpler than modern organisms and were certainly not more complex.

12. **The correct answer is (C).** The roots of plants help to hold the soil in place and prevent soil erosion; the ground can absorb water. Eroded lands do not absorb water readily. Water may run off, carrying with it some of the topsoil. This reduces the quality of the land. Where plants are present, the run-off is reduced or diminished, and the ground absorbs water.

13. **The correct answer is (A).** A *stimulus* is anything that can cause a *reaction* or response by the organism. The reaction may be involuntary, such as batting the eye when an object approaches, or voluntary, such as moving from an area of discomfort.

14. **The correct answer is (B).** Crossbreeding between strains with the desired traits, followed by selection of the offspring for future breeding and establishing the herd, is the best way to accomplish the breeder's goal. Inbreeding is just as likely to bring out undesirable hidden traits.

15. **The correct answer is (A).** The inhaling and the exhaling of air by the human lungs demonstrates Boyle's Law. Inhaling results from the expansion of the chest cavity (increase in volume and decrease in air pressure) and exhaling results from compression of the chest cavity (decrease in volume and increase in air pressure). These changes are accomplished by movement of the ribs and diaphragm.

16. **The correct answer is (D).** Pith typically consists of *parenchyma* cells, which store starch in typical green plants. Spongy cells, characteristic of dicot leaves, also store starch, but temporarily.

17. **The correct answer is (C).** The Hubble Telescope is able to produce sharper images of objects than other telescopes because it is in orbit around Earth and does not have its view obstructed by atmosphere. Images seen through telescopes on Earth's surface are always obscured to some degree by the scattering of light as it passes through the atmosphere and by the passage of air currents created by heating of the atmosphere.

18. **The correct answer is (D).** A symptom of diabetes is sugar (glucose) in the urine. *Benedict's solution* is a reagent used to test for the presence of reducing sugars such as glucose.

19. **The correct answer is (B).** Buffer Systems resist significant changes in pH. When a strong acid or a strong base is added to a buffer system, they produce a weak acid and a salt or a weak base and water, respectively. In each case the pH would change only slightly.

20. **The correct answer is (B).** Each turn of the Krebs cycle generates 2 moles of CO_2 and four pairs of H_2.

21. **The correct answer is (A).** A small amount of living tissue can be removed from a specific organ of a patient and examined by a pathologist to give the attending physician information needed for diagnosis. This excision and diagnostic study of living tissue is a *biopsy*, a useful diagnostic tool—especially for diseases of a cancerous nature.

22. **The correct answer is (C).** Water constitutes about 75–85 percent of the typical living cell. No activities associated with life can occur without water.

23. **The correct answer is (D).** Fats are *emulsified*, or broken down into small droplets, by bile secreted from the liver into the small intestine. The enzyme lipase then digests the fat droplets into fatty acids and glycerin. These products are not absorbed through capillary walls directly into the bloodstream, but enter the small lymph vessels, or *lacteals*, located in the villi of the intestine.

24. **The correct answer is (B).** The results of the penny toss approximate a 1:2:1 ratio, which is the same ratio that is obtained from a monohybrid cross:

$$Aa \times Aa \rightarrow 1AA:2Aa:1aa.$$

25. **The correct answer is (D).** In the light phase of photosynthesis, H_2O is dissociated into $H_2 + O_2$. The O_2 comes entirely from the water molecules. The resulting H_2 is then used to reduce CO_2 to simple sugar.

26. **The correct answer is (A).** Tissue culture is the technique of growing tissues or cells in solutions of water and nutrients. This technique is especially useful in studying growth, differentiation, and morphology.

27. **The correct answer is (B).** Incineration is an effective method of sterilization; holding a loop in a flame sterilizes the loop, preventing contamination of surfaces on work areas, etc., and the possible spread of infectious bacteria.

28. **The correct answer is (C).** Cellular respiration oxidizes digested food molecules and produces CO_2 and H_2O as end products. It is a downhill reaction and occurs in both plant and animal cells.

29. **The correct answer is (D).** *Combustion*, or burning, is a rapid reaction giving off much heat and light in a short period of time. The energy is expended more rapidly; thus, the reaction occurs at a higher temperature since the temperature of the combustible material must be raised to a combustion point. Cellular respiration occurs more slowly, at lower temperatures, and is controlled by enzymes. If cellular respiration occurred at combustion temperatures, cells would be destroyed.

30. **The correct answer is (B).** *Trypsin*, an enzyme found in pancreatic juice, digests proteins, peptones, and proteoses to peptides. The digestion of peptides to amino acids also occurs in the small intestine under the control of the enzyme erepsin. Some protein digestion (to peptones and proteoses) occurs in the stomach, under the control of the enzyme pepsin. Ptyalin and maltase act on carbohydrates; steapsin, on fats.

31. **The correct answer is (D).** Thrombocytes disintegrate when ruptured, as when blood flows from an injured blood vessel, releasing thrombokinase (thromboplastin), which acts to convert prothrombin to thrombin. Thrombin acts on fibrinogen in the plasma, converting it to insoluble fibrin, the material that forms the clot. Inadequacy of thrombokinase would prevent the first step of clotting, the formation of thrombin from prothrombin.

32. **The correct answer is (C).** *Cone cells* are photoreceptor cells found in the retina of the eye. They are responsible for color vision. Cone cells are functional only in bright light; therefore, color is not perceived in dim light.

33. **The correct answer is (C).** The *iris* is a circular muscle that regulates the diameter of the *pupil*, the aperture that allows light to enter the posterior chamber of the eye where the light-sensitive retina is located. The *cornea* allows light to enter the eye but does not regulate the amount of light entering. The *ciliary body* is a muscle that changes either the position or shape of the lens to focus the light coming through the pupil. The *conjunctiva* is a thin, protective layer of epithelium that covers the exposed surface of the eyeball.

34. **The correct answer is (A).** Most of the carbon dioxide is transported in the blood plasma in the form of sodium bicarbonate ($NaHCO_3$). *Erythrocytes*, *leucocytes*, and *platelets* (thrombocytes) are blood cells suspended in the plasma.

35. **The correct answer is (D).** *Adrenalin*, a hormone secreted by the adrenal glands, causes increases in blood pressure, heart rate, breathing, glucose blood levels, etc., preparing the body for stressful situations.

36. **The correct answer is (A).** *Auxins* are plant growth hormones; *testosterone* and *estrogen* are animal sex hormones. ATP (adenosine triphosphate) is an energy-transport compound found in cells.

37. **The correct answer is (D).** Bread mold is a fungus, while ferns are vascular plants. Both bread mold and ferns, however, produce spores as asexual reproductive cells. A *mycelium* is a mass of fungal hyphae and is not a part of the fern-plant body. *Pinnules* are the "leaflets" of a fern frond and are not part of a fungus.

38. **The correct answer is (A).** *Transpiration* is the loss of gaseous water from a plant through epidermal stomata of the aerial parts of the plant, especially the leaves. Water forms a continuous column in the xylem tissue. The pull of water effected by transpiration is a factor in the rise of *sap* (water plus dissolved materials). The process is much the same as drinking liquid through a straw.

39. **The correct answer is (B).** Xylem and phloem serve the purpose of transporting materials in vascular tissues. Upward translocation of plant sap is accomplished mainly through vessels (in angiosperms) and tracheids of xylem. Downward translocation is accomplished through the sieve tubes of phloem.

40. **The correct answer is (C).** The cotyledons of dicotyledonous plants (such as beans) store food for use by the plant embryo as it develops into a seedling that can carry on photosynthesis. The *plumule* is composed of the embryonic or first leaves of the embryo; the *hypocotyl* is the lower embryonic stem; and the *testa* is the seed coat.

41. **The correct answer is (A).** Normal cells have a high power of self-affinity (tendency to adhere to their own kind). Cancer cells loose this ability, as demonstrated by the spreading of cancer from one organ to another (malignancy).

42. **The correct answer is (A).** The *stigma* is the top portion of the pistil on which pollen lands in pollination. The *style* is the neck-like portion of the pistil, located between the stigma and the ovary, the basal part. *Ovules* are potential seeds.

43. **The correct answer is (B).** Intensive research has demonstrated the basic structure of cell membranes is a mosaic of proteins in an outer and inner layer of phospholipids.

44. **The correct answer is (B).** The enzyme sucrase adds a molecule of water (hydrolysis to the band that binds the monosaccharides forming sucrose) to decompose the dissaccharide to simple sugars.

45. **The correct answer is (B).** The movement of continents relative to one another is mostly the result of the spreading apart of sea floor between continental masses caused by the extrusion of molten rock through cracks in the sea floor. Fluctuations in Earth's magnetic field and Coriolis force are real events, but neither has any effect on continental drift. Fragmentation of large land masses to make smaller ones has sometimes been a part of continental drift, but it qualifies as a result rather than a cause.

46. **The correct answer is (C).** The generic formula for carbohydrates is $(CH_2O)^n = 1C:2H:1O$ (1:2:1).

47. **The correct answer is (A).** There are three morphological types, or shapes, of bacteria: spherical-shaped bacteria are called *cocci*; rod-shaped bacteria are called *bacilli*; curved or spiral-shaped bacteria are usually known as *spirilla*.

48. **The correct answer is (A).** Bacteria are classified as gram positive or gram negative; this depends on their ability to retain crystal violet, the primary stain of the gram stain. Those bacteria that cannot be decolorized with ethanol, but retain crystal violet, are classified as gram positive. Those that can be decolorized are gram negative. The difference is due to the chemical composition of the cell wall.

49. **The correct answer is (D).** A *bacteriophage* is a kind of virus that attacks and destroys the bacterial cell. The viruses can pass their DNA into the bacterial cells and cause the cells to manufacture vital DNA and viral protein.

50. **The correct answer is (C).** A *marsupial* is a viviparous mammal that gives birth to immature embryos; the development of the young is completed in the female's pouch, located on her ventral side. Nourishment for the embryo is from the mammary glands, the nipples of which are located in the pouch.

51. **The correct answer is (B).** Reptiles are the first vertebrates in evolutionary development that spend the early or developmental part of their lives, as well as adult stages, on land. They do not possess gills for breathing in water as do the larval stages of amphibians.

52. **The correct answer is (A).** Enzymes are macromolecular proteins that serve as biological catalysts that lower activation energy requirements in cellular reactions.

53. **The correct answer is (B).** Most eukaryotic cells are in the range of 10 microns to 100 microns.

54. **The correct answer is (D).** *Sickle cell anemia* is caused by inheriting the defective form of a gene that codes for part of the protein portion of the hemoglobin molecule. The number of erythrocytes produced and the amount of hemoglobin in each erythrocyte are normal, but the altered structure of the hemoglobin molecules causes them to stick together in a manner that distorts erythrocytes into an abnormal crescent shape, making them less able to carry oxygen. Other types of anemia are due to insufficient hemoglobin within erythrocytes, too few erythrocytes, or erythrocytes that are abnormally small.

55. **The correct answer is (C).** All named are members of the phylum Arthropoda, but only the sow bug is a crustacean. The characteristics of the class Crustacea are two pairs of antennae, three pairs of mouth parts, and a three-part body. Most crustaceans are aquatic, gilled animals, but a few live on land. The sow bug is one of these.

56. **The correct answer is (C).** Leucoplasts are cellular plastids that store starches and are found only in plant cells.

57. **The correct answer is (A).** The hydra and corals are coelenterates, diploblastic animals characterized by a gastrovascular cavity.

58. **The correct answer is (B).** Many insects have developed an immunity to or tolerance of DDT, so it does not kill them. However, DDT can accumulate in the bodies of insects and then be transferred to the tissues of birds, fishes, and other insect predators. These predators can accumulate DDT and, when consumed by their predators, pass on the DDT. Thus, this harmful insecticide can be passed up the food chain with the concentration in animal tissues increasing at each level, and it can have harmful effects on higher animals that consume the lower DDT-containing animals.

59. **The correct answer is (A).** Lysosomes store powerful hydrolysis enzymes.

60. **The correct answer is (A).** All environments have limited amounts of food and space, allowing animal populations to increase up to these limits, and regulating the populations by the number of individuals per unit of space (density-dependent).

61. **The correct answer is (C).** Any relationship between two individual species is *symbiosis*. The word *symbiosis* means "life together." There are several kinds of symbiotic relationships, including commensalism, parasitism, and mutualism. A *mutualistic* relationship is one in which strong bonds exist between the two species, and each member benefits from the relationship. This kind of symbiotic relationship exists between termites and the protozoans (flagellates) of their intestinal tract. There is evidence that some bacteria in the termite's intestinal tract also play a role in the relationship. The flagellates and bacteria digest the cellulose that the termites consume.

62. **The correct answer is (C).** The Human Genome Project, which is funded by the National Institutes of Health and the Department of Energy, was initiated in 1990 and is expected to be completed (identify about 3 billion base pairs) by the beginning of the next millennium.

63. **The correct answer is (A).** The human genomic contains 22 pairs of autosomes and 1 pair of sex chromosomes in each somatic cell.

64. **The correct answer is (C).** Chorionic villus sampling (CVS) involves inserting a catheter into the uterus to take samples of the fetal chorion.

65. **The correct answer is (D).** DNA fingerprinting analyses produce identical band patterns from all tissues of an individual and can be done with less than 100 microliters of tissue. These techniques have been done on samples from Egyptian mummies over 2,000 years old.

66. **The correct answer is (B).** All bands in the child's blood were inherited from either the father or the mother. Inasmuch as the father, in this case, produced half of the bands and contributed to an additional one quarter of them, paternity can be assigned with high statistical confidence.

67. **The correct answer is (B).** Carbon dioxide and water, in the presence of light and the chlorophylls, yield glucose and oxygen. The water is absorbed by the root system of green plants and translocated through xylem to the leaves and other parts, which are the photosynthetic organs. Carbon dioxide enters the plants through epidermal stomates.

68. **The correct answer is (A).** Salk vaccine is prepared from inactivated polio virus. Viruses are obligate intracellular parasites; therefore, a method for growing viruses outside the human body had to be discovered and refined. Viruses typically are cultured in chick embryos.

69. **The correct answer is (C).** Ringworm is caused by fungi known as dermatophytes. These are sometimes known as the *Tineas*.

70. **The correct answer is (D).** *Photosynthesis* is the process characteristic of green plants by which carbon dioxide and water react to produce glucose and oxygen. The carbon dioxide used in the process enters the tissue from the air, passing in through stomata of the epidermis; oxygen produced by the reaction passes through the stomata into the air. This process occurs only in the presence of light, and therefore continuous carbon dioxide removal occurs only in the presence of light.

71. **The correct answer is (D).** Mendel's Laws clearly stated the concepts of dominance and segregation (first law—Law of Segregation) and of independent assortment (second law—Law of Independent Assortment), but did not deal with the concept of hybrid vigor.

GENERAL SCIENCE
TEST 6

1. **The correct answer is (C).** The gingko is native to the Orient but has been imported into the United States and now is in widespread use as an ornamental tree.

2. **The correct answer is (C).** Evidence indicates that a primitive reptile known as a therapsid is the ancestor of mammals. These early reptiles of the Triassic period had acquired some mammalian characteristics such as warm-bloodedness, hair, and mammary glands. They are sometimes referred to as "premammals."

3. **The correct answer is (C).** *Electrophoresis* is a technique that takes advantage of the fact that molecules in solution will migrate through a porous gel when an electrical current is passed through it. A mixture of differently sized molecules is placed into a depression at one end of the gel, and the current is turned on. Smaller molecules will travel farther through the gel than larger molecules, with the result that bands of molecules will accumulate at various distances from the starting point according to their size. These bands can be made visible by staining, allowing the results of one electrophoretic separation to be compared to another.

4. **The correct answer is (B).** Fossil evidence indicates that there was an isolation of ape-like forms, including hominids (human-like creatures), during the Pliocene period. These seemingly originated from the same "branch" of the evolutionary "tree." Lemurs, New World monkeys, and Old World monkeys apparently evolved earlier.

5. **The correct answer is (A).** It was found that if a mixture of methane, ammonia, and hydrogen is continuously bombarded with spark discharges as an energy source, amino acids are formed. If inorganic phosphate is added to the mixture, ATP, the energy compound of cells, is formed also. The earth, at its very early age, had the inorganic substances, and the sun could have provided the energy source.

6. **The correct answer is (D).** The *condenser* is an adjustable lens that focuses light before it reaches the specimen. This enhances the sharpness of the image produced by the magnifying lenses of the microscope. The *objective* and the *ocular* are the lenses used to create a magnified image of the light after it has passed through the specimen. A *micrometer* is a device used to measure objects viewed through the microscope.

7. **The correct answer is (C).** Triple bonds, sharing six electrons between two carbon atoms, provide each with a complete octet.

8. **The correct answer is (B).** As the moon revolves around the earth, it rotates on its axis so that only one side of the moon faces earth. Because the moon makes one rotation with one revolution around the earth, one side of the moon never faces the earth.

9. **The correct answer is (B).** In all ecosystems, producers (green plants or algae) convert CO_2 and H_2O into sugars, which serve as food for consumers (animals) whose bodies are ultimately degraded by decomposers (bacteria and fungi). Water, although vital, is an inorganic substance.

10. **The correct answer is (C).** Carbon monoxide has a greater affinity than oxygen for hemoglobin. This binding blocks hemoglobin from binding oxygen for transport to body cells for metabolic needs.

11. **The correct answer is (A).** A deficiency of vitamin B_{12} leads to *pernicious anemia*, a condition in which red blood cells fail to mature. Vitamin B_{12} is essential for the formation of red blood cells.

12. **The correct answer is (A).** Scolar quantities have only magnitude; vectors have magnitude and direction.

13. **The correct answer is (B).** The catalytic converter uses platinum to convert carbon monoxide and hydrocarbons to carbon dioxide and water, resulting in reduced air pollution.

14. **The correct answer is (C).** In a cathode-ray tube, such as found in television sets (picture tube), a *cathode* (negative terminal) and an *anode* (positive terminal) are present. There is no material between the two through which electricity (electrons) can flow from one terminal to another: a vacuum exists in the tube. A heated cathode generates electrons, which become excited by heat and can acquire enough energy to leave the cathode. Once they do, they are attracted to the anode because of the difference in charges (electrons have a negative charge) and flow across the gap toward the anode. In other appliances, the material through which the electricity flows may produce some resistance; in a picture tube, the electrons are flowing across a space in a vacuum and encounter no resistance.

15. **The correct answer is (A).** The small-intestine lining is characterized by millions of *villi*, small, thin-walled projections into the lumen. Each villus is supplied with capillaries and a lacteal. The large number of villi greatly increase the absorptive area of the small intestine, and the blood vessels and lacteal are close to the food supply. Thus, digested foods are absorbed with ease through the thin-walled villus and thin capillary walls into the bloodstream or, in the case of fats, into the opened ends of the lacteals.

16. **The correct answer is (D).** Coal is the major source of SO_2 because gasoline, natural gas, and paper waste contain only small amounts of sulfur.

17. **The correct answer is (C).** The moon shines by the reflected light of the sun. Because the moon rotates on its axis as it revolves around the earth, one side of the moon never faces the earth. This side, the dark side of the moon, can never reflect the sun's light onto the earth.

18. **The correct answer is (A).** Poison ivy has a clear juice rather than a milky sap. Three-leaflet clusters, white berries, and shiny leaves are all characteristic of poison ivy.

19. **The correct answer is (B).** The divalent ($C\Phi^{++}$) cupric ion is the species capable of receiving electrons.

20. **The correct answer is (A).** A chemical reaction at equilibrium has a $\Delta G = 0$, meaning no exchange in free energy.

21. **The correct answer is (D).** Air is a mixture of gases; dry air consists of about 78 percent nitrogen and 21 percent oxygen. The remaining 1 percent consists of other gases, including carbon dioxide.

22. **The correct answer is (D).** Enzymes are proteins that catalize reactions of substances known as substrates.

23. **The correct answer is (A).** The reverse outside-inside concentration and membrane crossing of Na^+ and K^+ are the major ion responsible for resting potetids and action potentials.

24. **The correct answer is (C).** Exergonic reactions are downhill reactions.

25. **The correct answer is (C).** As oxygen accepts electrons from the ETS, it acquires a $++$ valence, which attracts $2H^+$ to form HOH.

26. **The correct answer is (B).** Air pressure at sea level is 14.7 pounds/square inch. This pressure, at 0 degrees C supports a barometer mercury column of 76 centimeters, or 30 inches. This is equivalent to one atmosphere of pressure.

27. **The correct answer is (C).** Radioactive elements suggest that the earth is 4.5 billion years old.

28. **The correct answer is (B).** A *high* indicates an area of high air pressure, while a *low* indicates an area of low air pressure. Weather can be predicted by measuring differences between pressures. A high usually indicates fair weather, whereas low pressure areas indicate storms and bad weather.

29. **The correct answer is (D).** The retina of the eye contains rods and cones; these are the photoreceptors of the eye, so named because of their shape. Rods are concerned with perception of gray to black in dim light, while cones respond to light of high intensity and are concerned with color perception. Nerve fibers from these receptors eventually converge to form the optic nerves leading to the brain.

30. **The correct answer is (C).** Malaria is a parasitic disease caused by protistans in the genus *Plasmodium*. Some of the life cycle stages of *Plasmodium* are passed in mosquitoes of the genus *Anopheles*, which transmit the disease.

31. **The correct answer is (B).** Archimedes' Principle indicates that an object will displace its weight in water. Thus, a 1,000-ton ship would displace 1,000 tons of water.

32. **The correct answer is (D).** A photoelectric cell works on the principle that light can be used to produce electric currents in some metals. When light energy strikes the metal (usually cesium) in the photoelectric cell, it is converted into electric energy. The cesium emits electrons. The greater the amount of light striking the metal, the more electric energy produced.

33. **The correct answer is (B).** A camera lens is convex; light passing through such a lens is bent toward the center of the lens. Light reflected near the object and passing through the thinner outer edges of a convex lens bends more than light passing through the thicker areas, and light passing through the exact center of the lens does not bend at all. Because light reflected from an object is focused through such a lens and bent, rather than passing in a straight line, as it would if passing through plain glass, the image formed is reversed and is smaller than the original object.

34. **The correct answer is (C).** Natural selection

35. **The correct answer is (B).** The flour beetle belongs to the Order Coleoptera which, with approximately 340,000 described species, is the largest order of insects. The housefly belongs to the Order Diptera, containing approximately 100,000 described species. The grasshopper belongs to the Order Orthoptera, containing approximately 20,000 species. The cockroach belongs to the Order Blattaria, containing only 3,700 species.

36. **The correct answer is (D).** The H^+ has no electrons, which enables it to use two unshared electrons from N to form a coordinate covalent bond.

37. **The correct answer is (B).** Photosynthesis is an endergonic reaction which uses $CO_2 + H_2O$ to produce simple sugar and O_2. It is driven by radiant energy from sunlight.

38. **The correct answer is (A).** Unicellular eukaryotes, including colonial forms, belong to the Kingdom *Protista*. The other organisms in this question belong to phyla in the Kingdom *Animalia*, of which all members are multicellular. Phylum *Annelida* includes segmented worms, such as the earthworm. Phylum *Porifera* includes sponges. Phylum *Arthropoda* includes animals such as insects, spiders, crabs, crayfish, and millipedes that have a chitinous exoskeleton and jointed appendages.

39. **The correct answer is (C).** Spiders are characterized by a two-part body and four pairs of legs, while insects have a three-part body and three pairs of legs.

40. **The correct answer is (B).** The CO_2 from the burning of fossil fuels prevents heat from escaping the earth's surface, thus raising temperatures.

41. **The correct answer is (A).** Hydrogen is the lightest element known, having an atomic weight of 1.008. The atom contains one proton, no neutrons, and one electron.

42. **The correct answer is (B).** Nitrogen composes nearly four fifths of the air; oxygen nearly one fifth. The remainder of air consists of other gases.

43. **The correct answer is (C).** Light travels at a speed of about 186,000 miles per second; the sun is approximately 93,000,000 miles from the earth. Thus, calculations (93,000,000 miles divided by 186,000 miles per second) show that it takes about 500 seconds, or a bit more than eight minutes, for light from the sun to reach the earth.

44. **The correct answer is (D).** Emergent properties of matter cause atoms that react to form compounds to lose their original properties and gain properties of the new substance.

45. **The correct answer is (B).** The earth makes one complete rotation on its axis (360 degrees) in 24 hours; 45 degrees is one eighth of 360 degrees. Therefore, it would take one eighth of 24 hours, or 3 hours, for the earth to rotate 45 degrees.

46. **The correct answer is (C).** The thyroid regulates metabolic rate under normal conditions. A deficiency of thyroid hormone will cause a low basal metabolism, while an excess of the hormone will increase the metabolic rate.

47. **The correct answer is (B).** A *peptide bond* is the covalent bond that links the nitrogen atom on the end of one amino acid molecule with the carbon atom on the opposite end of another amino acid molecule. A peptide bond is formed by removing a molecule of water from the two amino acid molecules (see the explanatory answer for question 23 in Chemistry and Physics Test 2 for an explanation of dehydration synthesis). Therefore, inserting a water molecule between two amino acids linked by a peptide bond will break the bond by putting a hydrogen atom back onto the nitrogen atom of one amino acid and a hydroxyl ion $(OH-)$ back onto the terminal carbon atom of the other amino acid. Breaking a bond between two molecules by inserting a water molecule between them is called *hydrolysis* and is a common way of digesting large organic molecules such as starches and proteins.

48. **The correct answer is (B).** The 23.5 inclination of the earth on its axis causes it to tilt toward and away from the sun as it revolves around the sun.

49. **The correct answer is (D).** Passive immunity involves administering an antibody (an antitoxin, in the case of diphtheria) to the patient. This immunity is temporary, since the patient's body is not stimulated to form antibodies, as it would be if an antigen were administered. The temporary immunity is considered *passive* because the body is not active in forming antibodies. If an antigen stimulates the body to form its own antibodies against it, the immunity produced is *active*. Passive immunity provides temporary protection to one who has been exposed to a disease, or a method of treatment until the patient's body has started producing its own antibodies if the disease has been contracted. Active immunity imparts more lasting protection.

50. **The correct answer is (C).** Group O blood lacks antigen A and antigen B. Although it can form antibodies against both A and B, it cannot stimulate the formation of antibodies against A and B. Persons of group O are known as *universal donors*. Group AB blood has both antigens A and B but cannot form antibodies against either. Persons of group AB are known as *universal recipients*. Since group O has neither antigen, and AB cannot form either antibody, the only safe transfusion of those listed is choice (C). Persons of group A contain antigen A and can form antibodies against antigen B; blood group B contains antigen B and can form antibodies against A.

51. **The correct answer is (A).** Synergism is a phenomenon in which the whole is greater than the sum of the individual parameters.

52. **The correct answer is (B).** Xylem, characterized in angiosperms by vessels, conducts material upward in the plant. Most of the material conducted upward is water that has been absorbed from the soil by the root system. The water contains dissolved minerals and may contain, especially in deciduous perennials in the spring, sugar that has been formed by the digestion of starch stored in the lower plant parts.

53. **The correct answer is (A).** After the common multiplier (M) was removed from $mgh = \frac{1}{2}mV^2$, the equation was multiplied by 2 to eliminate the $\frac{1}{2}$, and the square root of both sides was extracted.

54. **The correct answer is (D).** Total potential energy was connected to kinetic energy.

55. **The correct answer is (A).** Genes are composed of segments of nucleotide bases of DNA molecules.

56. **The correct answer is (C).** Distillation involves *evaporation*, or changing the water from a liquid to a gaseous state (usually by heating), and collecting and *condensing* the gaseous water back to a liquid. The water, because it is in a gaseous state, is separated from any impurities since they cannot evaporate with the water.

57. **The correct answer is (B).** On the Fahrenheit scale, the boiling point of water is 212 degrees; the freezing point is 32 degrees. Subtracting 32 degrees from 212 degrees results in a difference of 180 degrees, the number of degrees between the boiling and the freezing points of water.

58. **The correct answer is (B).** *Static electricity* is a non-moving electrical charge that accumulates on the surface of an object. A substance that contains an equal number of *protons* (positively charged particles) and *electrons* (negatively charged particles) is electrically neutral. If electrons are gained or lost, the substance becomes charged. When one object loses electrons and becomes positively charged, another must gain electrons and become negatively charged. If electrons are not in motion, the electricity is static. However, warm, moist air is a good conductor of electricity; moisture collects on the surfaces of objects and conducts electrons away from the surface, preventing the object from becoming charged. Cold air acts as a good insulator, preventing the movement of electrons away from the object. Therefore, static electricity can best be felt on a cold, dry day, when the electrons can accumulate on an object or surface.

59. **The correct answer is (A).** Jupiter is the largest planet known in our solar system, and is known to have twelve moons, or satellites, revolving around it. Neptune and Pluto are the greatest distance from the earth: two moons are identified for Neptune, and knowledge about Pluto, the most distant planet, is incomplete. Mercury is difficult to study because of its closeness to the sun. The glare of the sun makes observations difficult during the day and the planet is very low in the sky at night. However, with present explorations and studies of our solar system resulting in the accumulation of more knowledge, changes in previously held concepts are taking place.

60. **The correct answer is (A).** Deserts of the earth generally occur on the west side of continents, as influenced by prevailing westerly winds and nearby mountains. As the earth rotates from west to east, winds that approach continents from the west side loose moisture in ascending mountains and evaporate moisture from the opposite side—resulting in dry regions known as deserts.

61. **The correct answer is (B).** Atmospheric moisture combines with oxides of carbon, nitrogen, and sulfur to produce acid rain, as illustrated by the following reactions:

$$H_2O + CO_2 \rightarrow H_2CO_3$$
$$H_2O + 2NO_2 \rightarrow 2HNO_3$$
$$H_2O + SO_2 \rightarrow H_2SO_3$$

62. **The correct answer is (B).** As water is warmed, its solubility of oxygen decreases, resulting in a lower O_2 content and producing unfavorable conditions for animals.

63. **The correct answer is (D).** The pesticide DDT was banned from the United States during the 1970s because research studies had shown it to be present in milk, fatty tissues, and the eggs of eagles and other birds. It was also proven to be a biological concentration—building up to higher concentration in succeeding levels of food chains.

64. **The correct answer is (C).** The human body is composed primarily of oxygen, carbon, hydrogen, and nitrogen, which comprise approximately 96 percent of the body's mass, with about 15 other elements comprising the rest.

65. **The correct answer is (B).** Glucose and fructose are isomers because they are composed of identical numbers of carbon, hydrogen, and oxygen atoms, with different structural arrangements and different functional groups. The carbon-oxygen bonding in glucose and fructose form aldehydes and ketones, respectively.

66. **The correct answer is (D).** The approximate percentages of oxygen, carbon, nitrogen, and potassium in the human body are: 65, 18.5, 3.5, and 0.5, respectively.

67. **The correct answer is (B).** Density is defined as mass per unit volume $(D = \dfrac{m}{v})$. The mathematical relationship shows that when equal masses of two substances of different densities are compared, the one with greater density occupies less space (volume).

68. **The correct answer is (D).** The same four bases A, T, C, and G are in all living organisms. Organisms differ according the numbers and arrangements.

FINAL SCIENCE EXAMINATION

TEST 7

1. **The correct answer is (C).** All conditions are under genetic control; however, hereditary baldness is also under hormonal control. Baldness is expressed as a dominant characteristic in males but recessive in females because of the hormones present. Thus, a male and female may inherit the same genes for baldness, but the expression of the genes will depend on the sex hormones.

2. **The correct answer is (D).** Diploid cells in the testes undergo meiosis to reduce the chromosome number by one half to the haploid condition.

3. **The correct answer is (B).** There are only four basic kinds of tissues: epithelial, connective, muscle, and nerve. Gland cells are among the epithelial tissues that cover the internal and external surfaces of various parts of the body.

4. **The correct answer is (A).** The speed of sound in air varies slightly with temperature, increasing slightly as temperature increases. For convenience, the speed of sound in air is referred to as 1,100 feet per second. This is an approximate value that can be used despite various conditions. 1,100 feet is approximately one fifth of a mile (1 mile = 5,280 feet).

5. **The correct answer is (C).** A member of the acetylene series is unsaturated, with a triple bond between two carbons. The formula for acetylene, for example, is $H-C \equiv C-H$; because of the triple bond between two carbons, the number of hydrogens is reduced by two. Thus, the general formula is $Cn_2H_2n - 2$.

6. **The correct answer is (A).** A molecule of glucose uses two molecules of ATP to supply activation energy to initiate the glycolytic pathway.

7. **The correct answer is (D).** Prothrombin is produced in insufficient quantities if there is a deficiency of vitamin K; prothrombin produces thrombin, which acts as an enzyme to convert fibrinogen to fibrin, the mesh that traps blood cells, forming the clot. Thus, if vitamin K is deficient, prothrombin is deficient, and clotting is delayed or does not occur.

8. **The correct answer is (D).** Each nucleotide of a DNA molecule contains a molecule of deoxyribose sugar, a nitrogen base, and a phosphate group, which is attached to the 3' carbon of one sugar molecule and the 5' carbon of a second sugar.

9. **The correct answer is (A).** The wavelength of energy in the electromagnetic spectrum ranges from 10^{-3} nM to 10^{14} nM, with visible light between 350 nM and 700 nM.

10. **The correct answer is (D).** The buoyancy of an object in water or air is determined by its *density* relative to the surrounding medium: thus, objects less dense than the surrounding medium will float, and those more dense will sink. Salt water is denser than fresh water because of the much greater amount of dissolved substances. Therefore, a person will float more easily in salt water because there is a greater difference between the density of the person's body and that of the water.

11. **The correct answer is (B).** Two parameters are directly proportional if their ratio is a mathematical constant $(K = \dfrac{x}{y})$.

12. **The correct answer is (A).** Cellular proteins are synthesized at the ribosomes where codon triplets of m-RNA are paired with anticodon triplets of t-RNA to direct amino acid sequences.

13. **The correct answer is (C).** Insulin increases the permeability of the cell membrane to glucose, thus increasing the rate of glucose uptake by the cells from the bloodstream. Adrenalin promotes an increase in cardiac activity, respiratory rate, and the breakdown of glycogen (stored in the liver) to glucose, thus raising the glucose level of the blood. With physical activity, glucose is more rapidly utilized by cells, which must remove glucose from the blood, thus reducing the blood level of glucose.

14. **The correct answer is (B).** The digestion and absorption of most nutrients occurs in the *duodenum*, the first portion of the small intestine. Therefore, digestive juices are most active at this site.

15. **The correct answer is (C).** The term *cold-blooded* is commonly used in reference to animals such as reptiles that depend on external sources of heat to help regulate their body temperature. Cold-blooded animals, more properly called *ectotherms*, must bask in sunlight or lie on warm ground to raise their body temperature. Conversely, they must lie in the shade or shelter beneath an object such as a rock to cool off their bodies. By contrast, warm-blooded animals, more properly called *endotherms*, are more or less independent of external sources of heat, relying on a combination of heat generated by their metabolism and insulation on the surface of the body to keep their internal temperature constant.

16. **The correct answer is (C).** Chromosomes contain genetic material, or carry genes; the separation of the chromosomes of each pair is involved in *meiosis*, or reduction division, in the production of sexual reproductive cells. The *gametes* (egg and sperm) will each receive one half the chromosomes carried by the parent, or one chromosome of each pair carried by the parent. Thus, the gametes will be *haploid*. When fertilization occurs, the zygote becomes *diploid*, having received one chromosome of each pair from each parent. Therefore, each individual inherits one half of its chromosomes and genes from its father and one half from its mother.

17. **The correct answer is (A).** A *hertz* can be defined as the number of wavelengths per second. A wave or wavelength is the distance between successive values, for example, from crest to crest. The diagram shows four waves in the one-second period, or four hertz.

18. **The correct answer is (A).** Light consists of colors of varying wavelengths. Visible light ranges from red, with a wavelength of about 7,000 angstrom units, down to violet, with a wavelength of about 4,000 angstroms. Ultraviolet has shorter wavelengths (150–3,900 Å) and is bactericidal; the highest bactericidal activity occurs between 2,000 Å and 3,000 Å.

19. **The correct answer is (B).** The lens is concave; therefore, it is thicker at the edges. Light rays passing through a concave lens are refracted or bent outward, so they spread apart. A light ray passing through the center of the lens is not bent.

20. **The correct answer is (B).** The functional group for ethers is R-O-R.

21. **The correct answer is (A).** Visible light consists of different colors of light, producing a spectrum of red (with the longest wavelength), orange, yellow, green, blue, indigo, and violet (with the shortest wavelength).

22. **The correct answer is (D).** White light consists of the colors or wavelengths of the visible spectrum— red, orange, yellow, green, blue, indigo, and violet. An object appears to be a certain color when it is reflecting light of this wavelength, and absorbing all others. A white object is reflecting all of the colors or wavelengths at the same time.

23. **The correct answer is (C).** Liver glycogen, which is a polymer of glucose molecules, is called animal starch.

24. **The correct answer is (B).** Persons with sickle cell anemia carry a variant hemoglobin molecule in the red blood cells, instead of the normal hemoglobin A. The production of hemoglobin is under genetic control.

25. **The correct answer is (B).** All elements listed are found in cells. Carbon, hydrogen, and phosphorus are three of the six major elements from which most organic molecules are built. Potassium is one of the five essential minor elements.

26. **The correct answer is (C).** An *ampere* (amp) is a unit for measuring the rate of flow of electricity. A *watt* is the metric unit of power; it is the power produced by 1 amp in a I volt circuit. Thus, the formula *watt* = *amp* × *volt*, can be used, or *amp* = $\frac{watt}{volt}$. If the problem is worked using this formula, the answer is choice (C), 16 amps.

27. **The correct answer is (C).** Photosynthesis is the process by which an organic, energy-containing compound (sugar or glucose) is produced from inorganic materials. This is a process basic to the production of organic compounds that can be used for food. Algae and other green plants exhibit photosynthesis.

28. **The correct answer is (B).** A half of the dosage is 5×10^{-5}M.

29. **The correct answer is (D).** Cytokinesis is the stage in eukaryotic cell division in which the cytoplasm divides to produce daughter cells.

30. **The correct answer is (D).** Efficiency is the ratio of work-out per work-in.

31. **The correct answer is (B).** Eukaryotic cells have high efficiency, relative to mechanical device. They are capable of extracting approximately 50 percent of the energy in glucose molecules for biological work.

32. **The correct answer is (C).** Vector quantities must have both magnitude and direction for complete description. An object cannot have a velocity without direction.

33. **The correct answer is (A).** The equation $E = mc^2$ demonstrates mass and energy are interchangeable and that small amounts of mass can yield large amounts of energy under specific conditions.

34. **The correct answer is (B).** The overproduction of the thyroid hormones causes a condition known as exophthalmic goiter, or Graves' disease. The thyroid may or may not be enlarged, but increased metabolic rate, protrusion of eyes (exophthalmus), increased blood pressure, increased heart rate, loss of weight, etc., are symptoms of Graves' disease. This disease may be treated by surgical removal or destruction of part of the thyroid gland.

35. **The correct answer is (D).** A person of blood group AB has antigen A and antigen B, but cannot produce antibodies against A or B. Therefore, such a person can receive blood from any of the four blood groups and is often called a "universal recipient."

36. **The correct answer is (B).** The Schick Test, developed by Bela Schick, is administered by injecting a weak solution of the diphtheria toxin cutaneously. A reddening of the site of injection indicates susceptibility to diphtheria; lack of reddening indicates immunity and the presence of sufficient antitoxin to protect the person against diphtheria.

37. **The correct answer is (B).** *Evaporation* is the physical change of a substance from a liquid to a gas. The rate of movement of gas molecules into the air is more rapid in dry air or when the humidity is low, and decreases with increased humidity. The movement of air currents (wind) carries away the vapor above the surface of the liquid, thus increasing evaporation rate.

38. **The correct answer is (B).**

39. **The correct answer is (C).** Of the 17 atoms making up a molecule of $Al_2(SO_4)_3$, there are two atoms of aluminum, three atoms of sulfur, and twelve atoms of oxygen (four oxygens in each of the three sulfate ions). The weight of the oxygen is 192; the total weight of the molecule is 342. Thus, the percentage of oxygen by weight is $\frac{192}{342}$, or 56 percent.

40. **The correct answer is (D).** To determine genotype of a hybrid, a pure recessive is always used in a test backcross. Any dominant trait carried by the hybrid parent will be expressed in some of the offspring; the recessive traits will also be expressed in some of the offspring, since the recessive parent cannot produce a dominant to mask it. Ratios and phenotypes will indicate the genotype of the hybrid parent.

41. **The correct answer is (C).** A microscope field 2 mm in diameter is 2,000Φ. Paramecia (50Φ) could be placed 40 side-by-side across the field.

42. **The correct answer is (C).** Reptiles do not possess a diaphragm, but have the other structures listed.

43. **The correct answer is (C).** Sodium chloride is an ionic substance that dissociates in aqueous solutions, to give 2 times the number of particles per mole as molecular substances such as glucose.

44. **The correct answer is (B).** Inertia is the tendency of a body at rest or in motion to remain constant unless acted upon by an outside force.

45. **The correct answer is (B).** Permease are cellular proteins that transport substances across plasma membranes.

46. **The correct answer is (A).** In a food chain, algae are the primary "producers," occupying the bottom level of the food chain since they produce organic materials through photosynthetic processes. Insect larvae are some of the animals that can feed on algae; fish, which prey on animals such as insect larvae, are in turn consumed by humans.

47. **The correct answer is (A).** Grasses are usually pollinated by wind; the grass flower typically does not attract insects or birds. Since grasses are mostly land plants, water would not play a significant role in their pollination.

48. **The correct answer is (A).** The *ectoderm* is the outer germ layer, which gives rise to the nervous and integumentary systems of the embryo.

49. **The correct answer is (B).** Only green plants can produce organic materials (food) from inorganic materials (carbon dioxide and water) through the process of photosynthesis. Oxygen and a by-product are returned to the air by means of this process. Animals may consume green plants (direct dependence) or may consume animals that consume green plants (indirect dependence) for food and energy.

50. **The correct answer is (C).** Evolution. This illustrates the concept of survival-of-the-fittest from a bacterial population.

51. **The correct answer is (D).** One mole (gram molecular weight) of nitrogen is 28 grams, since two nitrogen atoms form a nitrogen molecule (N_2). One mole of gas occupies a volume of 22.4 liters at standard conditions.

52. **The correct answer is (B).** The frequency, or number of vibrations per second, determines pitch, or tone. The greater the frequency, the higher the pitch; the lower the frequency, the lower the pitch.

53. **The correct answer is (A).** In DNA and RNA molecules, adenine (A) must pair with thymine (T) or uracil (U). Guanine (G) always pairs with cytosine (C). This specificity is based on complementarity of molecular geometry, relative to the formation of double or triple bonds.

54. **The correct answer is (C).** The NH^+ species has a positive valence, which has affinity for a negative chloride (Cl^-) ion.

55. **The correct answer is (A).** Cancer of the cervix

56. **The correct answer is (B).** Boyle's Law illustrates the relationship between the pressure and volume of a mass of gas at a fixed temperature. The law can be simply stated: at a given fixed temperature and mass of gas, pressure, and volume are inversely proportional. For example, volume will increase as pressure decreases, or volume will decrease as pressure increases. Therefore, pressure $\times$ volume = a constant.

57. **The correct answer is (B).** Peas and beans are members of the legume family and have nitrogen-fixing bacteria in nodules on their roots. Nitrogen-fixing bacteria convert atmospheric gaseous nitrogen into nitrates, thus restoring nitrates to the soil. It is only in the form of nitrates that plants generally can obtain nitrogen from the soil.

58. **The correct answer is (A).** The male sex chromosome is referred to as the Y chromosome. It is inherited only by male offspring; thus, a male is XY and a female is XX, as far as inheritance of sex is concerned. Therefore, any gene located on the Y chromosome is inherited only by males since females will inherit an X from the male parent.

59. **The correct answer is (B).** Oxidation-reduction reactions are those in which one substance is oxidized by the loss of electrons, and another substance is reduced by the gain of electrons. In double replacement reactions, this does not occur. Ions are exchanged between reactants and do not lose or gain electrons.

60. **The correct answer is (B).** The cross indicates that the parents were heterozygous blacks (1 black and 1 white allele). The cross would yield 1 homozygous black, 2 heterozygous blacks, and 1 homozygous white offspring.

61. **The correct answer is (D).** The mitochondrion is called the powerhouse of the cell; most of the respiratory process involving the release of energy occurs in this organelle.

62. **The correct answer is (B).** Reproductive isolation is the major criterion for determination of speciation.

63. **The correct answer is (A).** Oxygen is a waste product of photosynthesis. Green plants use carbon dioxide and water as raw materials to produce sugar in the presence of chlorophyll and sunlight as follows:

$$CO_2 + H_2O \xrightarrow[\text{chlorophyll}]{\text{sunlight}} C_6H_{12}O_6 + O_2$$

64. **The correct answer is (C).** *Egestion* is the elimination of undigested wastes from the digestive tracts or cavity: enzymes are not involved in this process but are involved in the other processes named.

65. **The correct answer is (A).** Chloroplasts contain the chlorophylls, the green pigments, and are characteristic of green plants but not of animals.

66. **The correct answer is (A).** In the absence of oxygen, plants and microbes convert pyruvic acid into alcohol and carbon dioxide by a process called fermentation.

67. **The correct answer is (A).** The cell wall and plastids are characteristic of plant cells but not of animal cells. A nucleus may not be present in some cells, such as mature human red blood cells. But all cells have cytoplasm surrounded by a plasma or cell membrane.

68. **The correct answer is (A).** Digestion in humans occurs primarily in the lumen of the stomach and small intestine where macromolecules are degraded to small molecules capable of being absorbed.

69. **The correct answer is (B).** A virus does not exhibit reproduction, synthesis, and other characteristics of life outside a living host cell; thus, it is an obligate intracellular parasite.

70. **The correct answer is (A).** At the initiation of the reaction, all substances are reactants (A and B).

71. **The correct answer is (D).** The affinity of A and B is greater than that of C and D, resulting in a greater concentration of product than reactants at equilibrium.

72. **The correct answer is (D).** The reaction is shifted to the left.

73. **The correct answer is (C).** The human body is an open system—exchanging nutrients, CO_2 and O_2, nitrogenous waste, water, and heat with the external environment.

74. **The correct answer is (D).** 30,000

75. **The correct answer is (C).** Chromosome 21

READING COMPREHENSION

TECHNIQUES OF READING INTERPRETATION

Reading comprehension presents problems to many test-takers. To avoid this, make every effort to improve your ability to interpret reading passages.

First, understand that there are two aspects of success in reading interpretation:

1. reading speed

2. reading understanding

Too many individuals read with excellent comprehension but read too slowly. Remember, there is a time limit on your test. On the other hand, some people read rapidly, but, for reasons that we shall cite later, do not thoroughly understand what they are reading. Both speed of reading and comprehension of the material read are important during an exam. Let us, then, divide our discussion into two parts:

1. increasing reading speed

2. improving reading comprehension

GENERAL ADVICE

You were probably taught to read letter-by-letter. Gradually, as you matured, you learned to read word-by-word. As an adult, however, you should be able to read a complete phrase as quickly as you once read just one letter. If you cannot do this, or if you have trouble understanding what you read, you should practice reading intensively.

There is no need to be discouraged if this is the case. Most students can increase the speed of their reading significantly with little effort. The old idea that slow readers make up for their slowness by better comprehension of what they read has been proved untrue. Your ability to comprehend what you read should keep pace with your increase in speed. You can absorb as many ideas per page, and get many more ideas per unit of reading time, by applying specific techniques of reading.

It has been demonstrated that those who read best also read quickly. This is probably due to the fact that heavier concentration is required for rapid reading, and concentration is what enables a reader to grasp important ideas contained in the reading material.

A good paragraph generally has one central thought—that is, a *topic sentence*. Your main task is to locate and absorb that thought while reading the paragraph. The correct interpretation of the paragraph is based upon that thought, and not upon your personal opinions, prejudices, or preferences. If a selection consists of two or more paragraphs, its correct interpretation is based on the central idea of the entire passage. The ability to grasp the central idea of a passage can be acquired by practice—practice that will also increase the speed with which you read.

An important rule to follow in order to improve reading ability is to force yourself to increase your speed. Just as you once stopped reading letter-by-letter, now learn to stop reading word-by-word. Force yourself to read rapidly across the line of type, skimming it. Don't permit your eyes to stop for individual words; try instead to reconstruct the whole idea even if a word has been missed. Proceed quickly through the paragraph in this skimming fashion, without rereading or backtracking to a missed word.

If you find yourself failing to comprehend what you read, read the material over several times rapidly until you do understand. Do *not* slow down on rereading. At first, you may find yourself missing some of the ideas. With persistent practice, however, you will step up both your reading speed and your ability to comprehend.

You may need to overcome certain handicaps or unhelpful reading habits at once. Do not move your lips, pronounce words individually silently or aloud, or think of each word separately as you read. These habits can be overcome almost automatically if you learn to leap from phrase to phrase. You can synchronize your eye movements with your mind, both of which are nimbler than your lips.

Certain physical factors affect reading. You should always read sitting in a comfortable position, erect, with head slightly inclined. The light should be excellent, with both an indirect and a direct source available; direct light should come from behind you and slightly above your shoulder, in such a way that the type is evenly lit. Hold the reading matter at your own best reading distance and at a convenient height, so you don't stoop or squint. If you need reading glasses, you should certainly use them.

INCREASING READING SPEED: CAUSES OF AND CURES FOR SLOW READING

Cause 1: Word-by-word reading.
Our earliest reading, since it is done aloud, is, of necessity, word-by-word reading. Unfortunately, this method of reading sometimes becomes so firmly implanted that it persists as a bad reading habit.

Cure: Use the *eye-span method.*
Look at the first part of a sentence that consists of a thought-unit. Then, look for the next thought-unit, if there is another one in the same sentence—then, look for still another thought-unit. For example, consider this sentence:

Reading maketh a full man, conference a ready man, and writing an exact man. How many ideas are there in the sentence? Three. Now, employ the eye-span method in reading this sentence.

Reading maketh a full man,
    EYE-SPAN 1

conference a ready man,
    EYE-SPAN 2

and writing an exact man.
    EYE-SPAN 3

Cause 2: Vocalizing.
Some readers move their lips or whisper while they read "silently." This practice slows down silent reading time considerably.

Cure
You must consciously refrain from moving your lips or whispering during silent reading. Have someone watch you while you read. Are you vocalizing?

Cause 3: One-speed reading.
You should vary your reading speed according to what you are reading.

Cure
The pace of your reading should change not only from book to book, but even within a reading selection. Be flexible so that you can change speed from paragraph to paragraph, even from sentence to sentence. Adjust your reading rate according to the purpose for which you are reading. Scanning a passage for main ideas may be accomplished with rapid reading. Reading a novel for enjoyment would allow you to read at a medium rate. Reading to obtain detailed information would require you to read at a slower pace.

INCREASING READING COMPREHENSION
The following are good techniques to use on *any* reading interpretation question.

1. Read the selection through quickly to get the general sense.

2. Reread the selection, concentrating on the central idea.

3. Attempt to pick out the *topic sentence* in each paragraph.

4. If the selection consists of more than one paragraph, determine the *central idea* of the entire selection.

5. Examine the four choices for each test item carefully yet rapidly. Eliminate immediately those choices that are far-fetched, ridiculous, irrelevant, false, or impossible.

6. Eliminate those choices that may be true but have nothing to do with the sense of the selection.

7. Check those few choices that now remain as possibilities.

8. Refer back to the original selection and determine which one of these remaining possibilities is best in view of
   a. information *stated* in the selection
   b. information *implied* in the selection

9. Be sure to consider only the facts *given* or *definitely implied* in the selection.

10. Be especially careful of trick expressions or catch-words, which sometimes destroy the validity of a seemingly acceptable answer. These include the expressions "under all circumstances," "at all times," "always," "under no conditions," "absolutely," "completely," and "entirely."

Avoid Traps

Trap 1
Sometimes the questions cannot be answered on the basis of the stated facts. You may be required to make a deduction from the facts given. Making a deduction requires you to draw conclusions from something already known.

Trap 2
Some reading passages are designed to arouse the reader's emotion, or describe situations with which the reader can identify. Be certain to base an answer selection on the information presented in the passage. Eliminate your personal opinions.

Trap 3

Many questions, and the appropriate responses to these questions, are based on important details that are nestled in the paragraph. Reread the paragraph as many times as necessary (keeping an eye on your watch) to find significant facts that will provide answers to the questions.

Get Plenty of Practice
Read:

1. editorial pages of various newspapers

2. book, drama, and movie reviews

3. magazine articles

For each selection that you read, do the following:

1. Jot down the main idea of the article.

2. Look up the meanings of words of which you are unfamiliar or unsure.

A Sample Question
Here is a sample question followed by analysis. Try to understand the process of arriving at the correct answer.

> Too often, indeed, have scurrilous and offensive allegations by underworld figures been sufficient to blast the careers of irreproachable and incorruptible executives who, because of their efforts to serve the people honestly and faithfully, incurred the enmity of powerful political forces and lost their positions.

Judging from the contents of the preceding sentence, which conclusion might be most valid?

- **(A)** The large majority of executives are irreproachable and incorruptible.
- **(B)** Criminals often swear in court that honest officials are corrupt in order to save themselves.
- **(C)** Political forces are always clashing with government executives.
- **(D)** False statements by criminals sometimes cause honest officials to lose their positions or ruin their careers.

Interpretation
Choice (A) can generally be said to be a true statement, but it cannot be derived from the paragraph. Nothing is said in the paragraph about "the large majority" of executives.

Choice (B) may also be a true statement and can, to a certain extent, be derived from the paragraph. However, the phrase "in order to save themselves" is not relevant to the sense of the paragraph, and even if it were, this choice does not sum up its central thought.

Choice (C) cannot be derived from the paragraph. The catch-word "always" makes this choice entirely invalid.

Choice (D) is the best conclusion that can be drawn from the contents of the paragraph, in light of the four choices given. It is open to no exceptions and adequately sums up the central thought of the paragraph.

Analysis of the Reading Comprehension Test Item

There are standardized tests designed to assess reading comprehension skills and provide an evaluation of the test-taker's independent reading level, instructional reading level, frustration reading level, and reading rate. Reading comprehension test items usually elicit a response that would indicate the test-taker's ability to identify directly stated details; indirectly stated details; main ideas; inferences; and generalizations. Other target skills may include making judgments, drawing conclusions, and determining the author's purpose.

There are two types of reading comprehension test items. The first type is a long reading passage, usually a few paragraphs in length, followed by a series of questions. The second type is a short passage, usually a single paragraph in length, alongside one question. Several paragraphs in succession may treat the same topic, but the questions will always deal with the adjacent paragraph.

In order to determine your reading rate, the proctor will tell test-takers to stop after exactly 1 minute of exam time. Test-takers will then be asked to mark the point at which they were reading when they were told to stop, and this marking will be used for the determination.

Sample Questions 1

The sample long reading passage below, followed by a set of 6 questions, will help you to analyze comprehension test items and to understand why a particular response is the correct or appropriate one.

Studying the questions before reading a passage will cause you to be more alert when reading the passage; that is, you will be aware of what information in the passage will best help you answer the questions. Now read the 6 questions at the end of the passage and then read the passage and answer the questions. Note that the questions are followed by explanations that indicate the skill addressed and strategies to use in your approach to a particular type of question.

"The Land of Frost and Fire" is no misnomer for the elliptic island republic in the North Atlantic known as Iceland. The island is so called because erupting volcanoes and steaming hot springs lie adjacent to its glaciers and ice fields. The official name of the country in Icelandic is Lydveldid Island, or the Republic of Iceland.

The "frost" is frigidly evident in the island's numerous ice fields that traverse the hoary landscape. Approximately one eighth of the island is covered by glaciers. In the southeast, a glacier known as Vatnajokull makes an area of about 8,550 square kilometers (about 3,300 square miles). Iceland, just south of the Arctic Circle, has more than 120 glaciers.

Lydveldid Island's "fire" leaps from the many hot springs and spouting geysers that cloud the panorama of the seventeen-province republic. To add heat to the "fire" are some one hundred volcanoes, including at least twenty-five that have erupted and been recorded in the annals of the island's autocratic history. Lava and rocks erupting from volcanoes have contoured much of the land. The central highlands reflect the barren wilderness of lava fields. Hekla, in the southwest, is the best-known Icelandic volcano because of its many eruptions. The years 1766, 1940, 1947, and 1980 mark its explosive appearances.

Thermal springs are also common in Iceland. The springs occur as geysers, sizzling mud lakes, and various other forms. The most famous geyser here is Great Geysir, which is situated in southwest Iceland. The natives of this island of swift-flowing rivers boast of Geysir's spectacular and frequent eruptions occurring at irregular intervals of 5 to 36 hours. The torrid spring reportedly thrusts a column of boiling water upward to about 60 meters or 200 feet.

Volcanic in origin, Iceland is indeed a land of contrast. Dazzling ice and jet black lava covering most of Iceland's surface attest to the appropriateness of its nickname—"Land of Frost and Fire."

1. Where are Iceland's hot springs and geysers located?

   (A) In the central highlands
   (B) In the southwest
   (C) Next to the glaciers
   (D) In the southeast

The correct answer is (C). This is a directly stated detail question. When answering this type of question, always consider the *wh* word with which the question begins. *Who* can be answered by the name of a person. *When* is answered by a word or phrase that tells at what time or in what sequence something happens. *Why* is answered by a word or phrase that tells the reason something happens. *What* is usually answered by the name of a thing or event. *Which* is answered by choosing the correct person, place, or thing from two or more persons, places, or things. *Where* is answered by the name of a place or a phrase that describes the location of one person or thing in relation to another (spatial relationships). Finally, *how* should be considered with these question words. *How* is answered by the way in which something is done. Question 1 is a *where* question denoting a spatial relationship. The correct answer is (C). Since adjacent means "next to" and encompasses the location of both the glaciers and geysers, this is the appropriate response. Choices (A), (B), and (D) could be ruled out immediately because they do not describe the location of both the glaciers and the geysers.

2. An appropriate title for this passage would be

   (A) Volcanoes and Geysers.
   (B) Iceland: The Island Republic.
   (C) Iceland: A Land of Contrast.
   (D) Thermal Springs.

The correct answer is (C). This is a main idea question. This type of question requires the test-taker to consider what the passage is mostly about. Read the question first. Then scan the entire passage to find out what it is mostly about. A word of caution: Some answer choices are merely details from the passage. It is not difficult to choose (C) as the best title.

3. It is apparent that this passage is intended to

   (A) inform.
   (B) entertain.
   (C) persuade.
   (D) share an experience.

The correct answer is (A). The skill addressed in this question is identifying author's purpose. The test-taker must determine what the author is trying to accomplish by writing this selection. What kind of response does he or she want from the reader? If the reader can say that he or she enjoyed this passage or thought it was hilarious, obviously the passage was meant to entertain. If the reader's reaction is, "Well, I think I'll try that," or "I have to agree with that," then the passage was written to persuade. If the passage is a narration or a storytelling written in the first person (I, me, my, myself—all references to the writer), the passage is probably aimed at sharing an experience. If the reader's reaction is, "I didn't know that," or "I never heard of this before," there is a good chance that the author intended to inform.

4. The sentiments of people of Iceland toward the presence of geysers in their native land is one of
   (A) mixed emotions.
   (B) pride.
   (C) dread and fear.
   (D) indifference.

The correct answer is (B) This question requires the test-taker to infer a meaning or idea. In other words, "read between the lines." In the fourth paragraph of this passage, it is mentioned that the natives "boast of Geysir's spectacular and frequent eruptions." Usually, people boast about something when they are proud of it. The correct response would therefore be choice (B), "pride."

5. According to this passage, Iceland's form of government at one time reflected
   (A) total rule by the state.
   (B) rule by and for the people.
   (C) rule by royalty.
   (D) rule by dictator.

The correct answer is (D). This test question is an example of indirectly stated detail. In paragraph three of this passage the phrase "the annals of the island's autocratic history" appears. The adjective "autocratic," though irrelevant to the main idea of the passage, and even to the sentence in which it appears, does provide an informational detail. The term autocratic suggests government by one person having unlimited power. The correct answer, therefore, would be (D), "rule by dictator." In completing this type of question, the test-taker should scan the passage to eliminate answer choices that are obviously related to the main idea. In some cases, the reader should also be careful of negative words in the question (no, not, not any).

6. Iceland is a difficult place to
   (A) grow crops.
   (B) raise a family.
   (C) get an education.
   (D) start a business.

The correct answer is (A). Question 6 requires that you make a judgment or draw a conclusion. Since the passage does not mention family life, education, or industry, it would be safe to eliminate choices (B), (C), and (D). The passage also does not mention agriculture; however, it does describe the land as being "barren wilderness" and "covered by glaciers." These conditions are unsuitable for farming. Therefore, (A), "grow crops," is an appropriate answer.

Sample Questions 2

Below are two sample short reading passages and questions, followed by analyses of the test items. Try to determine the answers on your own before reading the explanation.

A

At birth, you more than likely weighed less than 10 pounds. As an adult you may weigh anywhere from 90 to 200 pounds or more. Obviously, there is much more of you as an adult. Despite your growth, the cells that make up your adult body are no larger than those that made up your body in infancy. This means that your adult body has billions more cells. You might question the source of these new cells. To satisfy your curiosity, they came from old cells via a process known as cell division.

31. The main idea of Paragraph A:

   (A) Most infants weigh less than 10 pounds.
   (B) Growth in human beings is accomplished by cell division.
   (C) Living cells increase in number by a process called cell division.
   (D) The cells that make up an adult body are larger than those of an infant body.

B

At a certain time during its existence, a cell divides into two cells. At the start of cell division, the nucleus becomes more dense and grainier than it was earlier. The grainy material, known as chromatin, eventually divides into short, cordlike structures called chromosomes. The chromosomes travel through the cell, forming a double line near the center of the cell.

32. As a result of the movement of chromosomes through the cell,

   (A) a grainy material is formed.
   (B) a cell divides into two cells.
   (C) the chromatin divides into short, cordlike structures.
   (D) a double line of them is formed near the center of the cell.

C

Boatmen who catch wild fish and shellfish are often more strictly regulated than seafood farmers, whose wholesome image has helped them resist government oversight. But after eight years of discussion, shrimp farmers around the world are considering adoption of a universal certification process that would require them to comply with standards on the siting of ponds, effluent treatment, the reduction of chemicals, and disease management. In exchange, their products would be labeled eco-friendly. By 2004, labels indicating whether seafood is farmed or wild will become mandatory in the U.S. (though they won't be required on restaurant menus). Jason Clay, 51, a senior fellow at World Wildlife Fund who helped develop the standards, is optimistic that they will be accepted. "As the industry gets more competitive, those who survive will be those who do it better and cleaner," he says.

—Copyright © 2002 Time Inc. Reprinted by permission.
From *Time*, Nov. 25, 2002. "A Fishy Business,"
by Terry McCarthy and Campbell River.

33. "Effluent" may be defined as

 (A) wealthy.
 (B) a fluid or liquid state.
 (C) flowing out from a larger body of water.
 (D) bubbling.

Question 31

The correct answer is (B). In question 31, you are clearly asked to find the main idea of Paragraph A. This means that you are to consider what the paragraph is mostly about. If you chose (B), "Growth in human beings is accomplished by cell division," you have cited the correct response. A review or second reading of the paragraph will show that choice (A) could be supported by the paragraph; however, you should question the word "most." This statement merely provides a detail that leads to the principal concept. Choice (C) is factual, but it only supplies a major detail to the overall concept. Choice (D), according to the paragraph, is incorrect information since the passage states that "despite your growth, the cells that comprise your adult body are no larger than those that made up your body in infancy." Choice (B) most clearly ties together the two remaining details, choices (A) and (C), and states what the paragraph is mostly about.

Question 32

The correct answer is (D). In question 32, the word "result" indicates a cause/effect response ("result" and "effect" are synonymous in this case). The paragraph clearly states that "the chromosomes travel through the cell, forming a double line near the center of the cell" (paraphrase: *causing* a double line to form). A review of the paragraph would prove that adding any of the activities described in choices (A), (B), or (C) to the question stem would not yield the proper sequence of the cell division process.

Question 33

The correct answer is (C). If you're thinking Paragraph C is definitely a short passage reading comprehension question, you're right. If you're saying to yourself, "but this looks like a verbal ability question," you're right again! Reading comprehension is closely related to and dependent upon the understanding of words that test authors often include; verbal ability questions are often integrated into reading comprehension test items. This type of question requires you to think in terms of the precise meaning of a word as used in the passage. We call the answer to this question "vocabulary in context." It may be beneficial to you to review Unit I: Verbal Ability of this study guide.

As for the answer to question 33, you should begin by eliminating choice (A). There is clearly no mention of money or financial assets in this passage. Choice (B) is also doubtful since only larger bodies of water are mentioned rather than the liquid state of matter. Choice (D) hints that the author is trying to trick you with the resemblance of the word effervescent to effluent. Recalling "Increased Word Power from Beginning to End" in the Verbal Ability unit, take the word "effluent" apart. Remember that the stem *flu* means flowing and that the prefix *e-* means out or out from.

READING IN THE CONTENT AREA

Efficient reading requires that the reader be flexible. As you read earlier in this unit ("Increasing Reading Speed"), it is necessary to adjust your reading rate according to the purpose for which you are reading. It is equally important to adapt your reading style to the material being read. Before investigating effective strategies to use in making such reading adjustments, it is necessary to examine and recognize the structure and patterns of writing unique to each subject area. This study of various reading materials will help you get a feel for their differences and determine which reading style to apply to any given reading task.

Reading comprehension test items are frequently designed to reflect the course content of the field of study targeted by the entrance examination. For instance, entrance exams for educational programs leading to health careers may feature reading passages that treat scientific topics and information.

Unlike the humanities—which deal with emotions, attitudes, and sympathies of human beings via the study of philosophy, religion, music, art, and literature—science is the accumulation of knowledge by means of the study, observation, and classification of data justifiable by general laws or concrete truths. Scientists look for and acquire information regarding forms and processes of nature. They search for an undistorted view of reality and, therefore, cannot allow their values, feelings, attitudes, beliefs, and prejudices—or those of society—interfere with their work.

Due to the nature of the subject matter, a scientist's writings follow a certain style. Descriptions are very exacting, factual, and detailed. They are void of background mood or setting, and are unemotional. As you read scientific material, you must concentrate on the following reading skills:

1. Developing vocabulary

2. Finding the main concepts

3. Determining and remembering supporting details

4. Understanding the organization or major pattern of writing in science (examination, classification, generalization, problem solution, comparison or contrast, sequence)

5. Drawing conclusions

A review of the Verbal Ability section of this book will provide strategies for understanding and developing specialized scientific vocabulary. One method encourages vocabulary expansion through the use of a glossary, dictionary, thesaurus, etc., as well as through context clues. Another encourages the recognition of words that stand for concepts instead of facts. Other approaches include the study of word roots and affixes and the recognition of symbols.

The design or style of the text in science reading materials makes finding the main concepts simple. There are usually titles, opening comments in boldface type, headings, a summary, and questions at the end of the chapter or chapter section. In your initial reading, read only the text features just listed. This will allow you to explore and get a sense of the main ideas presented in the chapter, article, or selection. It will also prepare you for a second and closer reading.

Once you have identified the main ideas in a scientific passage, the next step in understanding what you are reading is to determine the supporting details. Supporting details answer the who, what, why, where, and when surrounding the main idea. Ask yourself these questions once you have completed a paragraph. In science, you should also question how much or to what extent.

Understanding the organization or major pattern of writing in science is vital to your reading comprehension. First of all, you should concentrate on examining the material you are about to read *before* you actually read it. Know the topic(s) that will be addressed and sum up the vocabulary in the particular reading selection. Next, identify the writing pattern that stands out in the material. There are four patterns:

Classification places into groups and subgroups a variety of objects or areas. For instance, in the explanation of plant life, a writer may outline the classification of plants. The breakdown could begin with vascular and nonvascular and seedless nonvascular plants. From here the author could branch out to descriptions of mosses and liverworts, etc. In this pattern, watching for structural parts in order of importance is a must. Be aware of subheadings and all boldface type.

Process-description requires you to be aware of what the process is and exactly how it works. Studying illustrations and diagrams is helpful in this pattern.

Factual-statement involves the presentation of facts to define, compare or contrast, and illustrate. When reading for facts, remember that "fact" in the world of science means a statement that can be supported by scientific observation and experimentation and that has not yet been disproved. A fact defines something or explains its actions.

Problem-solving usually appears in science passages that give an account of past scientific problems and discoveries achieved through experimentation. There are 3 helpful questions that you should ask yourself when analyzing a problem-solving passage: (1) What is the problem or question? (2) How does the author answer or respond to the question? (3) How do I know the question was answered?

Drawing conclusions is basic to the study of the sciences. A sound conclusion is a judgment based on facts. Consider what you need to know in order to make a sound judgment about something you read. Check the given facts. Think about what these facts are based on (experimentation, observation, etc.) to make certain of their reliability. Then consider the facts that are not given. Reread the passage to gather information that may be implied rather than stated. This method should help you in your test-taking venture. Speaking of tests, by now you have probably drawn some conclusions about the entrance exam you are about to take, and about the specialized vocabulary that may appear on it. However, do not conclude that scientific reading material is extremely difficult; instead, think of it as a kind of reading material that requires a very different approach.

ANSWER SHEET

TEST 1

1. Ⓐ Ⓑ Ⓒ Ⓓ
2. Ⓐ Ⓑ Ⓒ Ⓓ
3. Ⓐ Ⓑ Ⓒ Ⓓ
4. Ⓐ Ⓑ Ⓒ Ⓓ

5. Ⓐ Ⓑ Ⓒ Ⓓ
6. Ⓐ Ⓑ Ⓒ Ⓓ
7. Ⓐ Ⓑ Ⓒ Ⓓ
8. Ⓐ Ⓑ Ⓒ Ⓓ

9. Ⓐ Ⓑ Ⓒ Ⓓ
10. Ⓐ Ⓑ Ⓒ Ⓓ
11. Ⓐ Ⓑ Ⓒ Ⓓ
12. Ⓐ Ⓑ Ⓒ Ⓓ

13. Ⓐ Ⓑ Ⓒ Ⓓ
14. Ⓐ Ⓑ Ⓒ Ⓓ
15. Ⓐ Ⓑ Ⓒ Ⓓ

TEST 2

1. Ⓐ Ⓑ Ⓒ Ⓓ
2. Ⓐ Ⓑ Ⓒ Ⓓ

3. Ⓐ Ⓑ Ⓒ Ⓓ
4. Ⓐ Ⓑ Ⓒ Ⓓ

5. Ⓐ Ⓑ Ⓒ Ⓓ
6. Ⓐ Ⓑ Ⓒ Ⓓ

7. Ⓐ Ⓑ Ⓒ Ⓓ
8. Ⓐ Ⓑ Ⓒ Ⓓ

TEST 3

1. Ⓐ Ⓑ Ⓒ Ⓓ
2. Ⓐ Ⓑ Ⓒ Ⓓ
3. Ⓐ Ⓑ Ⓒ Ⓓ

4. Ⓐ Ⓑ Ⓒ Ⓓ
5. Ⓐ Ⓑ Ⓒ Ⓓ

6. Ⓐ Ⓑ Ⓒ Ⓓ
7. Ⓐ Ⓑ Ⓒ Ⓓ

8. Ⓐ Ⓑ Ⓒ Ⓓ
9. Ⓐ Ⓑ Ⓒ Ⓓ

TEST 4

1. Ⓐ Ⓑ Ⓒ Ⓓ
2. Ⓐ Ⓑ Ⓒ Ⓓ
3. Ⓐ Ⓑ Ⓒ Ⓓ

4. Ⓐ Ⓑ Ⓒ Ⓓ
5. Ⓐ Ⓑ Ⓒ Ⓓ
6. Ⓐ Ⓑ Ⓒ Ⓓ

7. Ⓐ Ⓑ Ⓒ Ⓓ
8. Ⓐ Ⓑ Ⓒ Ⓓ

9. Ⓐ Ⓑ Ⓒ Ⓓ
10. Ⓐ Ⓑ Ⓒ Ⓓ

TEST 5

1. Ⓐ Ⓑ Ⓒ Ⓓ
2. Ⓐ Ⓑ Ⓒ Ⓓ

3. Ⓐ Ⓑ Ⓒ Ⓓ
4. Ⓐ Ⓑ Ⓒ Ⓓ

5. Ⓐ Ⓑ Ⓒ Ⓓ
6. Ⓐ Ⓑ Ⓒ Ⓓ

7. Ⓐ Ⓑ Ⓒ Ⓓ
8. Ⓐ Ⓑ Ⓒ Ⓓ

TEST 6

1. Ⓐ Ⓑ Ⓒ Ⓓ
2. Ⓐ Ⓑ Ⓒ Ⓓ

3. Ⓐ Ⓑ Ⓒ Ⓓ
4. Ⓐ Ⓑ Ⓒ Ⓓ

5. Ⓐ Ⓑ Ⓒ Ⓓ
6. Ⓐ Ⓑ Ⓒ Ⓓ

TEST 1

15 QUESTIONS ▪ TIME—35 MINUTES

Directions: Carefully read the following paragraphs and then answer the accompanying questions, basing your answer on what is stated or implied in the paragraphs. When you have decided which choice is best, fill in the corresponding space on your answer sheet. There is only one best answer for each question.

Taking It to Heart

A

Prior to 1628, when William Harvey published his book on the circulation of the blood and the operation of the heart, no one really knew or understood the function of the heart or how it worked. There was some speculation about it having something to do with the blood; however, people generally thought of it as the place in the body from which love and courage were generated.

B

Until Harvey's discovery, no one was aware that the heart is one of the toughest muscles in the human body and one of the most awesome pumps in the world. It is the heart that pumps the blood throughout the body night and day. This mighty muscle, though only the size of a clenched fist, does enough work in one 24-hour period to lift a man weighing 150 pounds to an altitude of almost 1,000 feet into the air.

C

Actually, the heart is two pumps, side by side—one on the right and one on the left. The right pump sends blood from the veins to the lungs. Then it pumps blood through the lungs to the pump on the left, which sends it through the body.

1. Based upon paragraph A, which of these statements is true?
   - **(A)** One function of the heart is to generate love and courage in a human being.
   - **(B)** The purpose and function of the heart was not understood until 1628.
   - **(C)** Harvey published a book that dealt with performing operations on the heart.
   - **(D)** The fact that the heart is instrumental in the circulation of the blood is merely speculation.

2. According to paragraph B, it is understood that
   - **(A)** the heart is a muscle that pumps blood throughout the body.
   - **(B)** Harvey discovered the heart.
   - **(C)** the heart can lift a man weighing 150 pounds to a height of 1,000 feet.
   - **(D)** all muscles in the human body perform as pumps.

3. The main idea of paragraph C is that
   - **(A)** the right pump of the heart sends blood from the veins to the lungs.
   - **(B)** the pumps that make up the heart are situated side by side.
   - **(C)** the left pump sends the blood through the body.
   - **(D)** the heart is two pumps that work to send blood throughout the body.

GO ON TO THE NEXT PAGE

D

Although the right- and left-hand sides of the heart are two different pumps with no direct connection between them, they squeeze and relax in just about the same rhythm. Together they pump approximately 13,000 quarts of blood through the body daily.

E

The most amazing thing about the heart is that it continues beating throughout life, resting only a fraction of a second after each beat. Considering that this entails 100,000 beats per day, the durability of this organ is undoubtedly phenomenal.

4. Paragraph D makes the point that
    (A) the human body contains 13,000 quarts of blood.
    (B) despite the fact that they squeeze and relax in just about the same rhythm, the two pumps do not have a connection.
    (C) the rhythm of the two pumps is synchronized.
    (D) the two pumps operate as one.

5. Which statement is supported by paragraph E?
    (A) The third part of the heartbeat is a period of rest.
    (B) A steady heartbeat is characteristic of a strong and healthy heart.
    (C) The heart beats about 70 times per minute.
    (D) You can easily detect your own heartbeat.

The Skin You're In

F

The first thing you see when you look at the human body is the skin. The average adult human body is covered with about 18 square feet of skin. Skin varies in thickness. It is very thin over the eyelids and considerably thicker on the palms of the hands and the soles of the feet.

G

The skin is composed of two layers. The outer layer of skin is called the epidermis. This name comes from ancient Greek meaning "outer layer." This layer is made up of dead, flattened cells that are continually sloughing off as we move around. The bottom of the epidermis is made of live cells that die and replace those that wear off on the surface. Throughout the body's lifetime, the under layer of skin continually creates new cells. This is the reason why cuts and scrapes heal in a short period of time.

H

Beneath the outer layer is another layer called the dermis. This is a much deeper layer made entirely of living cells. There are several small blood vessels and nerve endings in the dermis. There are coiled tubes in this layer that open into the epidermis layer through openings called pores. The pores are openings to the coiled tubes or sweat glands. Hairs, which grow out of the skin, are rooted in the dermis. They grow out of openings called hair follicles. Oil glands in the skin connected with the hair roots constantly oil the outer skin, keeping it supple and strong.

6. From paragraph F, the reader can conclude that
    (A) the skin is the one organ readily visible on the human body.
    (B) adults have thicker skin than children.
    (C) skin on the human body is thicker on parts of the body most likely to come in contact with foreign objects and surfaces.
    (D) 18 square feet of skin would be adequate to cover and protect all adult human beings.

7. From paragraph G, it may be inferred that

(A) that the production of new cells constitutes healing in the human being.

(B) the ancient Greeks were probably the first to study skin.

(C) the bottom of the epidermis is comprised of flattened cells that gradually wear away.

(D) skin is the organ responsible for growth in the human body.

8. Which statement is supported by paragraph H?

(A) The skin needs oil to remain pliant and durable.

(B) The coiled tubes in the epidermis are actually pores.

(C) Dry skin may be an indication of a problem in the hair follicle.

(D) The epidermis provides the body with adequate temperature control.

I

The functions of the skin are numerous. The skin is a protective covering for the body that is airtight and waterproof. When it is unbroken it is a barrier to harmful bacteria. The coloring matter of the skin, known as pigment, serves to screen out certain harmful rays of the sun. The skin helps to regulate the temperature of the body and also functions as a sense organ. There are many nerve endings in the skin that caution us to stay away from things that are too hot or too cold and cause us to have a sense of touch. They enable us to detect sensation in our immediate surroundings and transmit impulses to the brain where the sensations are identified.

9. According to paragraph I, it is understood that

(A) skin coloring is the result of harmful rays of the sun.

(B) sensations are directly perceived by the skin.

(C) the function of the skin is merely that of a protective covering.

(D) the skin is a deterrent to harmful bacteria only if it is unbroken.

Nursing Interventions

J

The term "nursing interventions" encompasses and describes activities that reflect nursing responsibility in the execution of health treatment. More specifically, it refers to nursing treatments, nursing observations, health teaching, and medical treatment performed by nurses. A nursing intervention is a single course of action intended to fulfill the unmet human needs that are ascertained from the patient's problem. A nursing diagnosis is, therefore, a prerequisite to implementing the appropriate care to meet the needs of the patient. It is apparent that in order to determine and initiate nursing intervention, one must have a scientific background and extensive education in nursing.

10. The main idea of paragraph J is that

(A) the role of an individual who has a scientific and nursing education background, and who performs a single course of action to satisfy the unmet human needs of a patient, is known as nursing intervention.

(B) a nursing diagnosis is synonymous with nursing intervention.

(C) nursing responsibility includes health teaching.

(D) nursing assessment is necessary for effective nursing intervention.

GO ON TO THE NEXT PAGE

Blood Donors Available—No Thanks!
I'll Do It Myself!

K

With the advent of AIDS and other communicable diseases, people are reluctant to submit to blood transfusions as a measure of medical treatment, even in emergency situations. Many individuals are opting to store their own blood in case it is ever needed.

L

New blood cells are constantly being produced in the body. This is the reason that lost blood in a healthy person is replaced quickly. This rapid production of blood cells also enables a person to donate to others who might need blood. When blood is taken from one person and given to another, the procedure is called a homologous blood transfer. When a person's own blood is used for transfusion, having been stored in anticipation of surgery, the procedure is known as autologous blood transfer. This blood is collected prior to surgery.

M

Though the concept of being transfused with one's own blood is very comforting, there are many factors that discourage the use of this technology. First is the expense of storing the blood. It has been estimated that the cost of safely storing the blood comes to approximately $200 per year. Another drawback is that a patient may be thousands of miles away from his or her blood supply or blood bank when the need for blood arises.

11. The accelerated interest in autologous transfusion is due to
    - (A) a lack of blood donors.
    - (B) an attempt to stimulate rapid production of new blood cells.
    - (C) the time-saving element in the event of emergency surgery.
    - (D) a rise in fear of communicable diseases.

12. This passage supports the concept that
    - (A) autologous transfer is a practical and easily accessible alternative to blood transfusion.
    - (B) any type of blood transfusion places a patient in a high-risk health situation.
    - (C) hemoglobin carries oxygen and carbon dioxide throughout the body.
    - (D) lost blood, even in a healthy person, is replaced only after a long period of time.

13. From this passage it may be inferred that
    - (A) saline is a cleansing or sterilizing agent.
    - (B) the storing of one's own blood supply is affordable for all.
    - (C) homologous transfusion requires blood typing and matching.
    - (D) the option of autologous transfusion is not feasible in instances of elective surgery.

N

In an attempt to satisfy patients' requests to be transfused with their own blood, regardless of the medical emergency, doctors have developed two forms of autologous blood transfusion. One form utilizes suction devices to collect blood lost during surgery. After this blood has been cleansed, it may be put back into the body. Blood lost during surgery can also be collected with sponges. The sponges are then squeezed out into a container of saline solution, a kind of salt solution. This blood is processed within 15 minutes and is again introduced into the patient's circulation. Doctors believe that by using both methods they can retrieve up to 90 percent of blood that would otherwise be lost.

O

Despite these efforts to make autologous blood transfer feasible for most patients, there still remain those situations that make it virtually impossible to collect blood. For instance, in the case of an auto accident victim, much blood is often lost before medical treatment is obtainable. To help in an incident such as this, doctors are researching ways to develop artificial hemoglobin that would temporarily transport oxygen and carbon dioxide throughout the body. Another solution being explored is the reproduction of a hormone that causes the body to produce blood cells much more rapidly than it would normally. This would mean that the body could replace most of its own blood and therefore reduce the need for transfusion. Even though researchers are doing extensive work to develop new techniques to protect people from blood tainted by disease, reserving one's own blood for future use seems to be the safest method of transfusion for now.

14. A fact expressed in this passage is that

    (A) artificial hemoglobin could permanently supply the body with oxygen and carbon dioxide.

    (B) suction devices and sponges are two surgical implements used in the collection of blood lost during surgery.

    (C) laser surgery is being used more frequently in an effort to minimize blood loss during surgery.

    (D) autologous transfusion, in the event of surgery, requires that the blood always be collected prior to surgery.

15. This article suggests that

    (A) homologous transfusions are on the decline.

    (B) the effort by researchers to protect patients from blood contaminated by disease cannot guarantee safe blood transfusion.

    (C) autologous transfusion is impractical.

    (D) surgical patients who are transfused autonomously are assured a more rapid recovery.

STOP If you finish before time is called, you may check your work on this section only. Do not turn to any other section in the test.

TEST 2

8 QUESTIONS ■ TIME—12 MINUTES

Directions: Carefully read the following passage and then answer the accompanying questions, basing your answers on what is stated or implied in the passage. When you have decided which choice is best, fill in the corresponding space on your answer sheet. There is only one best answer for each question.

Live and Learn

A

It has been a difficult year. As our country and the world continue to cope with the aftermath of September 11, 2001, some people have boldly chosen to take their lives back. Many others, though, are finding it extremely difficult to move on.

1. Paragraph A implies that the events of September 11, 2001 were

    (A) devastating.
    (B) unavoidable.
    (C) pragmatic.
    (D) intolerable.

2. The event(s) alluded to impacted

    (A) nationally.
    (B) globally.
    (C) positively.
    (D) moderately.

B

It is troubling that thousands of lives were taken in a heartbeat, and now we're witnessing a domino effect across the globe as a result of the attacks on America. It's no secret that the U.S. is an ally of Israel and that this position has been the fuel for terrorist attacks on our soil. But war in the Middle East has been brewing for years, so now we explore other issues that contribute to the conflict.

3. According to the writer, the loss of lives was

    (A) instantaneous.
    (B) by heart malfunction.
    (C) ephemeral.
    (D) predictable.

C

Are immigration and integration in Palestine to blame? What about U.S. dollars going to Israel? Or Muslim extremists? Whatever the reasons, every nation is adjusting its policies to ready themselves for what might be coming. Recently, the United States and a bloc of Southeast Asian nations signed a treaty aimed at making the region—a second front in the war against terrorism—more responsive to future threats. Sadly, it took a tragedy of this magnitude to get America to realize that it's not invincible and that we really are living in an interdependent world.

4. It is suggested that the attacks of 9/11 may be directly related to

    (A) the on-going Middle East oil dispute.
    (B) the absence of a treaty between the United States and Southeast Asian nations.
    (C) Palestinians' hatred of the United States.
    (D) U.S. aid to and friendship with Israel.

5. America's realization of its vulnerability

    (A) has prompted Middle East peace talks.
    (B) has resulted in more gun control laws.
    (C) is a significant outcome of 9/11.
    (D) has resulted in relaxed national security.

6. The author mentions "domino effect" to describe

(A) the falling of the towers.

(B) the mass physical destruction that came out of this event.

(C) the far-reaching consequences that stem from 9/11.

(D) the political turmoil that was caused by 9/11.

D

The nation's economy is in a serious slump. The failures of such high-performing companies as Enron, and the government investigations of others, including AOL Time Warner and MCI WorldCom, Inc., which was charged with fraud after the company admitted to hiding almost $4 billion in costs, has contributed to the stock market nosedive.

E

The ripple effects of the U.S. economic woes are widespread. Stress is on the rise for good reasons. The Dow Jones industrial average recently reached its largest weekly decline (nearly 700 points) since last September. Retirees are having to re-enter the work force, and who doesn't know someone who's recently lost his or her job? People continue to file claims for unemployment insurance, and a study released roughly four months after the attacks predicted that the effects of the more than 1.6 million jobs that will probably be lost in 2002 will reverberate through the U.S. economy for years to come.

F

The jobless are penny-pinching and postponing vacations, which is a dire dilemma for many tourism-dependent nations. Caribbean countries like Jamaica and St. Lucia are expected to lose $3 billion tourism revenue—money that is normally used for health care and other services and accounts for roughly 70 percent of the gross domestic product of many Caribbean countries.

G

Everyone has been affected by September 11 in one way or another. Even though we've struggled through the past year, we, as Americans, are truly blessed. What is most important now is to accept what has taken place, and to learn and grow from it. It takes faith, and it is that faith that has guided our people for centuries. So take pride in this country and help make it a better place for you and your children.

—Reprinted with permission of Upscale from Founder's Desk, Live and Learn, by Bernard Bronner, Founder. Upscale, October 2002.

7. The tragedy of 9/11 has

(A) left all of humankind emotionally scarred.

(B) drastically changed our lives and the way we view life.

(C) helped the economy rally.

(D) strengthened relations between the United States and the Middle East.

8. The attitude of the author is one of

(A) defeat.

(B) hopefulness.

(C) indifference.

(D) despair.

STOP   If you finish before time is called, you may check your work on this section only. Do not turn to any other section in the test.

TEST 3

9 QUESTIONS ▪▫ TIME—12 MINUTES

Directions: Carefully read the following passage and then answer the accompanying questions, basing your answers on what is stated or implied in the passage. When you have decided which choice is best, fill in the corresponding space on your answer sheet. There is only one best answer for each question.

Is It Your Fault If You're Fat?

A

Why are more Americans overweight and developing diabetes? Is it fast food? No regular meals and precious little exercise? Our love affair with the TV and computer? The wrong advice about what to eat?

B

Very likely it's all these things—combined with something about the genetic make-up in many of us. Genes may program some to feel hungry when they aren't and others to be less able to tell when they are full.

1. The generalization could be made that obesity is caused

    (A) by eating fast foods.
    (B) lack of exercise.
    (C) lack of education as to which foods to eat.
    (D) lifestyle and genetic make-up.

2. People are programmed to feel hungry (when they actually are not) by

    (A) therapists.
    (B) genes.
    (C) nutritional counseling.
    (D) dining trends.

C

Some extreme obesity in children is caused by an identifiable, single gene defect. Obesity is no more their "fault" than developing cystic fibrosis is the "fault" of a child who has the CF gene. Admittedly, perhaps only 5 percent of obesity is purely genetic. But research suggests that multiple genes control appetite and metabolism, and defects in one or more may make someone more prone to being overweight. Fat cells, particularly in the abdomen, in turn release substances that can make people more prone to insulin resistance, which leads to Type 2 diabetes.

D

Some people are genetically blessed and never gain much weight. Those with gene defects must expend huge effort to overcome messages their bodies are sending their brains to eat more.

3. People who are more prone to insulin resistance are

    (A) candidates for stomach problems.
    (B) those with no weight problem.
    (C) those who are likely to develop Type 2 diabetes.
    (D) in danger of becoming obese.

4. When great effort is put forth, people with gene defects can

    (A) overcome urges to eat more.
    (B) overcome diabetes.
    (C) live a normal life.
    (D) be overweight.

5. The author's purpose in this passage is to
- **(A)** inform.
- **(B)** persuade.
- **(C)** entertain.
- **(D)** analyze.

E

For example, research at Rockefeller University and elsewhere suggests that people who lack leptin or lack receptors to make their cells sensitive to leptin have uncontrolled hunger, overeat, and become extremely obese. The melanocortin pathway in the brain has recently been identified by scientists at Beth Israel Deaconess Medical Center and elsewhere as another target influencing both obesity and anorexia.

F

In addition, some researchers have shown that the absence of a peptide called MSH, which suppresses eating, leads to obesity. Research at Joslin Diabetes Center in Boston and elsewhere suggests that another peptide, MCH, which stimulates eating, may also play a role.

6. Researchers have found that
- **(A)** an overabundance of leptin causes obesity.
- **(B)** the absence of a certain substance in the body results in uncontrolled eating.
- **(C)** MHS is a peptide.
- **(D)** overeating is a habit.

7. Obesity may be defined as
- **(A)** fat.
- **(B)** a state of being significantly overweight.
- **(C)** a genetic condition.
- **(D)** a disease related to overeating.

G

Ghrelin, a stomach hormone that signals hunger, is another potential target. Interestingly, extremely obese individuals who undergo stomach bypass surgery (stomach stapling) may be less inclined to eat afterwards because food no longer passes through the section of the stomach that produces ghrelin.

H

Some overeating may be triggered by stress, boredom, or depression. For example, food smells may stimulate production of certain peptides that make one want to eat—even if not hungry. Behavior modification may be needed to combat these stimulants of weight gain.

I

As our genes haven't changed in the last 20–30 years, societal influences are still the major culprit for growing obesity. We are more sedentary. Super-sizing meals makes it harder not to eat for those trying mightily to ignore the errant signals their bodies are sending. Until we can identify who has what gene defects, and the medications are developed to treat them, we must remember that it is much easier to prevent weight gain than to lose weight once gained. Your body adjusts quickly to these extra calories.

J

Life as overweight adults often has its roots in life as a child. For the moment, the best approach to obesity, and the type 2 diabetes it causes, is prevention—in ourselves and our children. As nationwide studies show, even modest weight loss—15 pounds—and 30 minutes of daily exercise, are the best ways to prevent diabetes in those most likely to develop it.

GO ON TO THE NEXT PAGE

8. The main idea of this passage is
   (A) overeating can be controlled with diet and exercise.
   (B) diabetes is related to obesity.
   (C) current research reveals a number of contributing factors to obesity.
   (D) there are cures for obesity.

9. From this passage one can draw the conclusion that
   (A) being overweight is unhealthy.
   (B) children, too, can have weight problems.
   (C) being fat may not necessarily be the fault of the obese individual.
   (D) obesity can be attributed solely to genetics.

STOP If you finish before time is called, you may check your work on this section only. Do not turn to any other section in the test.

TEST 4

10 QUESTIONS   ▪   TIME—13 MINUTES

Directions: Carefully read the following passage and then answer the accompanying questions, basing your answers on what is stated or implied in the passage. When you have decided which choice is best, fill in the corresponding space on your answer sheet. There is only one best answer for each question.

With the recent use of DNA (deoxyribonucleic acid) as a means of providing evidence in a number of world-renowned criminal cases, the general public views this carrier of genetic information as a modern day scientific discovery. However, a glimpse at the history of DNA will prove the notion of a "modern day miracle" quite to the contrary.

To investigate the discovery of DNA, one would have to research the laboratory and work of the Swiss biochemist, Johan Friedrich Miescher, back in 1868. Miescher had been involved in the study of the cell nucleus, the round control center that contains the chromosomes as well as other elements. He believed that cells were made of protein and attempted to break down this protein with a digestive enzyme. As Miescher continued this investigation, he was perplexed by the fact that the enzyme would break down the cell but not the nucleus. He then launched an investigation of the substance that comprised the cell. As he analyzed it, he saw that it contained large amounts of a strange material that was very unlike protein. Miescher chose to call this substance nuclein. He had no idea of its significance, nor did he recognize that he had discovered what came to be known in later years as nucleic acid. Nucleic acid is the chemical family to which DNA belongs.

In 1944 a team of scientists from the Rockefeller Institute proved for the first time that DNA was the carrier of hereditary information. Oswald T. Avery, Colin M. MacLeod, and Maclyn McCarty accomplished this by extracting some of the DNA in pure form from a bacterium and substituting it for a defective gene in another related bacterium.

Some ten years later, the intricate molecular structure of DNA was described by Harvard biochemist James D. Watson and physicist Francis Crick of Great Britain. However, prior to this, scientist Rosalind Franklin discovered that the DNA molecule was a strand of molecules in a spiral form. Dr. Franklin demonstrated that the spiral was so large that it was most likely formed by two spirals. Ultimately, Franklin determined that the structure of DNA is similar to the handrails and steps of a spiral staircase.

Equipped with the work and findings of Rosalind Franklin and others, Watson and Crick were able to construct a model of a DNA molecule. This model depicted the sides or "handrails" of the DNA molecules as being made up of two twisted strands of sugar and phosphate molecules. The "stairs" that hold the two sugar phosphate strands apart are made up of molecules called nitrogen bases.

All of this data supports the fact that DNA is by no means a "new discovery"; however, what is the significance of it at all? Why is DNA important to you? The answer is that all of the characteristics you possess are affected by the DNA in your cells. It controls the color of your eyes, the color of your hair, and whether or not you have a tolerance for dairy products. These characteristics are known as traits. The way your traits appear depends on the kinds of proteins your cells make. DNA stores the blueprints for making the proteins. Your DNA is uniquely different from that of anyone else on earth, and you are identifiable by these proteins.

GO ON TO THE NEXT PAGE

1. It could be concluded that

   (A) Watson and Crick discovered DNA.
   (B) the strands of DNA take the form of a double hexagon.
   (C) DNA is as unique to individuals as a fingerprint.
   (D) Miescher's analysis of nuclein resulted directly in the discovery of DNA.

2. From this passage, it may be deduced that enzymes are

   (A) unstable.
   (B) ineffective.
   (C) catalysts.
   (D) solutions.

3. It may be inferred that an individual's DNA determines

   (A) whether or not he or she can digest milk.
   (B) whether or not he or she is immune to the common cold.
   (C) an individual's choice of residential location.
   (D) a person's inclination toward dishonesty.

4. The types of protein produced by a cell are controlled by the DNA contained in its

   (A) nitrogen bases.
   (B) nucleus.
   (C) cell wall.
   (D) sugar phosphate bands.

5. It is implied that proteins are

   (A) the control center of the cell.
   (B) the blueprint of the cell.
   (C) the storage center of the cell.
   (D) the building blocks of a cell.

6. A reference to the "spiral staircase" constitutes a description of

   (A) the molecular structure of proteins.
   (B) the molecular structure of digestive enzymes.
   (C) the molecular structure of RNA.
   (D) the molecular structure of DNA.

7. Digestive enzymes are effective in breaking up

   (A) nuclein.
   (B) DNA.
   (C) all chemical compounds.
   (D) protein.

8. The word "nucleus" refers to

   (A) the round control center of the cell.
   (B) the walls of the cell.
   (C) a strand of molecules.
   (D) a helix.

9. The scientific disciplines used in determining the structure of the DNA molecule include biology, chemistry, and

   (A) genealogy.
   (B) serology.
   (C) physics.
   (D) embryology.

10. As described in this passage, "model" means

    (A) an exhibitor of fashion.
    (B) a physical form representing a concept.
    (C) a miniature version of an existing object.
    (D) a person on whom an artist bases his or her rendition.

STOP   If you finish before time is called, you may check your work on this section only. Do not turn to any other section in the test.

TEST 5

8 Questions ▪▫ Time—8 Minutes

Directions: Carefully read the following passage and then answer the accompanying questions, basing your answers on what is stated or implied in the passage. When you have decided which choice is best, fill in the corresponding space on your answer sheet. There is only one best answer for each question.

Computer Watch Your Step

A

Can a computer spot a criminal or a terrorist infiltrating an airport tarmac? Face-recognition programs are useless if a person's face is obscured, unlit, or just too far away. So a number of researchers are trying to identify a person simply by the way he or she walks.

B

One approach is to collect video images of the surveillance area and analyze everybody passing through. "We've been trying to measure things like stride length and body shapes," says Aaron Bobick, a computer vision researcher at Georgia Tech in Atlanta. Video cameras still require good light and a clear view, however, so Gene Greneker at the Georgia Tech Research Institute is experimenting with radar. "It can see through clothes, at night, at long ranges," he says.

1. The title of this article
   (A) cautions computers to watch their step.
   (B) cautions readers to watch their step.
   (C) implies that computers will be able to observe the way people walk.
   (D) implies that computers are a threat.

2. "Surveillance" means
   (A) hidden.
   (B) obscure.
   (C) large surface.
   (D) official watch.

3. It is implied that
   (A) radar may be an alternative to problems encountered with video cameras.
   (B) good light and clear vision are attainable with video cameras.
   (C) computer vision researchers at Virginia Tech are advancing surveillance technology.
   (D) it will be a long time before this technology is available.

4. The video cameras
   (A) sweep a designated area.
   (B) view the perimeter of the area to be inspected.
   (C) collect images that pass through the surveillance area.
   (D) have zoom lenses that capture close-ups of people in the surveillance area.

GO ON TO THE NEXT PAGE ➤

C

Greneker and his team use a device that sends out a signal and measures the echo. If the return waves shift to higher frequencies, that means they reflected off something approaching. "There are different shifts for different body parts, because they are moving at different velocities," Greneker says. A computer program analyzes these shifts and creates a radar fingerprint for each person's walk. So far researchers have collected gait profiles of about 100 test subjects, which the program can identify up to 80 percent of the time. That is not nearly good enough for airport security, but Bobick is convinced gait recognition can be made to work. "If I show you moving light displays of people walking, you can distinguish one person from the next. We know the information is there."

—Reprinted with permission from *Discover*, "Computer Watch Your Step" by Fenella Saunders, Discover Special Issue: The Year in Science, January 2003.

5. The device used by Greneker and his team
   (A) lowers the frequencies.
   (B) sends out a signal and measures the echo.
   (C) shifts different body parts.
   (D) changes the velocities.

6. The identification accuracy is
   (A) very high.
   (B) moderately low.
   (C) average.
   (D) moderately high.

7. The researchers have
   (A) approved the device for airport security.
   (B) not been able to distinguish one person from the next.
   (C) completed their study.
   (D) gathered gait profiles of subjects.

8. "Gait" most nearly means
   (A) style of walking.
   (B) fence.
   (C) door.
   (D) speed of walking.

STOP If you finish before time is called, you may check your work on this section only. Do not turn to any other section in the test.

TEST 6

6 QUESTIONS ▪□ TIME—8 MINUTES

Directions: Carefully read the following passage and then answer the accompanying questions, basing your answers on what is stated or implied in the passage. When you have decided which choice is best, fill in the corresponding space on your answer sheet. There is only one best answer for each question.

A

During my stay at an expensive hotel in New York City, I woke up in the middle of the night with an upset stomach. I called room service and ordered some soda crackers. When I looked at the charge slip, I was furious. I called room service and fumed, "I know I'm in a luxury hotel, but $11.50 for six crackers is outrageous!"

B

"The crackers are complimentary," the voice at the other end coolly explained. "I believe you are complaining about your room number."

—Reprinted with permission from the January 2003 *Reader's Digest*, "Life in these United States" by Robert Menchim.

1. The purpose of this reading selection is to

    (A) persuade.
    (B) explain.
    (C) entertain.
    (D) inform.

2. It may be assumed that

    (A) the writer does not have sufficient reading comprehension skills.
    (B) the format of the bill included several numbers and was difficult to interpret.
    (C) room service had made an error.
    (D) the hotel guest is frugal.

3. The word "complimentary" means that the crackers were

    (A) well suited to the hotel guest.
    (B) served with other crackers.
    (C) free.
    (D) not to be ordered.

4. The author's tone in the call to room service is

    (A) humorous.
    (B) one of outrage.
    (C) sarcastic.
    (D) bland.

5. The author implies that

    (A) the anticipated services were costly at this particular hotel.
    (B) all New York hotels are expensive.
    (C) the hotel was substandard.
    (D) the hotel was not one of his choice.

6. An appropriate title for this story would be

    (A) You Get What You Pay For.
    (B) Quality and Price Are Synonymous.
    (C) A Room at the Top.
    (D) Look Before You Leap.

STOP   If you finish before time is called, you may check your work on this section only. Do not turn to any other section in the test.

ANSWER KEY

Test 1

1. **B**	5. **C**	9. **D**	13. **A**
2. **A**	6. **C**	10. **A**	14. **B**
3. **D**	7. **A**	11. **D**	15. **B**
4. **B**	8. **A**	12. **C**	

Test 2

1. **A**	3. **A**	5. **C**	7. **B**
2. **B**	4. **D**	6. **C**	8. **B**

Test 3

1. **D**	4. **A**	6. **B**	8. **C**
2. **B**	5. **A**	7. **B**	9. **C**
3. **C**			

Test 4

1. **C**	4. **B**	7. **D**	9. **C**
2. **C**	5. **D**	8. **A**	10. **B**
3. **A**	6. **D**		

Test 5

1. **C**	3. **A**	5. **B**	7. **D**
2. **D**	4. **C**	6. **D**	8. **A**

Test 6

1. **C**	3. **C**	5. **A**
2. **B**	4. **B**	6. **A**

PART III

PRACTICE FOR ALLIED HEALTH SCHOOL ENTRANCE EXAMINATIONS

VERBAL ABILITY

ANSWER SHEET

TEST 1: SYNONYMS

1. Ⓐ Ⓑ Ⓒ Ⓓ	8. Ⓐ Ⓑ Ⓒ Ⓓ	15. Ⓐ Ⓑ Ⓒ Ⓓ	22. Ⓐ Ⓑ Ⓒ Ⓓ	29. Ⓐ Ⓑ Ⓒ Ⓓ
2. Ⓐ Ⓑ Ⓒ Ⓓ	9. Ⓐ Ⓑ Ⓒ Ⓓ	16. Ⓐ Ⓑ Ⓒ Ⓓ	23. Ⓐ Ⓑ Ⓒ Ⓓ	30. Ⓐ Ⓑ Ⓒ Ⓓ
3. Ⓐ Ⓑ Ⓒ Ⓓ	10. Ⓐ Ⓑ Ⓒ Ⓓ	17. Ⓐ Ⓑ Ⓒ Ⓓ	24. Ⓐ Ⓑ Ⓒ Ⓓ	31. Ⓐ Ⓑ Ⓒ Ⓓ
4. Ⓐ Ⓑ Ⓒ Ⓓ	11. Ⓐ Ⓑ Ⓒ Ⓓ	18. Ⓐ Ⓑ Ⓒ Ⓓ	25. Ⓐ Ⓑ Ⓒ Ⓓ	32. Ⓐ Ⓑ Ⓒ Ⓓ
5. Ⓐ Ⓑ Ⓒ Ⓓ	12. Ⓐ Ⓑ Ⓒ Ⓓ	19. Ⓐ Ⓑ Ⓒ Ⓓ	26. Ⓐ Ⓑ Ⓒ Ⓓ	33. Ⓐ Ⓑ Ⓒ Ⓓ
6. Ⓐ Ⓑ Ⓒ Ⓓ	13. Ⓐ Ⓑ Ⓒ Ⓓ	20. Ⓐ Ⓑ Ⓒ Ⓓ	27. Ⓐ Ⓑ Ⓒ Ⓓ	34. Ⓐ Ⓑ Ⓒ Ⓓ
7. Ⓐ Ⓑ Ⓒ Ⓓ	14. Ⓐ Ⓑ Ⓒ Ⓓ	21. Ⓐ Ⓑ Ⓒ Ⓓ	28. Ⓐ Ⓑ Ⓒ Ⓓ	35. Ⓐ Ⓑ Ⓒ Ⓓ

TEST 2: ANTONYMS

1. Ⓐ Ⓑ Ⓒ Ⓓ	7. Ⓐ Ⓑ Ⓒ Ⓓ	13. Ⓐ Ⓑ Ⓒ Ⓓ	19. Ⓐ Ⓑ Ⓒ Ⓓ	25. Ⓐ Ⓑ Ⓒ Ⓓ
2. Ⓐ Ⓑ Ⓒ Ⓓ	8. Ⓐ Ⓑ Ⓒ Ⓓ	14. Ⓐ Ⓑ Ⓒ Ⓓ	20. Ⓐ Ⓑ Ⓒ Ⓓ	26. Ⓐ Ⓑ Ⓒ Ⓓ
3. Ⓐ Ⓑ Ⓒ Ⓓ	9. Ⓐ Ⓑ Ⓒ Ⓓ	15. Ⓐ Ⓑ Ⓒ Ⓓ	21. Ⓐ Ⓑ Ⓒ Ⓓ	27. Ⓐ Ⓑ Ⓒ Ⓓ
4. Ⓐ Ⓑ Ⓒ Ⓓ	10. Ⓐ Ⓑ Ⓒ Ⓓ	16. Ⓐ Ⓑ Ⓒ Ⓓ	22. Ⓐ Ⓑ Ⓒ Ⓓ	28. Ⓐ Ⓑ Ⓒ Ⓓ
5. Ⓐ Ⓑ Ⓒ Ⓓ	11. Ⓐ Ⓑ Ⓒ Ⓓ	17. Ⓐ Ⓑ Ⓒ Ⓓ	23. Ⓐ Ⓑ Ⓒ Ⓓ	29. Ⓐ Ⓑ Ⓒ Ⓓ
6. Ⓐ Ⓑ Ⓒ Ⓓ	12. Ⓐ Ⓑ Ⓒ Ⓓ	18. Ⓐ Ⓑ Ⓒ Ⓓ	24. Ⓐ Ⓑ Ⓒ Ⓓ	30. Ⓐ Ⓑ Ⓒ Ⓓ

TEST 1: SYNONYMS

35 QUESTIONS ▬▭ TIME—20 MINUTES

(Please review Unit 1 through Synonyms before attempting this test.)

Directions: In each sentence below, one word is italicized. For each sentence, select the option that best (or most nearly) corresponds in meaning with the italicized word.

1. It has been recommended that this system be used in place of *traditional* types.

    (A) unfamiliar
    (B) usual
    (C) flexible
    (D) general

2. In our society, irresponsible behavior often leads to a monetary *penalty*.

    (A) arrangement
    (B) gratification
    (C) punishment
    (D) precaution

3. He spent the *allotted* study time completing his assignments.

    (A) authorized
    (B) designated
    (C) agreed
    (D) alerted

4. The Senate passed the farmland *preservation* bill.

    (A) maintenance
    (B) stratagem
    (C) exordium
    (D) incumbency

5. It was apparent that he had attempted to *concoct* an alibi.

    (A) inculcate
    (B) conceal
    (C) reveal
    (D) fabricate

6. The City Council could have avoided this *scenario* by passing the ordinance.

    (A) preliminary plan
    (B) obliteration
    (C) veneration
    (D) deficiency

7. The Superior Court judge *imposed* the sentence.

    (A) indicated
    (B) granted
    (C) perpetuated
    (D) inflicted

8. The researchers will run a *comparative* series of tests.

    (A) objective
    (B) relative
    (C) subjective
    (D) scientific

9. Geologists *assure* us that our earth is a few billion years old.

    (A) guarantee
    (B) instruct
    (C) inform
    (D) advise

10. He was determined to *foil* the scheme of his opponent.

    (A) heighten
    (B) secure
    (C) disencumber
    (D) thwart

11. The examiner *purported* to be an official representative.

   (A) addressed
   (B) claimed
   (C) propitiated
   (D) conciliated

12. The ship carried refugees of every *persuasion*.

   (A) mediocrity
   (B) sort
   (C) prospectus
   (D) compendium

13. The child could not *recollect* the incident.

   (A) remember
   (B) dubitate
   (C) interrogate
   (D) illumine

14. The Supreme Court *rescinded* the law.

   (A) complicated
   (B) inveigled
   (C) revoked
   (D) accepted

15. The implementation of the plan was given *scant* consideration.

   (A) audacious
   (B) fervid
   (C) little
   (D) clothed

16. The key speaker, in his lengthy presentation, *scoffed* at religion.

   (A) exonerated
   (B) amplified
   (C) confuted
   (D) mocked

17. She completed the *sprint* with a sudden surge of energy.

   (A) relaxation
   (B) adventure
   (C) run
   (D) convergence

18. The content of the message was *urgent*.

   (A) privileged
   (B) amendable
   (C) pressing
   (D) absolved

19. A *simulated* rescue mission was conducted by the forest rangers.

   (A) pretended
   (B) superficial
   (C) stimulated
   (D) simultaneous

20. A *histamine* is released from the tissues when the cells are injured.

   (A) a histone
   (B) an amine
   (C) a stimulant
   (D) an isoenzyme

21. Her quickening gait seemed regulated by the *pulse* of the big city.

   (A) utility
   (B) pace
   (C) reverence
   (D) solace

22. The language of the publication is *unsophisticated* but informative.

   (A) ponderous
   (B) elaborate
   (C) simple
   (D) superficial

23. All the evidence presented pointed to *willful* execution of a crime.

   (A) deliberate
   (B) eminent
   (C) amicable
   (D) remorseful

24. There is no *provision* for deadlines in the contract.

   (A) improvement
   (B) convenience
   (C) aggregation
   (D) stipulation

GO ON TO THE NEXT PAGE

25. The furnishings *impart* an air of elegance to the room.

(A) communicate
(B) indemnify
(C) reinforce
(D) disguise

26. She exhibited great *valor* in handling the emergency.

(A) ingeniousness
(B) courage
(C) discretion
(D) optimism

27. Various courses were *fused* in the revision of the curriculum.

(A) required
(B) implicated
(C) combined
(D) involved

28. Production of complex molecules is accomplished by *replication*.

(A) duplication
(B) synthesis
(C) fixation
(D) reproduction

29. The task of choosing one from so many qualified applicants *bewildered* the employer.

(A) perplexed
(B) aggravated
(C) subdued
(D) infuriated

30. The revision of the city plan incorporated adjustments in the projected *modes* of transportation.

(A) increments
(B) expenditures
(C) means
(D) modifications

31. The politician sought to *aggrandize* himself at the expense of the people.

(A) exhaust
(B) subjugate
(C) sacrifice
(D) exalt

32. The newcomer made an effort to *mingle* with the crowd.

(A) argue
(B) mix
(C) disrupt
(D) flout

33. If an organization's programs were described as *philanthropic*, the programs would be

(A) primitive
(B) deleterious
(C) extraneous
(D) benevolent

34. If the traits of a nation's leader were *covetous*, they were

(A) greedy
(B) exemplary
(C) disparate
(D) adventitious

35. Rabbits *breed* offspring rapidly.

(A) raise
(B) gather
(C) propagate
(D) destroy

S T O P If you finish before time is called, you may check your work on this section only. Do not turn to any other section in the test.

TEST 2: ANTONYMS

30 QUESTIONS ▪▫ TIME—15 MINUTES

(Please review Unit 1 on Antonyms before attempting this test.)

Directions: Read each question carefully and consider all possible answers. When you have decided which choice is best, fill in the corresponding space on your answer sheet. There is only one best answer for each question.

1. IMMUTABLE
   - (A) erudite
   - (B) abject
   - (C) changeable
   - (D) fantastic
   - (E) aura

2. DUCTILE
   - (A) feted
   - (B) alluvial
   - (C) stubborn
   - (D) abnormal
   - (E) belabor

3. FASTIDIOUS
   - (A) factitious
   - (B) absurd
   - (C) indifferent
   - (D) sloppy
   - (E) chary

4. TEMERITY
   - (A) affinity
   - (B) cherubim
   - (C) humility
   - (D) degenerate

5. ITINERANT
   - (A) animosity
   - (B) metaphor
   - (C) perpetrator
   - (D) resident
   - (E) cerebrum

6. TACITURN
   - (A) malevolent
   - (B) loquacious
   - (C) paltry
   - (D) opaque
   - (E) morbid

7. NEFARIOUS
   - (A) grotesque
   - (B) virtuous
   - (C) jovial
   - (D) pious
   - (E) cerement

8. OBSEQUIOUS
   - (A) harbinger
   - (B) bold
   - (C) heredity
   - (D) quaff
   - (E) falchion

9. OSTENTATION
   - (A) emulsion
   - (B) languid
   - (C) modesty
   - (D) kilogram
   - (E) bey

10. CONTENTION
    - (A) equation
    - (B) guild
    - (C) oblivion
    - (D) pacification
    - (E) bream

GO ON TO THE NEXT PAGE ➤

11. IMPUTATION
    (A) assiduous
    (B) radiant
    (C) challis
    (D) raiment
    (E) vindication

12. BENIGN
    (A) cayenne
    (B) relevant
    (C) robot
    (D) malevolent
    (E) precarious

13. COHERENT
    (A) perspicacious
    (B) zephyr
    (C) weal
    (D) chaotic
    (E) changeling

14. DEPREDATION
    (A) plethoric
    (B) gloss
    (C) restoration
    (D) usher
    (E) trochal

15. PROVOCATIVE
    (A) sedentary
    (B) capricious
    (C) vindictive
    (D) tawny
    (E) pacifying

16. SUBMISSION
    (A) authorized
    (B) defiance
    (C) assignment
    (D) defeat
    (E) belabor

17. AFFLUENT
    (A) immigrant
    (B) junction
    (C) insufficient
    (D) kin
    (E) clandestine

18. CHURLISH
    (A) exiguous
    (B) laudable
    (C) cheerful
    (D) maternal
    (E) civet

19. SYMMETRY
    (A) invocation
    (B) madrigal
    (C) distortion
    (D) satyr
    (E) cilia

20. DULCET
    (A) extrinsic
    (B) optimistic
    (C) unanimous
    (D) acerbate
    (E) chiffonade

21. PIQUANT
    (A) factitious
    (B) vain
    (C) insipid
    (D) vulture
    (E) chromatic

22. OPPORTUNE
    (A) dialectical
    (B) mutable
    (C) clinch
    (D) weird
    (E) inexpedient

23. PETULANT
    (A) irascible
    (B) cheerful
    (C) uncouth
    (D) abnormal
    (E) closure

24. SAVORY
    (A) apathy
    (B) clandestine
    (C) pliant
    (D) unpalatable
    (E) capillary

25. SATIATED

   (A) satirical
   (B) centaur
   (C) gorgeous
   (D) delectable
   (E) hungry

26. RECLUSIVE

   (A) empyreal
   (B) obscure
   (C) gregarious
   (D) rustication
   (E) chilblain

27. COURTEOUS

   (A) flaccid
   (B) emollient
   (C) insolent
   (D) scrupulous
   (E) chaffinch

28. USURP

   (A) succinct
   (B) predict
   (C) pacify
   (D) clematis
   (E) donate

29. ACRIMONIOUS

   (A) alluvial
   (B) apocalyptic
   (C) concourse
   (D) harmonious
   (E) carcanet

30. SKEPTIC

   (A) cryptic
   (B) bigot
   (C) discursive
   (D) eminent
   (E) caricature

S T O P   If you finish before time is called, you may check your work on this section only. Do not turn to any other section in the test.

ANSWER KEY

TEST 1: SYNONYMS

1. **B**	10. **D**	19. **A**	28. **A**
2. **C**	11. **B**	20. **B**	29. **A**
3. **B**	12. **B**	21. **B**	30. **C**
4. **A**	13. **A**	22. **C**	31. **D**
5. **D**	14. **C**	23. **A**	32. **B**
6. **A**	15. **C**	24. **D**	33. **D**
7. **D**	16. **D**	25. **A**	34. **A**
8. **B**	17. **C**	26. **B**	35. **C**
9. **A**	18. **C**	27. **C**	

TEST 2: ANTONYMS

1. **C**	9. **C**	17. **C**	24. **D**
2. **C**	10. **D**	18. **C**	25. **E**
3. **D**	11. **E**	19. **C**	26. **C**
4. **C**	12. **D**	20. **D**	27. **C**
5. **D**	13. **D**	21. **C**	28. **E**
6. **B**	14. **C**	22. **E**	29. **D**
7. **B**	15. **E**	23. **B**	30. **B**
8. **B**	16. **B**		

QUANTITATIVE ABILITY

ANSWER SHEET

TEST 1: NONVERBAL ARITHMETIC

1. Ⓐ Ⓑ Ⓒ Ⓓ   4. Ⓐ Ⓑ Ⓒ Ⓓ   7. Ⓐ Ⓑ Ⓒ Ⓓ   10. Ⓐ Ⓑ Ⓒ Ⓓ   13. Ⓐ Ⓑ Ⓒ Ⓓ
2. Ⓐ Ⓑ Ⓒ Ⓓ   5. Ⓐ Ⓑ Ⓒ Ⓓ   8. Ⓐ Ⓑ Ⓒ Ⓓ   11. Ⓐ Ⓑ Ⓒ Ⓓ   14. Ⓐ Ⓑ Ⓒ Ⓓ
3. Ⓐ Ⓑ Ⓒ Ⓓ   6. Ⓐ Ⓑ Ⓒ Ⓓ   9. Ⓐ Ⓑ Ⓒ Ⓓ   12. Ⓐ Ⓑ Ⓒ Ⓓ

TEST 2: PROBLEM SOLVING

1. Ⓐ Ⓑ Ⓒ Ⓓ   4. Ⓐ Ⓑ Ⓒ Ⓓ   7. Ⓐ Ⓑ Ⓒ Ⓓ   10. Ⓐ Ⓑ Ⓒ Ⓓ   13. Ⓐ Ⓑ Ⓒ Ⓓ
2. Ⓐ Ⓑ Ⓒ Ⓓ   5. Ⓐ Ⓑ Ⓒ Ⓓ   8. Ⓐ Ⓑ Ⓒ Ⓓ   11. Ⓐ Ⓑ Ⓒ Ⓓ   14. Ⓐ Ⓑ Ⓒ Ⓓ
3. Ⓐ Ⓑ Ⓒ Ⓓ   6. Ⓐ Ⓑ Ⓒ Ⓓ   9. Ⓐ Ⓑ Ⓒ Ⓓ   12. Ⓐ Ⓑ Ⓒ Ⓓ   15. Ⓐ Ⓑ Ⓒ Ⓓ

TEST 3: ALGEBRA

1. Ⓐ Ⓑ Ⓒ Ⓓ   3. Ⓐ Ⓑ Ⓒ Ⓓ   5. Ⓐ Ⓑ Ⓒ Ⓓ   7. Ⓐ Ⓑ Ⓒ Ⓓ   8. Ⓐ Ⓑ Ⓒ Ⓓ
2. Ⓐ Ⓑ Ⓒ Ⓓ   4. Ⓐ Ⓑ Ⓒ Ⓓ   6. Ⓐ Ⓑ Ⓒ Ⓓ

TEST 4: QUANTITATIVE COMPARISONS

1. Ⓐ Ⓑ Ⓒ Ⓓ   5. Ⓐ Ⓑ Ⓒ Ⓓ   9. Ⓐ Ⓑ Ⓒ Ⓓ   13. Ⓐ Ⓑ Ⓒ Ⓓ   17. Ⓐ Ⓑ Ⓒ Ⓓ
2. Ⓐ Ⓑ Ⓒ Ⓓ   6. Ⓐ Ⓑ Ⓒ Ⓓ   10. Ⓐ Ⓑ Ⓒ Ⓓ   14. Ⓐ Ⓑ Ⓒ Ⓓ   18. Ⓐ Ⓑ Ⓒ Ⓓ
3. Ⓐ Ⓑ Ⓒ Ⓓ   7. Ⓐ Ⓑ Ⓒ Ⓓ   11. Ⓐ Ⓑ Ⓒ Ⓓ   15. Ⓐ Ⓑ Ⓒ Ⓓ   19. Ⓐ Ⓑ Ⓒ Ⓓ
4. Ⓐ Ⓑ Ⓒ Ⓓ   8. Ⓐ Ⓑ Ⓒ Ⓓ   12. Ⓐ Ⓑ Ⓒ Ⓓ   16. Ⓐ Ⓑ Ⓒ Ⓓ   20. Ⓐ Ⓑ Ⓒ Ⓓ

TEST 1: NONVERBAL ARITHMETIC

14 QUESTIONS ▪◻ TIME—20 MINUTES

Directions: Read each question carefully and consider all possible answers. When you have decided which choice is best, fill in the corresponding space on your answer sheet. There is only one best answer for each question.

1. What fraction of a whole is the shaded area in the figure below?

   (A) $\dfrac{1}{2}$

   (B) $\dfrac{3}{4}$

   (C) $\dfrac{2}{3}$

   (D) $\dfrac{2}{5}$

2. Which of the following equations demonstrates that the two figures are equivalent?

   (A) $\dfrac{3}{9} = \dfrac{1}{3}$

   (B) $\dfrac{9}{3} = \dfrac{3}{1}$

   (C) $\dfrac{3}{9} = \dfrac{3}{3}$

   (D) $\dfrac{9}{3} = \dfrac{1}{3}$

3. Select the answer that represents reduction of the fraction $\dfrac{630}{140}$ to the lowest term.

   (A) $\dfrac{70}{2}$

   (B) $\dfrac{70}{4}$

   (C) $\dfrac{2}{9}$

   (D) $\dfrac{9}{2}$

4. Which one of the following equations is correct for building up the fraction $\dfrac{3}{8}$ to have a denominator of 24?

   (A) $\dfrac{3}{8} = \dfrac{3 \times 3}{3 \times 8} = \dfrac{9}{24}$

   (B) $\dfrac{3}{8} = 3 \times \dfrac{24}{8} \times \dfrac{1}{24} \times \dfrac{9}{24}$

   (C) $8 \times \dfrac{3}{1} \times \dfrac{1}{24} = \dfrac{24}{24}$

   (D) $\dfrac{3}{24} = 3 \times \dfrac{1}{3} \times \dfrac{1}{8} = \dfrac{1}{24}$

5. Which of the following equations expresses the whole number 6 as an equivalent fraction with a denominator of 5?

   (A) $\dfrac{6}{5} = 6 \times \dfrac{5}{5} \times \dfrac{1}{5} = \dfrac{30}{25}$

   (B) $\dfrac{6}{5} = 6 \times \dfrac{1}{5} \times 1 = \dfrac{6}{5}$

   (C) $\dfrac{6}{1} = \dfrac{6 \times 5}{1 \times 5} = \dfrac{30}{5}$

   (D) $\dfrac{6}{1} = 5 \times \dfrac{1}{6} \times 1 = \dfrac{5}{6}$

6. The product of $\frac{5}{3} \times \frac{2}{7}$ equals

   (A) $\frac{6}{35}$

   (B) $\frac{35}{6}$

   (C) $\frac{21}{10}$

   (D) $\frac{10}{21}$

7. The product of $\frac{25}{36} \times \frac{16}{20}$ equals

   (A) $\frac{10}{8}$

   (B) $\frac{8}{10}$

   (C) $\frac{9}{5}$

   (D) $\frac{5}{9}$

8. $\frac{3}{4}$ divided by $\frac{5}{2}$ equals

   (A) $\frac{10}{3}$

   (B) $\frac{3}{10}$

   (C) $\frac{20}{6}$

   (D) $\frac{6}{20}$

9. Select the correct answer for $\frac{72}{50} \div \frac{200}{35}$.

   (A) $\frac{63}{250}$

   (B) $\frac{250}{63}$

   (C) $\frac{288}{35}$

   (D) $\frac{35}{288}$

10. A 12-ounce bottle has 7 ounces of liquid in it. What fraction of the bottle is filled?

    (A) $\frac{3}{4}$

    (B) $\frac{1}{2}$

    (C) $\frac{7}{12}$

    (D) $\frac{12}{7}$

11. What is the solution to the problem $\frac{2}{9} + \frac{5}{6} + \frac{3}{8}$?

    (A) $\frac{72}{60}$

    (B) $\frac{60}{72}$

    (C) $\frac{72}{49}$

    (D) $\frac{49}{72}$

12. When you multiply $2\frac{1}{2} \times 1\frac{1}{2}$, the answer is

    (A) $3\frac{1}{3}$

    (B) $3\frac{1}{2}$

    (C) $2\frac{1}{5}$

    (D) $2\frac{2}{6}$

GO ON TO THE NEXT PAGE

13. Change $2\dfrac{1}{2} \div 3\dfrac{1}{3}$ to a simple fraction. The answer is

(A) $\dfrac{3}{4}$

(B) $\dfrac{4}{3}$

(C) $\dfrac{1}{3}$

(D) $\dfrac{1}{4}$

14. Which one of the following options is a solution to the problem $5\dfrac{3}{4} + 6\dfrac{5}{9}$?

(A) $12\dfrac{5}{12}$

(B) $11\dfrac{15}{36}$

(C) $12\dfrac{11}{36}$

(D) $11\dfrac{8}{13}$

STOP   If you finish before time is called, you may check your work on this section only. Do not turn to any other section in the test.

TEST 2: PROBLEM SOLVING

15 QUESTIONS ▬▭ TIME—20 MINUTES

Directions: Read each question carefully and consider all possible answers. When you have decided which choice is best, fill in the corresponding space on your answer sheet. There is only one best answer for each question.

1. If there are 245 sections in a city containing five boroughs, the average number of sections for each of the five boroughs is

   (A) 50 sections.
   (B) 49 sections.
   (C) 47 sections.
   (D) 59 sections.

2. If, in that same city, a section has 45 miles of street to plow after a snowstorm, and nine plows are used, each plow will cover an average of how many miles?

   (A) 7 miles
   (B) 6 miles
   (C) 8 miles
   (D) 5 miles

3. If a crosswalk plow engine is run 5 minutes a day for ten days in a given month, how long will it run in the course of this month?

   (A) 50 minutes
   (B) $1\frac{1}{2}$ hours
   (C) 1 hour
   (D) 30 minutes

4. If the city uses 1,500 laborers in manual street cleaning and half as many more to load and drive trucks, the total number of laborers used is

   (A) 2,200
   (B) 2,520
   (C) 2,050
   (D) 2,250

5. Of 186 summonses issued, 100 were issued to first offenders. How many summonses were issued to other than first offenders?

   (A) 68
   (B) 90
   (C) 86
   (D) 108

6. A sanitation worker is 40 feet behind a sanitation truck. There is a second sanitation truck 90 feet behind the first truck. How much closer is the worker to the first truck than to the second?

   (A) 30 feet
   (B) 50 feet
   (C) 10 feet
   (D) 70 feet

7. If a flushing machine has a capacity of 1,260 gallons, how many gallons will it contain when it is two-thirds full?

   (A) 809 gallons
   (B) 750 gallons
   (C) 630 gallons
   (D) 840 gallons

8. If an employee earns $160.00 a week and has deductions of $8.00 for the pension fund, $12.00 for medical insurance, and $29.60 withholding tax, his take-home pay will be

   (A) $110.40
   (B) $108.60
   (C) $102.00
   (D) $98.40

GO ON TO THE NEXT PAGE

9. A city department uses 25 twenty-cent, 35 thirty-cent, and 350 forty-cent metered postage units each day. The total cost of stamps used by the department in a five-day period is

    (A) $29.50
    (B) $155.00
    (C) $290.50
    (D) $777.50

10. In 1975, a school bought 500 dozen pencils at $0.40 per dozen. In 1978, only 75 percent as many pencils were bought as were bought in 1975, but the price per dozen was 20 percent higher than the 1975 price. The total cost of the pencils bought in 1978 was

    (A) $180.00
    (B) $187.50
    (C) $240.00
    (D) $250.00

11. If the average cost of sweeping a square foot of a small town's street is $0.75, the cost of sweeping 100 square feet is

    (A) $7.50
    (B) $750
    (C) $75
    (D) $70

12. If a sanitation department scow is towed at the rate of 3 miles per hour, how many hours, will it need to go 28 miles?

    (A) 10 hours 30 minutes
    (B) 12 hours
    (C) 9 hours 20 minutes
    (D) 9 hours 15 minutes

13. If a man is 60 feet away from a sanitation truck, how many feet nearer is he to the truck than a second truck that is 100 feet away?

    (A) 60 feet
    (B) 40 feet
    (C) 50 feet
    (D) 20 feet

14. Six gross of special drawing pencils were purchased for use in a city department. If the pencils were used at the rate of 24 a week, the maximum number of weeks that the six gross of pencils would last is

    (A) 6 weeks.
    (B) 12 weeks.
    (C) 24 weeks.
    (D) 36 weeks.

15. A cogwheel having eight cogs plays into another cogwheel having 24 cogs. When the small wheel has made 42 revolutions, how many has the larger wheel made?

    (A) 14
    (B) 20
    (C) 16
    (D) 10

STOP If you finish before time is called, you may check your work on this section only. Do not turn to any other section in the test.

TEST 3: ALGEBRA

8 QUESTIONS ▪ TIME—20 MINUTES

Directions: Read each question carefully and consider all possible answers. When you have decided which choice is best, fill in the corresponding space on your answer sheet. There is only one best answer for each question.

1. In the equation $4a + 5 = 13$, a equals
   - (A) 4
   - (B) 2
   - (C) 7
   - (D) 6

2. In the equation $\dfrac{10}{m} - 8 = \dfrac{5}{3}$, m equals
   - (A) $\dfrac{10}{3}$
   - (B) $\dfrac{3}{10}$
   - (C) $\dfrac{30}{29}$
   - (D) $\dfrac{29}{30}$

3. In the equation $3c^2 = 75d^4$, c equals
   - (A) $\pm 5d^2$
   - (B) $\pm 5d^4$
   - (C) $\pm 25d^2$
   - (D) $\pm 25d^4$

4. If two moles of compound A react with 5 moles of compound B to form compound C, then how many moles of A are required to react completely with 7 moles of B to form compound C?
   - (A) 5.7
   - (B) 2.8
   - (C) 7.5
   - (D) 8.2

5. A car traveling at x mph takes 5 hours to go from city A to city B. Traveling at $x - 15$ mph, the car makes the return trip in $6\dfrac{2}{3}$ hours. What was the speed of the car on the return trip?
   - (A) 60 mph
   - (B) 55 mph
   - (C) 50 mph
   - (D) 45 mph

6. In 1997, item A cost $2,500. In 1998, the price of A went up 20 percent because of inflation, while in early 1999 there was a 10 percent increase in the price of A over its 1998 price. In June of 1999, A was put on sale with a 30 percent decrease in price. What was the sale price of A?
   - (A) 2,500
   - (B) 2,400
   - (C) 2,310
   - (D) 2,110

7. In the expression $\log_4 \dfrac{1}{16} = x$, what is the value of x?
   - (A) -2
   - (B) -4
   - (C) $+2$
   - (D) $+4$

8. What is the volume of a sphere of a radius 3 centimeters?
   - (A) 119.05 cc
   - (B) 113.04 cc
   - (C) 106.00 cc
   - (D) 101.08 cc

S T O P

If you finish before time is called, you may check your work on this section only. Do not turn to any other section in the test.

TEST 4: QUANTITATIVE COMPARISONS

20 QUESTIONS ▪▫ TIME—30 MINUTES

Common Information: In each question, information concerning one or both of the quantities to be compared is given in the ITEM column. A symbol that appears in any column represents the same thing in Column A as it does in Column B.

Figures: Assume that the position of points, angles, regions, and so forth, are in the order shown; that the lines shown as straight are indeed straight; that figures lie in a plane unless otherwise indicated. Figures accompanying questions are intended to provide information you can use in answering the questions. However, unless a note states that a figure is drawn to scale, you should solve the problems by using your knowledge of mathematics, NOT by estimating sizes by sight or by measurement.

Directions: For each of the following questions, two quantities are given: one in Column A and one in Column B. Compare the two quantities and mark your answer sheet with the correct, lettered conclusion. These are your options:

A   if the quantity in Column A is the greater;
B   if the quantity in Column B is the greater;
C   if the two quantities are equal;
D   if the relationship cannot be determined from the information given.

Column A	Column B		Column A	Column B

1.

5% of 34	The number that 34 is 5% of

2.

$$\angle 1 < \angle 2$$

IR	IT

SUMMARY DIRECTIONS

Select: A   if Column A is greater;
       B   if Column B is greater;
       C   if the two columns are equal;
       D   if the relationship cannot be determined from the information given.

Column A	**Column B**		**Column A**	**Column B**

3. $4 > x > -3$

$\dfrac{x}{3}$	$\dfrac{3}{x}$

6. $y =$ an odd integer

The numerical value of y^2	The numerical value of y^3

4.

$\dfrac{2}{3} + \dfrac{3}{7}$	$\dfrac{16}{21} - \dfrac{3}{7}$

7.

$8 + (6 \div 3) - 7(2)$	$6 + (8 \div 2) - 7(3)$

5.

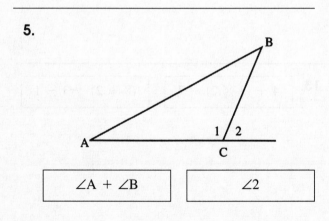

$\angle A + \angle B$	$\angle 2$

8.

$\dfrac{3}{4}$ of $\dfrac{9}{9}$	$\dfrac{9}{9} \times \dfrac{3}{4}$

GO ON TO THE NEXT PAGE

SUMMARY DIRECTIONS

Select: A if Column A is greater;
       B if Column B is greater;
       C if the two columns are equal;
       D if the relationship cannot be determined from the information given.

Column A	**Column B**

9.

NC	CY

10.

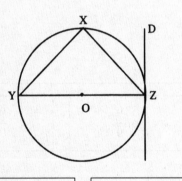

∠YXZ	∠DZY

Column A	**Column B**

11.

A given chord in a given circle	The radius of the same circle

12.

BC	FD

13.

$4 + (3 \times 2) - 7$	$(8 \div 2) + 3 - 1$

SUMMARY DIRECTIONS

Select: A   if Column A is greater;
          B   if Column B is greater;
          C   if the two columns are equal;
          D   if the relationship cannot be determined from the information given.

Column A	Column B

14.

50% of $\frac{4}{5}$	$\frac{4}{5}$ of $\frac{1}{2}$

17.

Column A	Column B

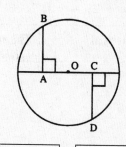

AB	CD

15.

AB	CD

18.

The number that 6 is 20% of	10% of 300

16.

0.01 ÷ .1	0.01 × .1

GO ON TO THE NEXT PAGE

SUMMARY DIRECTIONS

Select: A   if Column A is greater;
B   if Column B is greater;
C   if the two columns are equal;
D   if the relationship cannot be determined from the information given.

Column A	**Column B**		**Column A**	**Column B**

19. $3x + 2y = -1; 2x + 3y = 1$

The numerical value of x	The numerical value of y

20.

$CD \perp AB; \angle A > \angle B$

AC	CB

STOP   If you finish before time is called, you may check your work on this section only. Do not turn to any other section in the test.

ANSWER KEY

TEST 1: NONVERBAL ARITHMETIC

1. C	5. C	9. A	12. B
2. A	6. D	10. C	13. A
3. D	7. D	11. D	14. C
4. A	8. B		

TEST 2: PROBLEM SOLVING

1. B	5. C	9. D	13. B
2. D	6. C	10. A	14. D
3. A	7. D	11. C	15. A
4. D	8. A	12. C	

TEST 3: ALGEBRA

1. B	3. A	5. D	7. A
2. C	4. B	6. C	8. B

TEST 4: QUANTITATIVE COMPARISONS

1. B	6. D	11. D	16. A
2. A	7. A	12. D	17. B
3. D	8. C	13. B	18. C
4. A	9. B	14. C	19. B
5. C	10. C	15. A	20. B

EXPLANATORY ANSWERS

TEST 1: NONVERBAL ARITHMETIC

1. **The correct answer is (C).** Since the whole is divided into 3 units, the denominator is 3. There are 2 units shaded, so the numerator is 2. The shaded part is $\frac{2}{3}$ of the whole.

2. **The correct answer is (A).** The left-hand figure is divided into 9 parts, and is a square. The shaded part can be represented by the fraction $\frac{3}{9}$. The right-hand figure is divided in 3 parts, and is also a square. The fraction $\frac{1}{3}$ represents the shaded part; $\frac{3}{9}$ and $\frac{1}{3}$ represent the same part of the whole and are therefore equivalent, $\frac{3}{9} = \frac{1}{3}$.

3. **The correct answer is (D).**
$$\frac{630}{140} = \frac{63}{14} = \frac{63 \div 7}{14 \div 7} = \frac{9}{2}$$

4. **The correct answer is (A).** Multiply both parts by the same number. 8 multiplied by what number will give 24. Answer: divide 24 by 8 = 3. The denominator and the numerator are multiplied by 3 to get $\frac{9}{24}$.
$$\frac{3}{8} = \frac{3 \times 3}{3 \times 8} = \frac{9}{24}$$

5. **The correct answer is (C).** Use the same process as number 4.
$$\frac{6}{1} = \frac{6}{1} \times \frac{5}{5} = \frac{30}{5}$$

6. **The correct answer is (D).** Multiply numerators and denominators.
$$\frac{5}{3} \times \frac{2}{7} = \frac{5 \times 2}{3 \times 7} = \frac{10}{21}$$

7. **The correct answer is (D).** Reduce and perform the multiplication.
$$\frac{25}{36} \times \frac{\cancel{16}}{\cancel{20}} = \frac{25}{36} \times \frac{4}{5} \quad \text{(divide by 4)}$$
$$\frac{\cancel{25}}{36} \times \frac{4}{\cancel{5}} = \frac{5}{36} \times \frac{4}{1} \quad \text{(divide by 5)}$$
$$= \frac{5}{36} \times \frac{4}{1} \quad \text{(divide by 4)}$$
$$= \frac{5}{9} \times \frac{1}{1}$$
$$= \frac{5 \times 1}{9 \times 1}$$
$$= \frac{5}{9}$$

8. **The correct answer is (B).** Invert the divisor and change the operation to multiplication, reduce, and perform the multiplication.
$$\frac{3}{4} \div \frac{5}{2} = \frac{3}{4} \times \frac{2}{5}$$
$$\frac{3}{4} \times \frac{2}{5} \quad \text{(divide by 2)}$$
$$\frac{3}{2} \times \frac{1}{5} = \frac{3}{10}$$

9. **The correct answer is (A).** Use the same procedure as number 8.
$$\frac{72}{50} \div \frac{200}{35} = \frac{72}{50} \times \frac{35}{200}$$
$$\frac{72}{50} = \frac{35}{200} \quad \text{(divide by 8)}$$
$$\frac{9}{50} \times \frac{35}{25} \quad \text{(divide by 5)}$$
$$\frac{9}{50} \times \frac{7}{25} = \frac{63}{250}$$

10. **The correct answer is (C).** The bottle (whole) is divided into 12 ounces (the denominator) of which 7 ounces (the numerator) is filled. Thus, $\frac{7}{12}$ of the bottle is filled.

11. **The correct answer is (D).** Find the lowest common denominator (LCD), build up each fraction to have 72 as denominator, and perform addition and subtraction as indicated.

The least common multiple (LCM) of 9 and 6 is 18.

LCM of 18 and 8 is 72

Therefore, LCD = 72

$$\frac{2}{9} = \frac{2}{9} \times \frac{8}{8} = \frac{16}{72}$$

$$\frac{5}{6} = \frac{5 \times 12}{6 \times 12} = \frac{60}{72}$$

$$\frac{3}{8} = \frac{3 \times 9}{8 \times 9} = \frac{27}{72}$$

$$\frac{2}{9} + \frac{5}{4} - \frac{3}{8} = \frac{16}{72} + \frac{60}{72} - \frac{27}{72} = \frac{76}{72} - \frac{27}{72} = \frac{49}{72}$$

12. **The correct answer is (B).** Change both mixed numbers into improper fractions and multiply:

$$2\frac{1}{3} \times 1\frac{1}{2} = \frac{7}{3} \times \frac{3}{2}$$

$$\frac{7}{3} \times \frac{3}{2} = \frac{7}{2} = 3\frac{1}{2}$$

13. **The correct answer is (A).** Use the same procedure as in number 12, then change ÷ to × and invert the second fraction.

$$2\frac{1}{2} \div 3\frac{1}{3} = \frac{5}{2} \div \frac{10}{3}$$

$$\frac{\overset{1}{\cancel{5}}}{2} \times \frac{3}{\underset{2}{\cancel{10}}} = \frac{1}{2} \times \frac{3}{2} = \frac{3}{4}$$

14. **The correct answer is (C).** Add the whole numbers and fractional parts separately. Change improper fraction to a mixed number. Find common denominators for fractional parts, then add.

$$5\frac{3}{4} + 6\frac{5}{9} = 5 + \frac{3}{4} + 6 + \frac{5}{9}$$

$$= 11 + \frac{3}{4} + \frac{5}{9}$$

$$= 11 + \frac{27}{36} + \frac{20}{36}$$

$$= 11 + \frac{47}{36}$$

$$= 11 + 1 + \frac{11}{36}$$

$$= 12 + \frac{11}{36}$$

$$= 12\frac{11}{36}$$

Test 2: Problem Solving

1. **The correct answer is (B).** To find the *average* number of sections per borough, divide:

    245 sections divided by 5 boroughs = 49

49 sections/borough

2. **The correct answer is (D).** Total miles = 45

    number of plows = 9

To find the *average* number of miles, divide:

    45 miles by 9 plows = 5 miles/plow

Average = 5 miles

3. **The correct answer is (A).**

    Total time per day = 5 minutes
    Total days per month = 10 days
    Total time per month =

$$\frac{5 \text{ minutes}}{\text{day}} \times \frac{10 \text{ days}}{\text{month}} = \frac{50 \text{ minutes}}{\text{month}}$$

4. **The correct answer is (D).**

    Total number for street cleaning =   1,500
    half that number load and drive = + 750
    _____
                                          2,250

2,250 laborers used

5. **The correct answer is (C).**

$$
\begin{array}{ll}
\text{Total issued} = & 186 \\
\text{subtract:} & \\
\text{first offenders} = & -100 \\
\hline
\text{other-than-first offenders} & 86
\end{array}
$$

6. **The correct answer is (C).** The second truck is 90 feet − 40 feet = 50 feet from the man. The first truck is 40 feet from the man. The first truck is 50 feet − 40 feet = 10 feet closer than the second truck.

7. **The correct answer is (D).** Total capacity = 1,260 gallons

$$
\frac{2}{3} \text{ of } 1{,}260 = \frac{2}{3} \times 1{,}260
$$
$$
= \frac{2{,}520}{3}
$$
$$
= 840 \text{ gallons}
$$

8. **The correct answer is (A).**

$$
\begin{array}{ll}
\text{Total earnings} = & \$160.00 \\
\text{Deductions} = & \$8.00 \text{ pension}
\end{array}
$$

$$
\begin{array}{ll}
= & \$12.00 \text{ medical insurance} \\
= & \$29.60 \text{ withholding tax} \\
\hline
= & \$49.60 \text{ total deductions}
\end{array}
$$

The take-home pay can be found by subtracting the total deduction from the salary.

$$
\$160.00 - \$49.60 = \$110.40
$$

Take-home pay = $110.40

9. **The correct answer is (D).**

Stamps per day	*Cost per day*
25/day × $0.20 =	5.00
35/day × $0.30 =	10.50
350 × $0.40 =	140.00
Total cost/day	$155.50

For five days, 5 × $155.50 = $777.50

Total cost = $777.50

10. **The correct answer is (A).** Total number of pencils bought in 1975 was 500 dozen at $0.40 a dozen; in 1978, 75 percent of the 500 dozen were bought at a 20 percent increase in price.

First, find how many pencils were bought in 1978. Do this by multiplying:

$$
500 \times 0.75 = 375 \text{ dozen were bought in 1978}
$$

Now find the price per dozen. You know that it was 20 percent more than $0.40:

$$
\$0.40 \times 0.20 \text{ increase} = \$0.08 \text{ or } 8¢ \text{ increase in price}
$$

So the price per dozen is:

$$
40¢ + 8¢ = 48¢ \text{ or } \$0.48
$$

To find the cost, multiply the number of dozens of pencils by the cost per dozen.

$$
375 \text{ dozen} \times \$0.48/\text{dozen} = \$180
$$

Total cost for 1978 = $180

11. **The correct answer is (C).** If it costs $0.75 to sweep one square foot, to find the cost for 100 square feet, multiply:

$$
100 \text{ square feet} \times 0.75 \text{ per square foot} = \$75
$$

Total cost = $75

12. **The correct answer is (C).** It takes 1 hour to tow a scow 3 miles. Find the time to tow the scow 28 miles by dividing:

$$
28 \text{ miles} \div 3 \text{ miles/hour} = 9\frac{1}{3} \text{ hours}
$$

$$
\frac{1}{3} \text{ hour} \times 60 \text{ minutes/hour} = 20 \text{ minutes}
$$

Note: 1 hour = 60 minutes. To change hours to minutes multiply the fraction of an hour by

$$
\frac{60 \text{ minutes}}{\text{hour}}.
$$

It takes 9 hours, 20 minutes to tow the scow 28 miles.

13. **The correct answer is (B).**

Truck to the other truck	100 feet
Truck to the man	− 60 feet
	40 feet

The difference is 40 feet.

14. **The correct answer is (D).** One gross = 144 pencils

6 gross = 144/gross × 6 gross = 864 pencils (on hand)

If 24 pencils are used each week, divide to find the number of weeks they will last:

864 divided by 24/week = 36 weeks

Supplies would last 36 weeks.

15. **The correct answer is (A).** If the cogs on two wheels are sized and spaced the same, the smaller of the two wheels will turn faster than the larger one—the fewer cogs a wheel has, the more revolutions it makes. The number of cogs is, therefore, inversely proportional to the number of revolutions.

The smaller wheel will make 3 revolutions for every 1 revolution the larger wheel makes. So when the smaller wheel makes 42 revolutions, the larger wheel will make 42 divided by 3 = 14 revolutions.

TEST 3: ALGEBRA

1. **The correct answer is (B).** $4a + 5 - 5 = 13 - 5$

$$4a = 8$$
$$\frac{4a}{4} = \frac{8}{4}$$
$$a = 2$$

2. **The correct answer is (C).**

$$\frac{10}{m} - 8 = \frac{5}{3} \qquad \text{(multiply by } 3m\text{)}$$

$$3m \times \frac{10}{m} - (3m)(8) = \frac{(3m)(5)}{3}$$

$$\frac{30m}{m} - 24m = \frac{15m}{3}$$

$$30 - 24m = 5m$$
$$30 = 29m$$
$$m = \frac{30}{29}$$

3. **The correct answer is (A).**

$$\frac{3c^2}{3} = \frac{75d^4}{3}$$
$$c^2 = 25d^4$$
$$\sqrt{c^2} = \sqrt{25d^4}$$
$$c = \pm 5d^2$$

4. **The correct answer is (B).** In a chemical reaction, the quantities of reactants/products are directly proportional.

Let $x_1 = 2$ moles of A and $y_1 = 5$ moles of B.

Then x_2 = number of moles of A and $y_2 = 7$ moles of B such that:

$$\frac{5}{2} = \frac{7}{x_2}; \; x_2 = 2.8 \text{ moles of A.}$$

5. **The correct answer is (D).** Since displacement = (speed)(time), $d = vt$, speed and time are inversely proportional for a constant displacement. Let $v1 = x$ mph and $t1 = 5$ hours; $v2 = x - 15$ mph and $t2 = 6\frac{2}{3}$ hours $= \frac{20}{3}$ hours. Since both displacements are the same:

$$5x = 6\frac{2}{3}(x - 15)$$
$$5x = \frac{20}{3}(x - 15)$$
$$3(5x) = 3\left(\frac{20}{3}\right)(x - 15)$$
$$15x = 20(x - 15)$$
$$15x = 20x - 300$$
$$300 = 5x$$

$x = 60$ mph, speed from A to B

$x - 15 = 45$ mph is the speed on the return trip

6. **The correct answer is (C).** Sale price (1999) = $2,310

1997: Cost of A = $2,500

1998: Cost of A = $2,500 + $\frac{20}{100}$ × $2,500 = $3,000

1999: Cost of A = $3,000 + $\frac{10}{100}$ × $3,000 = $3,300

Sale Price (1999) = $3,300 − $\frac{30}{100}$ × $3,300 = $2,310

7. **The correct answer is (A).**

$$\log_4 \frac{1}{16} = x$$
$$4^x = \frac{1}{16}$$
$$x = -2$$

8. **The correct answer is (B).** $v = \frac{4}{3}\pi r^3$

   Because $r = 3$ and $\pi = 3.14$

   $$v = \frac{4}{3}\pi r^3$$
   $$= \frac{4}{3}(3.14)(3^3)$$
   $$= \frac{4}{3}(3.14)(27)$$
   $$= \frac{4(3.14)(27)}{3}$$
   $$= 4(3.14)(9)$$
   $$= 113.04 \text{ cc}$$

TEST 4: QUANTITATIVE COMPARISONS

1. **The correct answer is (B).** 5% of 34 = 34 × 0.05 = 1.7

   The number that 34 is 5% of = 5% of n = 34

   $0.05n = 34$

   $n = \dfrac{34}{0.05}$ $.05\overline{)34.00}$

   $n = 0.05$ $\dfrac{30}{40}$

   $n = 680$ $\dfrac{40}{0}$

                    $\dfrac{0}{}$

2. **The correct answer is (A).** In a triangle, the greater side lies opposite the greater angle. $\angle 2 > \angle 1$ (given) IR > IT

3. **The correct answer is (D).** Since x could be any number from -3 to 4, the values of the fractions are impossible to determine.

4. **The correct answer is (A).**

   $$\frac{2}{3} + \frac{3}{7} = \frac{14}{21} + \frac{9}{21}$$
   $$= \frac{23}{21}$$
   $$\frac{16}{21} - \frac{3}{7} = \frac{16}{21} - \frac{9}{21}$$
   $$= \frac{7}{21}$$

5. **The correct answer is (C).**

   $\angle 2 = \angle A + \angle B$ (an exterior angle of a triangle is equal to the sum of the two interior remote angles)

6. **The correct answer is (D).** There is not enough information given; y could equal 1, which would make both quantities equal; or y could be greater than 1, which would make y^3 greater than y^2. If y were a negative integer, then y^2 would be greater than y^3.

7. **The correct answer is (A).**

   $$8 + (6 \div 3) - 7(2) = 8 + 2 - 14$$
   $$= 10 - 14$$
   $$= -4$$
   $$6 + (8 \div 2) - 7(3) = 6 + 4 - 21$$
   $$= 10 - 21$$
   $$= -11$$
   $$-4 > -11$$

8. **The correct answer is (C).** $\dfrac{3}{4}$ of $\dfrac{9}{9} = \dfrac{3}{4} \times \dfrac{9}{9} = \dfrac{3}{4}$

9. **The correct answer is (B).**

   NC = NY given

   $\angle C = \angle Y$ angles opposite equal sides are equal

   $\angle N < \angle C$ given

   $\angle N < \angle Y$ substitution

   CY < NC the greater side lies opposite the greater angle

10. **The correct answer is (C).**

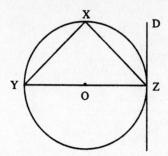

∠YXZ = 90° an angle inscribed in a semi-circle equals 90°

∠DZY = 90° a radius is perpendicular to a tangent at their point of contact

11. **The correct answer is (D).** Impossible to determine from the information given. The radius could be less than, equal to, or greater than the chord.

12. **The correct answer is (D).** Since there are three unknown sides on both triangles, the length of BC or FD is impossible to determine.

13. **The correct answer is (B).**

$$4 + 3 \times 2 - 7 = 4 + 6 - 7$$
$$= 10 - 7$$
$$= 3$$
$$8 \div 2 + 3 - 1 = 4 + 3 - 1$$
$$= 7 - 1$$
$$= 6$$

14. **The correct answer is (C).**

$$50\% \text{ of } \frac{4}{5} = .50 \times \frac{4}{5}$$
$$= \frac{1}{2} \times \frac{4}{5}$$
$$= \frac{2}{5}$$
$$\frac{4}{5} \text{ of } \frac{1}{2} = \frac{4}{5} \times \frac{1}{2}$$
$$= \frac{2}{5}$$

15. **The correct answer is (A).** The shortest line between two parallel lines is a line perpendicular to both lines. Therefore, if there are two transversals between parallel lines, the one whose angle of intersection with the parallel lines is further from 90° is the longer transversal.

$$\angle B = 90° - 78° = 12°$$
$$\angle D = 101° - 90° = 11°$$
$$\therefore AB > CD$$

16. **The correct answer is (A).**

$$0.01 \div 0.1 = 0.1$$
$$0.01 \times 0.1 = 0.001$$
$$.1 > .001$$

17. **The correct answer is (B).** If two perpendiculars are drawn from the circumference of a circle to a diameter of the same circle, the one that is closer to the center of the circle will be longer.

18. **The correct answer is (C).** The number that 6 is 20% of:

$$20\% \text{ of } n = 6$$
$$0.20n = 6$$
$$n = 6 \div 0.2$$
$$n = 30$$
$$10\% \text{ of } 300 = 10\% \times 300$$
$$= .10 \times 300$$
$$= 30$$

19. **The correct answer is (B).**

$$3x + 2y = -1$$
$$2x + 3y = 1$$

$3(3x + 2y = -1)$ (multiply the first equation by 3)
$2(2x + 3y = 1)$ (multiply the second equation by 2)

$$\begin{array}{rl} 9x + 6y = & -3 \\ -\ 4x + 6y = & 2 \\ \hline 5x = & -5 \\ x = & -1 \end{array}$$ (subtract the second equation from the first equation)

$$3x + 2y = -1$$
$$3(-1) + 2y = -1$$
$$-3 + 2y = -1$$
$$2y = 2$$
$$y = 1$$

(substitute the −1 for x in the one of the original equations and solve for y)

20. **The correct answer is (B).** ∠A > ∠B given CB > AC. In a triangle, the greater side lies opposite the greater angle.

SCIENCE

ANSWER SHEET

TEST 1: CELLS, STRUCTURE, AND FUNCTION

1. Ⓐ Ⓑ Ⓒ Ⓓ	9. Ⓐ Ⓑ Ⓒ Ⓓ	17. Ⓐ Ⓑ Ⓒ Ⓓ	25. Ⓐ Ⓑ Ⓒ Ⓓ	33. Ⓐ Ⓑ Ⓒ Ⓓ
2. Ⓐ Ⓑ Ⓒ Ⓓ	10. Ⓐ Ⓑ Ⓒ Ⓓ	18. Ⓐ Ⓑ Ⓒ Ⓓ	26. Ⓐ Ⓑ Ⓒ Ⓓ	34. Ⓐ Ⓑ Ⓒ Ⓓ
3. Ⓐ Ⓑ Ⓒ Ⓓ	11. Ⓐ Ⓑ Ⓒ Ⓓ	19. Ⓐ Ⓑ Ⓒ Ⓓ	27. Ⓐ Ⓑ Ⓒ Ⓓ	35. Ⓐ Ⓑ Ⓒ Ⓓ
4. Ⓐ Ⓑ Ⓒ Ⓓ	12. Ⓐ Ⓑ Ⓒ Ⓓ	20. Ⓐ Ⓑ Ⓒ Ⓓ	28. Ⓐ Ⓑ Ⓒ Ⓓ	36. Ⓐ Ⓑ Ⓒ Ⓓ
5. Ⓐ Ⓑ Ⓒ Ⓓ	13. Ⓐ Ⓑ Ⓒ Ⓓ	21. Ⓐ Ⓑ Ⓒ Ⓓ	29. Ⓐ Ⓑ Ⓒ Ⓓ	37. Ⓐ Ⓑ Ⓒ Ⓓ
6. Ⓐ Ⓑ Ⓒ Ⓓ	14. Ⓐ Ⓑ Ⓒ Ⓓ	22. Ⓐ Ⓑ Ⓒ Ⓓ	30. Ⓐ Ⓑ Ⓒ Ⓓ	38. Ⓐ Ⓑ Ⓒ Ⓓ
7. Ⓐ Ⓑ Ⓒ Ⓓ	15. Ⓐ Ⓑ Ⓒ Ⓓ	23. Ⓐ Ⓑ Ⓒ Ⓓ	31. Ⓐ Ⓑ Ⓒ Ⓓ	39. Ⓐ Ⓑ Ⓒ Ⓓ
8. Ⓐ Ⓑ Ⓒ Ⓓ	16. Ⓐ Ⓑ Ⓒ Ⓓ	24. Ⓐ Ⓑ Ⓒ Ⓓ	32. Ⓐ Ⓑ Ⓒ Ⓓ	40. Ⓐ Ⓑ Ⓒ Ⓓ

BIOLOGY

TEST 2

1. Ⓐ Ⓑ Ⓒ Ⓓ	5. Ⓐ Ⓑ Ⓒ Ⓓ	9. Ⓐ Ⓑ Ⓒ Ⓓ	13. Ⓐ Ⓑ Ⓒ Ⓓ	17. Ⓐ Ⓑ Ⓒ Ⓓ
2. Ⓐ Ⓑ Ⓒ Ⓓ	6. Ⓐ Ⓑ Ⓒ Ⓓ	10. Ⓐ Ⓑ Ⓒ Ⓓ	14. Ⓐ Ⓑ Ⓒ Ⓓ	18. Ⓐ Ⓑ Ⓒ Ⓓ
3. Ⓐ Ⓑ Ⓒ Ⓓ	7. Ⓐ Ⓑ Ⓒ Ⓓ	11. Ⓐ Ⓑ Ⓒ Ⓓ	15. Ⓐ Ⓑ Ⓒ Ⓓ	19. Ⓐ Ⓑ Ⓒ Ⓓ
4. Ⓐ Ⓑ Ⓒ Ⓓ	8. Ⓐ Ⓑ Ⓒ Ⓓ	12. Ⓐ Ⓑ Ⓒ Ⓓ	16. Ⓐ Ⓑ Ⓒ Ⓓ	

TEST 3

1. Ⓐ Ⓑ Ⓒ Ⓓ	5. Ⓐ Ⓑ Ⓒ Ⓓ	9. Ⓐ Ⓑ Ⓒ Ⓓ	13. Ⓐ Ⓑ Ⓒ Ⓓ	17. Ⓐ Ⓑ Ⓒ Ⓓ
2. Ⓐ Ⓑ Ⓒ Ⓓ	6. Ⓐ Ⓑ Ⓒ Ⓓ	10. Ⓐ Ⓑ Ⓒ Ⓓ	14. Ⓐ Ⓑ Ⓒ Ⓓ	18. Ⓐ Ⓑ Ⓒ Ⓓ
3. Ⓐ Ⓑ Ⓒ Ⓓ	7. Ⓐ Ⓑ Ⓒ Ⓓ	11. Ⓐ Ⓑ Ⓒ Ⓓ	15. Ⓐ Ⓑ Ⓒ Ⓓ	19. Ⓐ Ⓑ Ⓒ Ⓓ
4. Ⓐ Ⓑ Ⓒ Ⓓ	8. Ⓐ Ⓑ Ⓒ Ⓓ	12. Ⓐ Ⓑ Ⓒ Ⓓ	16. Ⓐ Ⓑ Ⓒ Ⓓ	20. Ⓐ Ⓑ Ⓒ Ⓓ

TEST 4: HUMAN ANATOMY AND PHYSIOLOGY

1. Ⓐ Ⓑ Ⓒ Ⓓ	21. Ⓐ Ⓑ Ⓒ Ⓓ	41. Ⓐ Ⓑ Ⓒ Ⓓ	61. Ⓐ Ⓑ Ⓒ Ⓓ	81. Ⓐ Ⓑ Ⓒ Ⓓ
2. Ⓐ Ⓑ Ⓒ Ⓓ	22. Ⓐ Ⓑ Ⓒ Ⓓ	42. Ⓐ Ⓑ Ⓒ Ⓓ	62. Ⓐ Ⓑ Ⓒ Ⓓ	82. Ⓐ Ⓑ Ⓒ Ⓓ
3. Ⓐ Ⓑ Ⓒ Ⓓ	23. Ⓐ Ⓑ Ⓒ Ⓓ	43. Ⓐ Ⓑ Ⓒ Ⓓ	63. Ⓐ Ⓑ Ⓒ Ⓓ	83. Ⓐ Ⓑ Ⓒ Ⓓ
4. Ⓐ Ⓑ Ⓒ Ⓓ	24. Ⓐ Ⓑ Ⓒ Ⓓ	44. Ⓐ Ⓑ Ⓒ Ⓓ	64. Ⓐ Ⓑ Ⓒ Ⓓ	84. Ⓐ Ⓑ Ⓒ Ⓓ
5. Ⓐ Ⓑ Ⓒ Ⓓ	25. Ⓐ Ⓑ Ⓒ Ⓓ	45. Ⓐ Ⓑ Ⓒ Ⓓ	65. Ⓐ Ⓑ Ⓒ Ⓓ	85. Ⓐ Ⓑ Ⓒ Ⓓ
6. Ⓐ Ⓑ Ⓒ Ⓓ	26. Ⓐ Ⓑ Ⓒ Ⓓ	46. Ⓐ Ⓑ Ⓒ Ⓓ	66. Ⓐ Ⓑ Ⓒ Ⓓ	86. Ⓐ Ⓑ Ⓒ Ⓓ
7. Ⓐ Ⓑ Ⓒ Ⓓ	27. Ⓐ Ⓑ Ⓒ Ⓓ	47. Ⓐ Ⓑ Ⓒ Ⓓ	67. Ⓐ Ⓑ Ⓒ Ⓓ	87. Ⓐ Ⓑ Ⓒ Ⓓ
8. Ⓐ Ⓑ Ⓒ Ⓓ	28. Ⓐ Ⓑ Ⓒ Ⓓ	48. Ⓐ Ⓑ Ⓒ Ⓓ	68. Ⓐ Ⓑ Ⓒ Ⓓ	88. Ⓐ Ⓑ Ⓒ Ⓓ
9. Ⓐ Ⓑ Ⓒ Ⓓ	29. Ⓐ Ⓑ Ⓒ Ⓓ	49. Ⓐ Ⓑ Ⓒ Ⓓ	69. Ⓐ Ⓑ Ⓒ Ⓓ	89. Ⓐ Ⓑ Ⓒ Ⓓ
10. Ⓐ Ⓑ Ⓒ Ⓓ	30. Ⓐ Ⓑ Ⓒ Ⓓ	50. Ⓐ Ⓑ Ⓒ Ⓓ	70. Ⓐ Ⓑ Ⓒ Ⓓ	90. Ⓐ Ⓑ Ⓒ Ⓓ
11. Ⓐ Ⓑ Ⓒ Ⓓ	31. Ⓐ Ⓑ Ⓒ Ⓓ	51. Ⓐ Ⓑ Ⓒ Ⓓ	71. Ⓐ Ⓑ Ⓒ Ⓓ	91. Ⓐ Ⓑ Ⓒ Ⓓ
12. Ⓐ Ⓑ Ⓒ Ⓓ	32. Ⓐ Ⓑ Ⓒ Ⓓ	52. Ⓐ Ⓑ Ⓒ Ⓓ	72. Ⓐ Ⓑ Ⓒ Ⓓ	92. Ⓐ Ⓑ Ⓒ Ⓓ
13. Ⓐ Ⓑ Ⓒ Ⓓ	33. Ⓐ Ⓑ Ⓒ Ⓓ	53. Ⓐ Ⓑ Ⓒ Ⓓ	73. Ⓐ Ⓑ Ⓒ Ⓓ	93. Ⓐ Ⓑ Ⓒ Ⓓ
14. Ⓐ Ⓑ Ⓒ Ⓓ	34. Ⓐ Ⓑ Ⓒ Ⓓ	54. Ⓐ Ⓑ Ⓒ Ⓓ	74. Ⓐ Ⓑ Ⓒ Ⓓ	94. Ⓐ Ⓑ Ⓒ Ⓓ
15. Ⓐ Ⓑ Ⓒ Ⓓ	35. Ⓐ Ⓑ Ⓒ Ⓓ	55. Ⓐ Ⓑ Ⓒ Ⓓ	75. Ⓐ Ⓑ Ⓒ Ⓓ	95. Ⓐ Ⓑ Ⓒ Ⓓ
16. Ⓐ Ⓑ Ⓒ Ⓓ	36. Ⓐ Ⓑ Ⓒ Ⓓ	56. Ⓐ Ⓑ Ⓒ Ⓓ	76. Ⓐ Ⓑ Ⓒ Ⓓ	96. Ⓐ Ⓑ Ⓒ Ⓓ
17. Ⓐ Ⓑ Ⓒ Ⓓ	37. Ⓐ Ⓑ Ⓒ Ⓓ	57. Ⓐ Ⓑ Ⓒ Ⓓ	77. Ⓐ Ⓑ Ⓒ Ⓓ	97. Ⓐ Ⓑ Ⓒ Ⓓ
18. Ⓐ Ⓑ Ⓒ Ⓓ	38. Ⓐ Ⓑ Ⓒ Ⓓ	58. Ⓐ Ⓑ Ⓒ Ⓓ	78. Ⓐ Ⓑ Ⓒ Ⓓ	98. Ⓐ Ⓑ Ⓒ Ⓓ
19. Ⓐ Ⓑ Ⓒ Ⓓ	39. Ⓐ Ⓑ Ⓒ Ⓓ	59. Ⓐ Ⓑ Ⓒ Ⓓ	79. Ⓐ Ⓑ Ⓒ Ⓓ	99. Ⓐ Ⓑ Ⓒ Ⓓ
20. Ⓐ Ⓑ Ⓒ Ⓓ	40. Ⓐ Ⓑ Ⓒ Ⓓ	60. Ⓐ Ⓑ Ⓒ Ⓓ	80. Ⓐ Ⓑ Ⓒ Ⓓ	100. Ⓐ Ⓑ Ⓒ Ⓓ

TEST 5: CHEMISTRY

1. Ⓐ Ⓑ Ⓒ Ⓓ	6. Ⓐ Ⓑ Ⓒ Ⓓ	10. Ⓐ Ⓑ Ⓒ Ⓓ	14. Ⓐ Ⓑ Ⓒ Ⓓ	18. Ⓐ Ⓑ Ⓒ Ⓓ
2. Ⓐ Ⓑ Ⓒ Ⓓ	7. Ⓐ Ⓑ Ⓒ Ⓓ	11. Ⓐ Ⓑ Ⓒ Ⓓ	15. Ⓐ Ⓑ Ⓒ Ⓓ	19. Ⓐ Ⓑ Ⓒ Ⓓ
3. Ⓐ Ⓑ Ⓒ Ⓓ	8. Ⓐ Ⓑ Ⓒ Ⓓ	12. Ⓐ Ⓑ Ⓒ Ⓓ	16. Ⓐ Ⓑ Ⓒ Ⓓ	20. Ⓐ Ⓑ Ⓒ Ⓓ
4. Ⓐ Ⓑ Ⓒ Ⓓ	9. Ⓐ Ⓑ Ⓒ Ⓓ	13. Ⓐ Ⓑ Ⓒ Ⓓ	17. Ⓐ Ⓑ Ⓒ Ⓓ	21. Ⓐ Ⓑ Ⓒ Ⓓ
5. Ⓐ Ⓑ Ⓒ Ⓓ				

TEST 6: CHEMISTRY AND PHYSICAL SCIENCE

1. Ⓐ Ⓑ Ⓒ Ⓓ   11. Ⓐ Ⓑ Ⓒ Ⓓ   21. Ⓐ Ⓑ Ⓒ Ⓓ   31. Ⓐ Ⓑ Ⓒ Ⓓ   41. Ⓐ Ⓑ Ⓒ Ⓓ

2. Ⓐ Ⓑ Ⓒ Ⓓ   12. Ⓐ Ⓑ Ⓒ Ⓓ   22. Ⓐ Ⓑ Ⓒ Ⓓ   32. Ⓐ Ⓑ Ⓒ Ⓓ   42. Ⓐ Ⓑ Ⓒ Ⓓ

3. Ⓐ Ⓑ Ⓒ Ⓓ   13. Ⓐ Ⓑ Ⓒ Ⓓ   23. Ⓐ Ⓑ Ⓒ Ⓓ   33. Ⓐ Ⓑ Ⓒ Ⓓ   43. Ⓐ Ⓑ Ⓒ Ⓓ

4. Ⓐ Ⓑ Ⓒ Ⓓ   14. Ⓐ Ⓑ Ⓒ Ⓓ   24. Ⓐ Ⓑ Ⓒ Ⓓ   34. Ⓐ Ⓑ Ⓒ Ⓓ   44. Ⓐ Ⓑ Ⓒ Ⓓ

5. Ⓐ Ⓑ Ⓒ Ⓓ   15. Ⓐ Ⓑ Ⓒ Ⓓ   25. Ⓐ Ⓑ Ⓒ Ⓓ   35. Ⓐ Ⓑ Ⓒ Ⓓ   45. Ⓐ Ⓑ Ⓒ Ⓓ

6. Ⓐ Ⓑ Ⓒ Ⓓ   16. Ⓐ Ⓑ Ⓒ Ⓓ   26. Ⓐ Ⓑ Ⓒ Ⓓ   36. Ⓐ Ⓑ Ⓒ Ⓓ   46. Ⓐ Ⓑ Ⓒ Ⓓ

7. Ⓐ Ⓑ Ⓒ Ⓓ   17. Ⓐ Ⓑ Ⓒ Ⓓ   27. Ⓐ Ⓑ Ⓒ Ⓓ   37. Ⓐ Ⓑ Ⓒ Ⓓ   47. Ⓐ Ⓑ Ⓒ Ⓓ

8. Ⓐ Ⓑ Ⓒ Ⓓ   18. Ⓐ Ⓑ Ⓒ Ⓓ   28. Ⓐ Ⓑ Ⓒ Ⓓ   38. Ⓐ Ⓑ Ⓒ Ⓓ   48. Ⓐ Ⓑ Ⓒ Ⓓ

9. Ⓐ Ⓑ Ⓒ Ⓓ   19. Ⓐ Ⓑ Ⓒ Ⓓ   29. Ⓐ Ⓑ Ⓒ Ⓓ   39. Ⓐ Ⓑ Ⓒ Ⓓ   49. Ⓐ Ⓑ Ⓒ Ⓓ

10. Ⓐ Ⓑ Ⓒ Ⓓ   20. Ⓐ Ⓑ Ⓒ Ⓓ   30. Ⓐ Ⓑ Ⓒ Ⓓ   40. Ⓐ Ⓑ Ⓒ Ⓓ   50. Ⓐ Ⓑ Ⓒ Ⓓ

TEST 1: CELLS, STRUCTURE, AND FUNCTION

40 QUESTIONS ▪▫ TIME—30 MINUTES

Directions: Read each question carefully and consider all possible answers. When you have decided which choice is best, fill in the corresponding space on your answer sheet. There is only one best answer for each question.

1. Which movement requires carrier proteins but no direct cellular energy?

   (A) Diffusion
   (B) Osmosis
   (C) Dialysis
   (D) Facilitated transport

2. The polymerase chain reaction (PCR) technique is more efficient than cloning for copying large quantities of a gene because it is performed

   (A) without DNA polymerase.
   (B) in vitro.
   (C) without primers.
   (D) in vivo.

3. Which term denotes the movement of glucose molecules from an area of lower concentration to an area of higher concentration?

   (A) Osmosis
   (B) Diffusion
   (C) Dialysis
   (D) Active transport

4. You place a cell in a solution of substance x and water. Substance x is always present in the cell, but you do not know the concentration ratio in either case. The cell increases in size. What is the tonicity of the solution in which you placed the cell?

   (A) Hypotonic
   (B) Isotonic
   (C) Hypertonic
   (D) None of the above

5. Substance x passes through a plasma membrane easily. What phrase best describes the probable nature of the substance?

   (A) It is hydrophilic and nonpolar.
   (B) It is hydrophobic and polar.
   (C) It is hydrophilic and polar.
   (D) It is hydrophobic and nonpolar.

6. Cells that contain more dissolved salts and sugars than the surrounding solution are called

   (A) isotonic.
   (B) hypertonic.
   (C) hypotonic.
   (D) osmosis.

7. Foods containing unsaturated fatty acids are more healthy than those with saturated ones because they contain

   (A) more hydrogen.
   (B) less oxygen.
   (C) more nitrogen.
   (D) less hydrogen.

8. You are watching an amoeba engulf another organism. This process is an example of

   (A) receptor-mediated endocytosis.
   (B) facilitated transport.
   (C) pinocytosis.
   (D) phagocytosis.

9. The concentration of glucose in blood cells is lower than the concentration of glucose in liver cells. During active transport, glucose moves from blood cells into the liver. Which organelle would you expect to find in large numbers in the liver?

   (A) Golgi bodies
   (B) Endoplasmic reticulum
   (C) Ribosomes
   (D) Mitochondria

10. If a red blood cell is placed in sea water, it will be in what kind of solution?

    (A) Isotonic
    (B) Hypotonic
    (C) Hypertonic
    (D) Facilitated diffusion

11. Plasmolysis is a term describing

    (A) cytoplasmic movement.
    (B) cells that become turgid.
    (C) cellular shrinkage, which occurs when cells are immersed in hypertonic solution.
    (D) amoeboid movement.

12. The movement of substances from lesser concentration to higher concentration is called

    (A) osmosis.
    (B) diffusion.
    (C) active transport.
    (D) pinocytosis.

13. Which particular structure is present in both eucaryotic and prokaryotic cells?

    (A) Membrane-bound nucleus
    (B) Mitochondria
    (C) Plastids
    (D) Cell membrane

14. In photosynthesis, the reactants CO_2 and H_2O, in the presence of sunlight and chlorophyll, combine chemically to produce glucose and O_2. The O_2 comes from

    (A) H_2O.
    (B) CO_2.
    (C) CO_2 and H_2O.
    (D) N_2.

15. The endoplasmic reticulum and the Golgi body are found in prokaryotes but not eukaryotes.

    (A) True
    (B) False

16. If a radioactive element with a half-life ($t\frac{1}{2}$) of 100 years has 31.5 kg remaining after 400 years of decay, the amount in the original sample was close to

    (A) 2,500 kg.
    (B) 500 kg.
    (C) 50 kg.
    (D) 5,000 kg.

17. As you try to mix water and oil in your salad dressing, they do not mix because

    (A) water is hydrophilic and oil is hydrophobic.
    (B) water is polar and oil is nonpolar.
    (C) both are hydrophilic.
    (D) None of the above

18. Plant cells differ from animal cells in that plant cells

    (A) have a glycoprotein covering their plasma membrane.
    (B) have a cell wall and animal cells do not.
    (C) have mitochondria and animal cells do not.
    (D) do not have a nucleus.

19. Which cell type is characterized by the lack of a true nucleus and the absence of membrane-bound organelles?

    (A) Animal cell type
    (B) Plant cell type
    (C) Fungal cell type
    (D) Prokaryotic cell

20. The cytoskeleton within the cell is thought to function

    (A) in a structural capacity.
    (B) in positioning certain enzymes in close proximity for increased efficiency.
    (C) as a means of enhancing secretion of metabolites within the cell.
    (D) Both (A) and (B)

GO ON TO THE NEXT PAGE

21. Which organelle is associated with hydrolytic enzymes and is sometimes referred to as a "suicide bag"?

(A) Golgi apparatus
(B) Lysosome
(C) Mitochondrion
(D) Ribosome

Questions 22 and 23 refer to the following structural formula.

$$H\ C \!\!\!\begin{array}{c} H \\[-2pt] | \\[-2pt] \\[-2pt] | \\[-2pt] H \end{array}\!\!\!-\!\!\!\begin{array}{c} H \\[-2pt] | \\[-2pt] C \\[-2pt] | \\[-2pt] NH_2 \end{array}\!\!\!-COOH$$

22. The above compound is a(an)

(A) amino acid.
(B) aldehyde.
(C) alpha-keto acid.
(D) alcohol.

23. In human digestion, this compound is the end product of

(A) fats.
(B) vitamins.
(C) proteins.
(D) carbohydrates.

24. The virus belongs to which one of the following kingdoms?

(A) Monera
(B) Plantae
(C) Protista
(D) None of the above

25. Organisms that live on dead organic matter are called

(A) parasites.
(B) carnivorous.
(C) autotrophs.
(D) saprophytes.

Questions 26 and 27 refer to the diagrams below.

I

II

26. A person who turns off the television does not also cause the refrigerator to stop because they are

(A) in circuit I; TV in series and refrigerator in parallel.
(B) in circuit II; TV in parallel and refrigerator in series.
(C) in circuit II; both the TV and refrigerator are in parallel circuits.
(D) in circuit I; both TV and refrigerator are in series.

27. Along a string of lights on a Christmas tree, if one half goes out, they all go out. Use the above diagram to determine which of the following illustrates this circuitry.

(A) Both I and II
(B) I
(C) II
(D) Neither I nor II

28. Pinocytosis is the process of

(A) enclosing a food source or other substance in a membrane and bringing it into a cell.
(B) enclosing a liquid substance in a membrane and bringing it into the cell.
(C) enclosing a manufactured substance in a membrane and secreting it from the cell.
(D) binding a substance and a receptor and bringing it into the cell.

29. The AIDS virus is transported in bodily fluids. The Surgeon General of the United States sends out information about the disease and its transmission. In one section, there is a recommendation that one should use latex (a form of plastic) condoms rather than those made of natural membranes. This recommendation is probably based upon the principal of

    (A) diffusion.
    (B) facilitated transport.
    (C) active transport.
    (D) varied selectivity, permeability of membranes.

30. The plasma membrane of the eukaryotic cell determines selectively which substances can enter and leave the cell. Such a membrane is said to be

    (A) impermeable.
    (B) selectively permeable.
    (C) isotonic.
    (D) hypotonic.

31. What primarily determines the shape of cells that lack cell walls?

    (A) Microtubules and microfilaments
    (B) Nucleus
    (C) Endoplasmic reticulum (ER)
    (D) Ribosomes

32. Which pair of organelles is responsible for energy supply to eukaryotic cells?

    (A) Ribosomes and mitochondria
    (B) Chloroplasts and mitochondria
    (C) Nuclei and ribosomes
    (D) Mitochondria and nuclei

Questions 33 and 34 relate to the following equation and graph of an enzyme-catalyzed cellular reaction.

33. The linear distance between P_1 and P_2 on the above graph is the initial velocity of the reaction, as expressed by the slope (m) of the line (see above formula), which is

    (A) 60
    (B) 10
    (C) 40
    (D) 6

34. Choose the correct statement, relative to 10 minutes of reaction time.

    (A) Enzyme has been denatured.
    (B) All ES has been converted to [P].
    (C) All enzyme [E] is occupied with substrate [S].
    (D) All product has been converted to substrate.

35. You collect some pond water and filter out the different organisms into separate jars. You add no food to the water, but one kind of organism is still alive long after the others have died. That species is best described as being

    (A) autotrophic.
    (B) hydrophilic.
    (C) autonomous.
    (D) heterotrophic.

GO ON TO THE NEXT PAGE

36. When you mix salt with water, what is the water called?

(A) Solute
(B) Solvent
(C) Solution
(D) Ionizer

Questions 37 and 38 refer to the diagram below.

Exponential growth (I):

$\Delta N/\Delta t = rN$–change in number per change in time

Logistic growth (II):

$\Delta N/\Delta t = rN(k–N/K)$

    r = intrinsic rate of increase

    K = carrying capacity of the environment

37. Choose the correct statement expressed by curve II, as N approaches K.

(A) r approaches maximum.
(B) K expands upward.
(C) $\Delta N/\Delta t$ approaches zero.
(D) Resources remain unlimited.

38. Choose the correct statement about curve I.

(A) It assumes unlimited resources.
(B) It expresses limited growth.
(C) It expresses a K value.
(D) It assumes limited resources.

39. With which organelle is the synthesis of ATP associated?

(A) Ribosome
(B) Plastid
(C) Mitochondrion
(D) Lysosome

40. The plasma membrane is soluble to

(A) lipids.
(B) proteins.
(C) acids.
(D) nucleic acids.

STOP   If you finish before time is called, you may check your work on this section only. Do not turn to any other section in the test.

BIOLOGY
TEST 2

19 QUESTIONS ▪ TIME—15 MINUTES

Directions: Read each question carefully and consider all possible answers. When you have decided which choice is best, fill in the corresponding space on your answer sheet. There is only one best answer for each question.

1. The process whereby muscle cells produce lactic acid is called
   - (A) aerobic respiration.
   - (B) glycolysis.
   - (C) fermentation.
   - (D) electron transport chain.

2. During aerobic respiration, which one of the following substances is released?
   - (A) 22 ATP
   - (B) 32 ATP
   - (C) 2 ATP
   - (D) 36 ATP

Questions 3 and 4 refer to the diagram below.

$\Delta G = \Delta H - T\Delta S$

In cellular metabolism, the energy available for doing biological work is called free energy (G). It is equal to the molecular energy, enthalpy (H) minus the disorder, entropy (S) times the absolute temperature (T).

3. Choose the correct statement describing reaction I.
   - (A) The reaction is exergonic.
   - (B) ΔG is negative.
   - (C) Glucose and O_2 have less energy than CO_2 and H_2O.
   - (D) The reaction is endergonic.

4. Choose the correct statement describing reaction II.
   - (A) ΔG is positive.
   - (B) CO_2 and H_2O have more energy than glucose and O_2.
   - (C) The reaction is exergonic.
   - (D) The reaction is endergonic.

5. In exergonic reactions, the energy is
   - (A) used.
   - (B) stored.
   - (C) released.
   - (D) lost.

6. Most human enzymes function best in the temperature range of
   - (A) 5–15 degrees C.
   - (B) 20–30 degrees C.
   - (C) 35–40 degrees C.
   - (D) 45–50 degrees C.

7. Vitamins are important to the human diet because they are incorporated into
   - (A) enzyme substitutes.
   - (B) ATP.
   - (C) co-enzymes.
   - (D) inhibitors.

GO ON TO THE NEXT PAGE

8. Stored energy is referred to as
   (A) activation energy.
   (B) kinetic energy.
   (C) potential energy.
   (D) electrical energy.

9. Noncyclic-photophosphorylation takes place inside the
   (A) stroma.
   (B) cytoplasm.
   (C) thylakoids.
   (D) Golgi bodies.

10. The products of the light reaction of photosynthesis are
    (A) carbohydrate + CO_2.
    (B) $NADPH_2$ + ATP + O_2.
    (C) PGAL + CO_2 + H_2O.
    (D) starch + CO_2.

11. The dark reaction of photosynthesis takes place in
    (A) thylakoids.
    (B) cytoplasm.
    (C) stroma.
    (D) grana.

Questions 12 and 13 refer to the following ecological pyramid of biomass and energy.

12. Select the correct population changes resulting from hunters reducing the hawk population.
    (A) Grasshoppers increase ÷ Field mice decrease ÷ Sunflowers increase
    (B) Field mice increase ÷ Grasshoppers increase ÷ Sunflowers increase
    (C) Field mice increase ÷ Grasshoppers decrease ÷ Sunflowers increase
    (D) Sunflowers decrease ÷ Grasshoppers decrease ÷ Field mice decrease

13. The second law of thermodynamic would suggest that the most energy-efficient feeding pattern would be if
    (A) field mice ate grasshoppers.
    (B) hawks ate sunflowers.
    (C) hawks ate field mice.
    (D) grasshoppers ate field mice.

14. Aerobic cellular respiration is more important to sustaining life than anaerobic because it produces
    (A) more pyruvic acid.
    (B) more sugar.
    (C) more energy.
    (D) more lactic acid.

15. Which organelle is responsible for oxygen production?
    (A) Mitochondria
    (B) Cilia
    (C) Golgi body
    (D) Chloroplasts

16. An organic catalyst that enhances the chemical reaction is called

    (A) a fat.
    (B) a lactic acid.
    (C) a polysaccharide.
    (D) an enzyme.

17. The first stage of aerobic cellular respiration is

    (A) electron transport chain.
    (B) Krebs cycle.
    (C) glycolysis.
    (D) light reaction.

18. Glycolysis occurs in the

    (A) nucleus.
    (B) mitochondrion.
    (C) plasma membrane.
    (D) cytoplasm.

19. For the aerobic pathway, electron transport systems are located in the

    (A) cytoplasm.
    (B) Golgi bodies.
    (C) lysosomes.
    (D) mitochondrion.

STOP   If you finish before time is called, you may check your work on this section only. Do not turn to any other section in the test.

TEST 3

20 QUESTIONS ▪▭ TIME—15 MINUTES

Directions: Read each question carefully and consider all possible answers. When you have decided which choice is best, fill in the corresponding space on your answer sheet. There is only one best answer for each question.

1. If body cells of cows contain a total of 40 chromosomes, sperm and egg cells of cows contain how many chromosomes total?

   (A) 10
   (B) 20
   (C) 25
   (D) 40

2. Codominance occurs when

   (A) both the alleles in a heterozygote are expressed phenotypically in an individual.
   (B) expression of 2 different alleles alternates from one generation to the next.
   (C) a heterozygote expresses an intermediate phenotype.
   (D) offspring exhibit several different phenotypic expressions of a single trait.

3. Mitosis in a single human cell usually results in the formation of

   (A) 2 diploid cells.
   (B) 2 haploid cells.
   (C) 4 diploid cells.
   (D) 4 haploid cells.

4. Meiosis in a single human cell usually results in the formation of

   (A) 2 diploid cells.
   (B) 2 haploid cells.
   (C) 4 diploid cells.
   (D) 4 haploid cells.

5. If you reproduce sexually, you produce gametes via

   (A) fertilization.
   (B) mitosis.
   (C) meiosis.
   (D) recombination.

6. If you reproduce asexually, you produce offspring via

   (A) fertilization.
   (B) mitosis.
   (C) meiosis.
   (D) recombination.

7. According to Mendel's Law of Segregation, an organism with the genotype Aa

   (A) produces only gametes containing the A allele.
   (B) produces only gametes containing the a allele.
   (C) half the time produces gametes containing A, and half the time, a.
   (D) three quarters of the time produces gametes containing A, and one quarter of the time, a.

8. What type of allele is expressed in the phenotype of only a homozygous individual?

   (A) Incompletely dominant
   (B) Haploid
   (C) Recessive
   (D) Dominant

9. The sex of a human child is determined by the sex chromosome from

   (A) the mother.
   (B) the father.
   (C) both parents.
   (D) neither parents.

10. Cell division occurs most rapidly in

   (A) heart tissue.
   (B) muscle tissue.
   (C) nervous tissue.
   (D) cancerous tissue.

11. If the sperm cells of a fish have 30 chromosomes, the body cell of the fish has

    (A) 80 chromosomes.
    (B) 60 chromosomes.
    (C) 120 chromosomes.
    (D) None of the above

12. A condition resulting from the presence of an extra twenty-first chromosome is

    (A) hemophilia.
    (B) the Rh-positive condition.
    (C) phenylketonuria.
    (D) Down syndrome.

13. A woman who is a heterozygous carrier for a sex-linked recessive gene will pass it to

    (A) all of her sons.
    (B) all of her daughters.
    (C) all children.
    (D) one half of her sons and one half of her daughters.

14. Persons who have hemophilia cannot produce

    (A) new red blood cells.
    (B) normally shaped red blood cells.
    (C) functional blood clotting factors.
    (D) white blood cells.

15. Which of the following is an example of a sex-linked genetic disorder?

    (A) Tay-Sachs disease
    (B) Cystic fibrosis
    (C) Turner's syndrome
    (D) Hemophilia

16. In the case of the sex-linked trait red-green color-blindness, which one of the following CANNOT occur?

    (A) A carrier mother passing the gene on to her son
    (B) A carrier mother passing the gene on to her daughter
    (C) A color-blind father passing the gene on to his son
    (D) A color-blind father passing the gene on to his daughter

17. The genotype for a man who has blue eyes and hemophilia is

    (A) $x^b y \ x^h y$
    (B) bb hh
    (C) bb $x^h y$
    (D) Bbh

18. If both parents have blood type AB, what will be the blood types of offspring?

    (A) A
    (B) AB
    (C) A, AB, and B
    (D) O

19. Which blood type would be a universal donor?

    (A) A
    (B) AB
    (C) B
    (D) O

20. Males who tend to be tall and have strong criminal records have which of the following sex chromosomes?

    (A) XXY
    (B) XY
    (C) XYY
    (D) XYXY

S T O P If you finish before time is called, you may check your work on this section only. Do not turn to any other section in the test.

TEST 4: HUMAN ANATOMY AND PHYSIOLOGY

100 QUESTIONS ▬▭ TIME—75 MINUTES

Directions: Read each question carefully and consider all possible answers. When you have decided which choice is best, fill in the corresponding space on your answer sheet. There is only one best answer for each question.

1. The _____ system picks up fluid leaked from blood vessels, houses white blood cells, and is highly involved in mechanisms of immunity.
   - (A) urinary
   - (B) endocrine
   - (C) integumentary
   - (D) lymphatic

2. The major muscle component of inspiration is the
   - (A) diaphragm.
   - (B) external intercostal muscles.
   - (C) internal intercostal muscles.
   - (D) abdominal muscles.

3. Skin, nails, and hair are components of the _____ system.
   - (A) integumentary
   - (B) lymphatic
   - (C) skeletal
   - (D) endocrine

4. Water reabsorption in the collecting duct of the kidneys is controlled by _____ from the posterior pituitary.
   - (A) oxytocin
   - (B) ADH
   - (C) epinephrine
   - (D) aldosterone

5. Most homeostatic control mechanisms are
   - (A) positive feedback mechanisms.
   - (B) negative feedback mechanisms.
   - (C) neural mechanisms.
   - (D) endocrine mechanisms.

6. The most important structure(s) in the routine control of respiration is(are) the
   - (A) trachea.
   - (B) irritant receptors.
   - (C) peripheral chemoreceptors.
   - (D) central chemoreceptors.

7. A _____ plane is a vertical plane that divides the body into left and right parts.
   - (A) frontal
   - (B) transverse
   - (C) sagittal
   - (D) coronal

8. Cardiac output is equal to
   - (A) heart rate.
   - (B) stroke volume.
   - (C) the product of stroke volume and heart rate.
   - (D) stroke volume divided by heart rate.

9. Movement of a solute across a biological membrane from an area of low concentration to an area of high concentration occurs via
   - (A) osmosis.
   - (B) diffusion.
   - (C) active transport.
   - (D) inertia.

10. The right ventricle pumps blood through the _____ valve into the _____.
    - (A) atrioventricular; pulmonary veins
    - (B) pulmonary semilunar; pulmonary veins
    - (C) atrioventricular; pulmonary arteries
    - (D) pulmonary semilunar; pulmonary arteries

11. The primary beta-2 catechol amine agonist is
    (A) acetylcholine.
    (B) epinephrine.
    (C) norepinephrine.
    (D) nicotine.

12. Action potentials result from an increased membrane permeability to
    (A) calcium.
    (B) sodium.
    (C) potassium.
    (D) chloride.

13. Food is prevented from entering the trachea during swallowing by the
    (A) glottis.
    (B) esophageal sphincter.
    (C) cardiac sphincter.
    (D) epiglottis.

14. Oxygen transported in blood is mainly
    (A) dissolved in plasma.
    (B) combined with hemoglobin.
    (C) CO_2.
    (D) carried as bicarbonate.

15. Pyramidal tract fibers originate in the
    (A) precentral gyrus.
    (B) postcentral gyrus.
    (C) thalamus.
    (D) spinal cord.

16. The transmitter substance at the neuromuscular junction is
    (A) acetylcholinesterase.
    (B) norepinephrine.
    (C) acetylcholine.
    (D) epinephrine.

17. _____ dilate or constrict to control the flow of blood into a particular capillary bed.
    (A) Arteries
    (B) Arterioles
    (C) Capillaries
    (D) Veins

18. Hormone secretion and neurotransmitter release use the process of _____ to move substances from the cell interior into the extracellular space.
    (A) phagocytosis
    (B) endocytosis
    (C) exocytosis
    (D) pinocytosis

19. The area innervated by all the axons in a single dorsal root is a(n)
    (A) receptive field.
    (B) dermatome.
    (C) sensory unit.
    (D) motor unit.

20. Stratified squamous anatomically describes a form of _____ tissue.
    (A) muscle
    (B) nerve
    (C) connective
    (D) epithelial

21. _____ forms most of the embryonic skeleton, connects the ribs of the sternum, and comprises the solid supportive structures of the nose and trachea.
    (A) Bone
    (B) Areolar connective tissue
    (C) Adipose tissue
    (D) Cartilage

22. _____ is the fibrous protein found in the stratum corneum that helps give the epidermis its protective properties.
    (A) Keratin
    (B) Melanin
    (C) Carotene
    (D) Hemoglobin

23. Pain information is carried by _____ afferents.
    (A) A Delta
    (B) C
    (C) A Alpha
    (D) A Delta and C

GO ON TO THE NEXT PAGE

24. Increased parasympathetic activity will result in

    (A) increased heart rate.
    (B) increased cardiac output.
    (C) vasoconstriction.
    (D) decreased heart rate.

25. The receptor for the stretch reflex is the

    (A) Golgi tendon organ.
    (B) free nerve ending.
    (C) hair cell.
    (D) muscle spindle.

26. The glomerular membrane is

    (A) more permeable than most other capillaries.
    (B) less permeable than most other capillaries.
    (C) highly permeable to proteins.
    (D) highly permeable to erythrocytes.

27. CO_2 in blood is mainly

    (A) dissolved in plasma.
    (B) carried as bicarbonate.
    (C) dissolved in RBCs.
    (D) combined with hemoglobin.

28. Glucose is returned in blood in the kidneys by

    (A) glomerular filtration.
    (B) tubular reabsorption.
    (C) tubular secretion.
    (D) reabsorption in the collection duct.

29. The outer surface of the diaphysis of a long bone is covered with a double-layered membrane called the _____. The inner layer of that membrane contains bone-forming cells called _____.

    (A) endosteum; osteoblasts
    (B) endosteum; osteoclasts
    (C) periosteum; osteoclasts
    (D) periosteum; osteoblasts

30. Atrial contraction is

    (A) initiated by the AV node.
    (B) most important in a resting subject.
    (C) initiated by the SA node.
    (D) responsible for most of the ventricular filling.

31. The first heart sound is a result of

    (A) closing of the pulmonary valve.
    (B) closing of the AV valves.
    (C) closing of the aortic valve.
    (D) contraction of the atria.

32. The portion of the skull overlying the region of the cerebral cortex primarily involved with visual process is the _____ bone.

    (A) frontal
    (B) parietal
    (C) occipital
    (D) temporal

33. Normally, most of the body's total blood is found in the

    (A) veins.
    (B) arteries.
    (C) capillaries.
    (D) heart.

34. The kneecap or patella is an example of a(n) _____ bone.

    (A) long
    (B) short
    (C) flat
    (D) irregular

35. The normal pacemaker of the heart is the

    (A) SA node.
    (B) AV node.
    (C) atria.
    (D) ventricle.

36. Blood pressure is highest in

    (A) arteries.
    (B) arterioles.
    (C) capillaries.
    (D) veins.

37. Water permeability is greatest in the _____ of the nephron.

    (A) collecting duct
    (B) distal convoluted tubule
    (C) loop of Henle
    (D) proximal convoluted tubule

38. Movement of particles across a biological membrane is enhanced by

(A) large particle size.
(B) lipid solubility.
(C) particle charge.
(D) lipophobic properties.

39. The division of the autonomic nervous system that functions during emergencies is the

(A) sympathetic.
(B) parasympathetic.
(C) craniosacral.
(D) somatic.

40. Sympathetic preganglionic neurons originate in the

(A) cervical spinal cord.
(B) thoracic spinal cord.
(C) sacral spinal cord.
(D) coccygeal spinal cord.

41. Cellular energy production takes place within

(A) rough endoplasmic reticulum.
(B) smooth endoplasmic reticulum.
(C) mitochondria.
(D) Golgi apparatus.

42. _____ is a bending movement that decreases the angle of a joint and brings two articulating bones closer together.

(A) Retraction
(B) Flexion
(C) Extension
(D) Rotation

43. New epidermal cells are formed in the stratum

(A) germinativum.
(B) corneum.
(C) spinosum.
(D) lucidum.

44. Women have a larger percentage of adipose tissue than men; this tissue is mainly found in the

(A) epidermis.
(B) dermis.
(C) subcutaneous layer.
(D) muscle.

45. Membranes that line body cavities that open to the outside are

(A) mucous.
(B) serous.
(C) synovial.
(D) cutaneous.

46. Epidermal cells are supplied with nutrition from blood vessels located within the

(A) epidermis.
(B) dermis.
(C) subcutaneous layer.
(D) All of the above

47. The terms visceral, nonstriated, and involuntary are descriptive of _____ muscle.

(A) skeletal
(B) smooth
(C) cardiac
(D) postural

48. Blood cell formation is a function of the _____ system.

(A) circulatory
(B) skeletal
(C) endocrine
(D) muscular

49. Blood calcium is elevated by

(A) calcitonin.
(B) parathyroid hormone.
(C) growth hormone.
(D) thyroxine.

50. A 7-year-old patient is perspiring freely on the forehead, palms, and soles, indicating activity of the

(A) eccrine glands.
(B) apocrine glands.
(C) sebaceous glands.
(D) ceruminous glands.

GO ON TO THE NEXT PAGE

51. Flexion of the elbow results from contraction of the _____ muscle, and flexion of the knee involves contraction of the _____ muscle.

    (A) biceps brachii; biceps femoris
    (B) triceps brachii; triceps femoris
    (C) biceps femoris; biceps brachii
    (D) triceps femoris; triceps brachii

52. Sweat glands that become functional at puberty are

    (A) apocrine.
    (B) eccrine.
    (C) sebaceous.
    (D) ceruminous.

53. An individual with higher than normal blood calcium (hypercalcemia) will compensate by elevating levels of

    (A) parathyroid hormone.
    (B) calcitonin.
    (C) Both (A) and (B)
    (D) Neither (A) nor (B)

54. The _____ system carries hormones to their sites of action.

    (A) endocrine
    (B) cardiovascular
    (C) respiratory
    (D) skeletal

55. The most rapidly conducting axons within the human nervous system are _____ and _____.

    (A) unmyelinated; small diameter
    (B) unmyelinated; large diameter
    (C) myelinated; small diameter
    (D) myelinated; large diameter

56. The basic unit of structure and function within the kidneys is the

    (A) glomerulus.
    (B) nephron.
    (C) ureter.
    (D) urethra.

57. The esophagus enters the stomach at the _____ region.

    (A) fundus
    (B) cardiac
    (C) body
    (D) pyloric

58. Release of _____ by the posterior pituitary will lead to contractions of the smooth muscle of the uterus.

    (A) ADH
    (B) ACTH
    (C) oxytocin
    (D) prolactin

59. Inhibition of ADH release will result in

    (A) high blood pressure.
    (B) increased urine output.
    (C) uterine contractions.
    (D) decreased urine output.

60. Ovulation occurs in response to

    (A) FSH.
    (B) ADH.
    (C) prolactin.
    (D) LH.

61. Heartburn results from reflux of gastric fluids into the esophagus. The structure that normally prevents this is the

    (A) pyloric sphincter.
    (B) cardiac spincter.
    (C) ileocecal valve.
    (D) epiglottis.

62. Fat is broken down in the duodenum by _____ from the gallbladder.

    (A) lipase
    (B) amylase
    (C) bile
    (D) HCl

63. Most digestion takes place in the

    (A) stomach.
    (B) duodenum.
    (C) ileum.
    (D) jejunum.

64. Visual receptors are located on the
    (A) lens.
    (B) cornea.
    (C) retina.
    (D) optic tract.

65. Most food absorption takes place in the
    (A) duodenum.
    (B) colon.
    (C) ileum.
    (D) stomach.

66. Centers for cardiovascular and respiratory control, vomiting, and coughing are found within the _____, the most inferior part of the brain stem.
    (A) midbrain
    (B) pons
    (C) medulla
    (D) thalamus

67. Bile is manufactured in the
    (A) duodenum.
    (B) liver.
    (C) gall bladder.
    (D) pancreas.

68. A patient who is abnormally short and retarded suggests
    (A) hyperthyroidism as an infant.
    (B) hypothyroidism as an infant.
    (C) adult hyperthyroidism.
    (D) adult hypothyroidism.

69. Receptors used for color vision are
    (A) hair cells.
    (B) rods.
    (C) cones.
    (D) retinae.

70. The inner lining of the digestive system is the _____ layer.
    (A) mucosal
    (B) submucosal
    (C) muscular
    (D) serosal

71. The _____ has both endocrine and exocrine functions.
    (A) adrenal cortex
    (B) pancreas
    (C) parathyroid
    (D) thyroid

72. Lacrimation refers to the production of
    (A) salvia.
    (B) mucous.
    (C) tears.
    (D) urine.

73. The sense of smell travels over cranial nerve number
    (A) I
    (B) II
    (C) III
    (D) IV

74. The gland adjacent to the urethra that enlarges in older males is the
    (A) testes.
    (B) seminal vesicle.
    (C) bulbourethral gland.
    (D) prostate.

75. Linear acceleration of the head is detected by receptors within the
    (A) semicircular canals.
    (B) utricles and saccules.
    (C) cochlea.
    (D) middle ear.

76. The most abundant protein in blood is
    (A) alpha globulin.
    (B) albumin.
    (C) gamma globulin.
    (D) fibrin.

77. Fertilization normally occurs within the
    (A) fallopian tube.
    (B) ovary.
    (C) uterus.
    (D) vagina.

GO ON TO THE NEXT PAGE

78. Depression is characterized by

    (A) high levels of norepinephrine.
    (B) low levels of serotonin.
    (C) high levels of serotonin.
    (D) high levels of norepinephrine.

79. Lymphatic vessels originate at

    (A) vascular capillaries.
    (B) lymphatic capillaries.
    (C) lymph nodes.
    (D) lymphocytes.

80. Human chorionic gonadotropin (HCG) is responsible for

    (A) maintaining the corpus luteum.
    (B) lowering estrogen levels.
    (C) lowering progesterone levels.
    (D) initiating menstruation.

81. Loss of the sense of sweet and sour tastes from the tongue indicate damage to the _____ nerve.

    (A) first
    (B) fifth
    (C) seventh
    (D) tenth

82. Salivation, lacrimation, urination, and defecation are primarily under control of the _____ division of the autonomic nervous system.

    (A) sympathetic
    (B) parasympathetic
    (C) somatic
    (D) voluntary

83. Sperm cells are stored in the _____ after leaving the seminiferous tubules.

    (A) epididymis
    (B) vas deferens
    (C) seminal vesicle
    (D) prostate

84. The hormone from the pancreas that is responsible for elevating blood glucose levels between meals is

    (A) insulin.
    (B) glucagon.
    (C) somatostatin.
    (D) epinephrine.

85. The most abundantly formed elements in blood are

    (A) white blood cells.
    (B) red blood cells.
    (C) globulins.
    (D) albumins.

86. The most rapid mechanism of pH adjustment involves

    (A) buffers.
    (B) the respiratory system.
    (C) the kidneys.
    (D) the liver.

87. Normal pH of blood is

    (A) 6
    (B) 7.4
    (C) 8
    (D) 1.0

88. Hematocrit is a measure of _____ levels.

    (A) white cell
    (B) plasma
    (C) blood
    (D) erythrocyte

89. Cardiac muscle, because of its constant activity, has a high oxygen demand, which must be met without interruption. Oxygen is supplied to cardiac muscle by

    (A) the blood being pumped through the chambers of the heart.
    (B) coronary arteries.
    (C) coronary veins.
    (D) pulmonary arteries.

90. Auditory receptors are

    (A) rods.
    (B) hair cells.
    (C) cones.
    (D) muscle spindles.

91. Blood containing the A antigen and the B antibody is type

    (A) A
    (B) B
    (C) AB
    (D) O

92. Hemoglobin forms abnormal long chains in

    (A) pernicious anemia.
    (B) iron deficiency anemia.
    (C) aplastic anemia.
    (D) sickle cell anemia.

93. Auditory receptors are found within the

    (A) outer ear.
    (B) middle ear.
    (C) auditory ossicles.
    (D) cochlea.

94. Female menopause is characterized by low levels of

    (A) GnRH.
    (B) LH.
    (C) FSH.
    (D) estrogen.

95. Hyperventilation resulting from hysteria may cause

    (A) respiratory acidosis.
    (B) respiratory alkalosis.
    (C) metabolic acidosis.
    (D) metabolic alkalosis.

96. The major component of plasma is

    (A) ions.
    (B) proteins.
    (C) water.
    (D) gases.

97. _____ acts as a contraceptive agent by inhibiting release of GnRH.

    (A) Sperm
    (B) Estrogen
    (C) Testosterone
    (D) LH

98. Coagulation is inhibited by

    (A) fibrin.
    (B) calcium.
    (C) thrombin.
    (D) heparin.

99. Ovulation is triggered by the release of

    (A) FSH.
    (B) LH.
    (C) GnRH.
    (D) estrogen.

100. Testosterone is produced by _____ cells.

    (A) prostate
    (B) seminiferous
    (C) epididymis
    (D) interstitial

STOP   If you finish before time is called, you may check your work on this section only. Do not turn to any other section in the test.

TEST 5: CHEMISTRY

21 QUESTIONS ▪▭ TIME—20 MINUTES

Directions: Read each question carefully and consider all possible answers. When you have decided which choice is best, fill in the corresponding space on your answer sheet. There is only one best answer for each question.

1. A high concentration of H^+ ions is characteristic of
   - (A) high pH.
   - (B) strong acid.
   - (C) alkaline base.
   - (D) Both (A) and (C)

2. Long chains of glucose molecules are involved in the structure of
   - (A) proteins.
   - (B) fats.
   - (C) cholesterol.
   - (D) polysaccharides.

3. When a solution has a pH of 7, it is
   - (A) a strong base.
   - (B) a strong acid.
   - (C) a weak base.
   - (D) neutral.

4. Which one of the following is NOT a carbohydrate?
   - (A) Maltose
   - (B) Cellulose
   - (C) Glycogen
   - (D) Cholesterol

5. An example of an organic compound is
   - (A) water (H_2O).
   - (B) ammonia (NH_3).
   - (C) salt (NaCl).
   - (D) glucose ($C_6H_{12}O_6$).

6. A covalent bond is believed to be caused by
   - (A) transfer of electrons.
   - (B) sharing of electrons.
   - (C) release of energy.
   - (D) None of the above

7. An atom has the electron configuration (2-8-8-2). This atom would tend to
   - (A) gain electrons.
   - (B) loose 2 electrons.
   - (C) be inert.
   - (D) None of the above

8. Which of the following is a dissaccharide?
   - (A) Glucose
   - (B) Maltose
   - (C) Fructose
   - (D) Chilin

9. Which one of the following is NOT a carbohydrate?
   - (A) Maltose
   - (B) Cellulose
   - (C) Glycogen
   - (D) Wax

10. The basic building blocks of proteins are
   - (A) polypeptides.
   - (B) glucose.
   - (C) amino acids.
   - (D) None of the above

11. If the atomic number of magnesium is 12, what will be the number of protons?
   - (A) 6
   - (B) 10
   - (C) 14
   - (D) 12

12. Which is NOT an inert element?
   - (A) Hydrogen
   - (B) Neon
   - (C) Oxygen
   - (D) Nitrogen

13. Atoms are electrically neutral. This means that an atom will contain

  (A) more protons than neutrons.
  (B) more electrons than protons.
  (C) an equal number of protons and electrons.
  (D) None of the above

14. Which is true of alkaline solutions?

  (A) More H^+ ion than OH ion
  (B) Same amount of H^+ ion + OH^- ion
  (C) More OH^- ion than H^+ ion
  (D) None of the above

15. A common detergent has pH 11.0, so the detergent is

  (A) neutral.
  (B) acidic.
  (C) alkaline.
  (D) None of the above

16. The basic building block of carbohydrate is

  (A) starch.
  (B) chitin.
  (C) sucrose.
  (D) glucose.

17. The number of different amino acids in proteins is

  (A) 20
  (B) 26
  (C) 50
  (D) 92

18. A nucleotide is

  (A) phospholipid, sugar, and base.
  (B) phosphate, sugar, and base.
  (C) phosphate, protein, and base.
  (D) phospholipid, sugar, and protein.

19. Polar bonds form when

  (A) electrons are shared unequally between atoms.
  (B) more than one pair of electrons is shared.
  (C) ions are formed.
  (D) an acid and base are combined.

20. Which of the following is an example of hydrogen bonding?

  (A) The bond between O and H in a single molecule of water
  (B) The bond between O of one water molecule and H of a second water molecule
  (C) The bond between O of one water molecule and O of a second water molecule
  (D) The bond between H of one water molecule and H of a second water molecule

21. The Central Dogma of Information Transfer states that information is passed in what sequence?

  (A) RNA to proteins to DNA
  (B) DNA to RNA to proteins
  (C) Proteins to RNA to DNA
  (D) RNA to DNA to proteins

STOP   If you finish before time is called, you may check your work on this section only. Do not turn to any other section in the test.

TEST 6: CHEMISTRY AND PHYSICAL SCIENCE

50 QUESTIONS ◼◻ TIME—45 MINUTES

Directions: Read each question carefully and consider all possible answers. When you have decided which choice is best, fill in the corresponding space on your answer sheet. There is only one best answer for each question. You may use the periodic table on page 197 if needed.

1. The compound that has the greatest polarity is

    (A) $CH_3—CH_2—O—CH_2—CH_3$
    (B) $CH_3—CH_2CH_2CH_2—CH_3$
    (C) $CH_3—CH_2—CH_2—CH_2—CH_2—Cl$
    (D) $CH_3—CH_2—CH_2—CH_2—CH_2—OH$

2. The formula that represents the strongest acid in the following group is

    (A) HCl
    (B) HCN
    (C) HNO_3
    (D) HCOOH

3. The sugar with the highest molecular weight of those listed is

    (A) fructose.
    (B) sucrose.
    (C) glucose.
    (D) None of the above; all have the same molecular weight.

4. A hydride ion and a hydrogen atom both have

    (A) the same number of electrons.
    (B) the same charge.
    (C) the same number of protons.
    (D) equal atomic radii.

5. The general formula for an aldehyde is

    (A) RCOOH
    (B) RCOOR
    (C) ROH
    (D) RCHO

6. The compound that will not be acidic when dissolved in water is

    (A) HBr
    (B) N_2O_5
    (C) CaO
    (D) NH_4Cl

7. Atoms that have the same atomic number but different atomic masses

    (A) are from different elements.
    (B) are isobars.
    (C) have different numbers of electrons.
    (D) are isotopes.

8. When electrolysis is done with molten NaCl, the substance produced at the anode is

    (A) chlorine.
    (B) hydrogen.
    (C) sodium.
    (D) oxygen.

9. The non-electrolyte in the following group is

    (A) acetic acid.
    (B) calcium chloride.
    (C) sodium bromide.
    (D) sugar.

10. Rubbing alcohol is

    (A) methyl alcohol.
    (B) ethyl alcohol.
    (C) phenol.
    (D) isopropyl alcohol.

11. Which of the following elements is a transition element?

    (A) Argon
    (B) Copper
    (C) Barium
    (D) Aluminum

12. When calcium reacts with chlorine to form calcium chloride, it

    (A) shares two electrons.
    (B) gains two electrons.
    (C) loses two electrons.
    (D) gains one electron.

13. The compound NaClO is called

    (A) sodium perchlorate.
    (B) sodium oxychloride.
    (C) sodium chlorate.
    (D) sodium hypochlorite.

14. Reaction kinetics deals with

    (A) equilibrium position.
    (B) reaction rates.
    (C) molecular reactant size.
    (D) None of the above

15. A 1-molar solution of K_3PO_4, potassium phosphate, contains in 1 liter

    (A) one mole of potassium ions.
    (B) one mole of oxygen atoms.
    (C) one mole of phosphorus atoms.
    (D) no ions.

16. In the compound propene, $H_2C=CH—CH_3$, the single bond between two carbon atoms is

    (A) stronger than the double bond.
    (B) shorter than the double bond.
    (C) equal to the double bond in bond strength.
    (D) longer than the double bond.

17. Of the following groups the least reactive are

    (A) the halogens.
    (B) the inert gases.
    (C) group IIA metals.
    (D) precious metals of group IB.

18. Per liter, compared to a 3 molar aqueous solution, a 3 molar aqueous solution contains

    (A) the same amount of solute.
    (B) more solute.
    (C) less solute.
    (D) a variable amount of solute.

19. For a molecular substance, a gram formula weight

    (A) is unrelated to the gram molecular weight.
    (B) is always equal to the mass corresponding to its empirical formula.
    (C) can always be calculated from its empirical formula alone.
    (D) is identical to its gram molecular weight.

20. If gas A has a molecular weight four times that of gas B,

    (A) the average speed of gas A is about 4 times that of gas B.
    (B) the average speed of gas B is about 4 times that of gas A.
    (C) the average speed of gas A is about twice that of gas B.
    (D) the average speed of gas B is about twice that of gas A.

21. Ice can be melted most effectively by _____ if 1 mole is used.

    (A) sucrose
    (B) calcium chloride
    (C) sodium chloride
    (D) methanol

22. Per atom, an element that has an atomic number of 19 contains

    (A) 19 electrons and 19 neutrons.
    (B) 19 electrons and 19 protons.
    (C) 19 protons and 19 neutrons.
    (D) a total of 19 protons and neutrons.

GO ON TO THE NEXT PAGE

23. In a volume of air at one atmosphere pressure at sea level, the partial pressure of nitrogen will be about

    (A) 490 mm of mercury.
    (B) 760 mm of mercury.
    (C) 106 mm of mercury.
    (D) 608 mm of mercury.

24. If the stirring of a solution results in precipitation of solute with no change in temperature, the solution must have been

    (A) saturated.
    (B) concentrated.
    (C) dilute.
    (D) supersaturated.

25. If the reaction : A + B → C + D is designated as first order, the rate depends on

    (A) the concentration of only one reactant.
    (B) the concentration of each reactant.
    (C) no specific concentration.
    (D) the temperature only.

26. The loss of an alpha particle from the radioactive atom $\frac{228}{88}$ would leave

    (A) $\frac{224}{86}$ Rn
    (B) $\frac{222}{86}$ Rn
    (C) $\frac{224}{88}$ Ra
    (D) $\frac{230}{90}$ Th

27. Which of the following is NOT a form of radioactive decay?

    (A) Electron capture
    (B) Beta emission
    (C) Alpha emission
    (D) Proton emission

28. The greatest amount of energy would be produced by the burning of one gram of

    (A) fat.
    (B) carbohydrate.
    (C) protein.
    (D) ribonucleic acid.

29. For the reaction: $H_2(g) + Br_2(g) \rightarrow 2HBr(g)$, the reaction can be driven to the left by

    (A) increasing the pressure.
    (B) increasing the hydrogen.
    (C) increasing hydrogen bromide.
    (D) decreasing hydrogen bromide.

30. Carbon-14 has a half life of 5.73×10 years. If a sample contained 1 gram of C-14, the time required to decay to only 0.0625 g would be

    (A) 11.46×10 years.
    (B) 5.73×10 years.
    (C) 22.92×10 years.
    (D) None of the above

31. The oxidation number of Mn in the compound K_2MnO_4 is

    (A) +7
    (B) +2
    (C) 0
    (D) +6

32. The element with the highest ionization energy of those below is

    (A) Mg
    (B) Sr
    (C) Ca
    (D) Ba

33. The least electronegative of the following elements is

    (A) Cl
    (B) F
    (C) Br
    (D) I

34. The element with the smallest atomic radius of the following is

    (A) Sr
    (B) Mg
    (C) Ba
    (D) Ra

35. Which of the following salts would be more soluble in 1.0M acid than in pure water?

    (A) KCl
    (B) $CaCO_3$
    (C) $CaCl_2$
    (D) KNO_3

36. Which of the following is NOT an acid/conjugate base pair?

(A) HCN/CN

(B) H_2CO_3/OH^-

(C) H_2SO_4/HSO_4^-

(D) H_3PO_4/$H_2PO_4^-$

37. In a titration of 40.0 ml of 0.20 M NaOH with 0.4 M HCl, what will be the final volume of the solution when the sodium hydroxide is completely neutralized?

(A) 42 ml

(B) 20 ml

(C) 60 ml

(D) 80 ml

38. When dissolved in water to form 0.2 M solutions, which of the following would have the highest pH?

(A) The salt of a strong acid

(B) A weak acid

(C) The ammonium salt of a strong acid

(D) The sodium salt of a weak acid

39. Consider the reaction $N_2(g) + 3H_2(g) \rightarrow 2NH_3(g)$ + heat. Indicate the incorrect statement.

(A) An increase in temperature will shift the equilibrium to the right.

(B) An increase in pressure applied will shift the equilibrium to the right.

(C) The addition of ammonia will shift the equilibrium to the left.

(D) The addition of H_2 will shift the equilibrium to the right.

40. All of the following are colligative properties of solutions EXCEPT

(A) vapor pressure.

(B) osmotic pressure.

(C) density.

(D) boiling point elevation.

41. What statement is incorrect?

(A) London dispersion forces are among those binding the units of molecular solids.

(B) Molten ionic compounds are conductors of electricity.

(C) Molecular solids have high melting points.

(D) Molecular solids are non-conductors.

42. Which of the following groups contain no ionic compounds?

(A) HCN, NO, $Ca(NO_3)_2$

(B) KOH, CCL_4, SF_6

(C) NaH, CaF_2, $NaNH_2$

(D) CH_2O, H_2S, NH_3

43. In a cubic lattice, an atom lying at the corner of a unit cell is shared by how many unit cells?

(A) 2

(B) 4

(C) 8

(D) 12

44. On the basis of the following boiling point data, which of the following liquids would be expected to have the highest vapor pressure at room temperature?

SUBSTANCE	BOILING POINT
(A) acetone	56.2°C
(B) ethanol	78.5°C
(C) water	100°C
(D) ethylene glycol	198°C

45. $\frac{34}{17}$ Cl has

(A) 17 protons, 17 electrons, and 17 neutrons.

(B) 17 protons, 19 electrons, and 17 neutrons.

(C) 17 protons, 18 electrons, and 17 neutrons.

(D) 34 protons, 34 electrons, and 17 neutrons.

46. Which of the following arrangements gives the correct trend of electronegativitism?

(A) I<Br<Cl<F

(B) Sr<Ca<Ra<Mg

(C) Al>Si>P>S

(D) Na<K<Li<H

GO ON TO THE NEXT PAGE

47. The number of unpaired electrons in the outer subshell of a phosphorus atom (atomic number: 15) is

  (A) 2
  (B) 0
  (C) 3
  (D) 1

48. An atom that has five 3 p electrons in its ground state is

  (A) Si
  (B) P
  (C) Cl
  (D) O

49. How many valence electrons are needed to complete the outer valence shell of sulfur?

  (A) 1
  (B) 2
  (C) 3
  (D) 4

50. Consider three 1-liter flasks at STP. Flask A contains NO gas; Flask B contains NH^3 gas; and Flask C contains N_2 gas. Which flask contains the greatest number of atoms?

  (A) Flask A
  (B) Flask B
  (C) Flask C
  (D) All contain the same number of atoms.

STOP   If you finish before time is called, you may check your work on this section only. Do not turn to any other section in the test.

ANSWER KEY

TEST 1: CELLS, STRUCTURE, AND FUNCTION

1. D	11. C	21. B	31. A
2. D	12. C	22. A	32. B
3. D	13. D	23. C	33. B
4. A	14. A	24. D	34. C
5. D	15. B	25. D	35. A
6. B	16. B	26. C	36. B
7. D	17. B	27. B	37. C
8. D	18. B	28. B	38. A
9. D	19. D	29. D	39. C
10. C	20. D	30. B	40. A

BIOLOGY

TEST 2

1. C	6. C	11. C	16. D
2. D	7. C	12. C	17. C
3. D	8. C	13. B	18. D
4. C	9. C	14. C	19. D
5. C	10. B	15. D	

TEST 3

1. B	6. B	11. B	16. C
2. A	7. C	12. D	17. C
3. A	8. D	13. D	18. C
4. D	9. B	14. C	19. D
5. C	10. D	15. D	20. C

TEST 4: HUMAN ANATOMY AND PHYSIOLOGY

1. D	26. A	51. B	76. B
2. A	27. B	52. A	77. A
3. A	28. B	53. B	78. B
4. B	29. D	54. B	79. B
5. B	30. C	55. D	80. A
6. D	31. B	56. B	81. C
7. C	32. C	57. B	82. B
8. C	33. A	58. C	83. A
9. B	34. B	59. B	84. B
10. D	35. A	60. D	85. B
11. B	36. A	61. B	86. A
12. B	37. D	62. C	87. B
13. D	38. B	63. B	88. B
14. B	39. A	64. C	89. A
15. A	40. B	65. C	90. B
16. C	41. C	66. C	91. A
17. B	42. B	67. B	92. D
18. C	43. A	68. B	93. D
19. B	44. C	69. C	94. D
20. D	45. A	70. A	95. B
21. D	46. B	71. B	96. C
22. A	47. B	72. C	97. B
23. D	48. B	73. A	98. D
24. D	49. B	74. D	99. B
25. D	50. A	75. B	100. D

Test 5: Chemistry

1. **B**	7. **B**	12. **B**	17. **A**
2. **D**	8. **B**	13. **C**	18. **B**
3. **D**	9. **D**	14. **C**	19. **A**
4. **D**	10. **C**	15. **C**	20. **B**
5. **D**	11. **D**	16. **D**	21. **B**
6. **B**			

Test 6: Chemistry and Physical Science

1. **D**	14. **B**	27. **D**	39. **A**
2. **A**	15. **C**	28. **A**	40. **C**
3. **B**	16. **D**	29. **C**	41. **C**
4. **C**	17. **B**	30. **C**	42. **D**
5. **D**	18. **C**	31. **D**	43. **C**
6. **C**	19. **D**	32. **A**	44. **A**
7. **D**	20. **D**	33. **D**	45. **A**
8. **A**	21. **B**	34. **B**	46. **A**
9. **D**	22. **B**	35. **B**	47. **D**
10. **D**	23. **D**	36. **B**	48. **C**
11. **B**	24. **D**	37. **D**	49. **B**
12. **C**	25. **A**	38. **D**	50. **B**
13. **D**	26. **A**		

EXPLANATORY ANSWERS

TEST 1: CELLS, STRUCTURE, AND FUNCTION

1. **The correct answer is (D).** In facilitated diffusion, large molecules and ions diffuse through channels within membrane proteins. The process requires no input of energy on the part of the cell, since materials move down a concentration gradient. Facilitated diffusion occurs more rapidly when the temperature is higher, and when the concentration gradient is steeper.

2. **The correct answer is (D).** The polymerase chain reaction (PCR) is an in vitro technique.

3. **The correct answer is (D).** In active transport, the transport proteins move a solute against its concentration gradient. Active transport does not proceed spontaneously. It requires an energy (ATP) input.

4. **The correct answer is (A).** A cell immersed in a solution with a lower concentration of dissolved materials (solutes) is in a hypotonic environment. The concentration of water is higher outside of the cell than inside. Under these conditions, water diffuses into the cell.

5. **The correct answer is (D).** Substance x is hydrophobic and nonpolar, so it can easily pass through the membrane due to the phospholipid structure of the membrane.

6. **The correct answer is (B).** A cell is hypertonic when it has higher solute concentration and less water concentration compared to the outside solution, which has more water and less solute (hypotonic), so the water will diffuse inside the cell.

7. **The correct answer is (D).** Oxidation is the loss of electrons or the loss of hydrogen from a substance. Therefore, the carbon-carbon double bonds of unsaturated fats are oxidized more easily than the simple bonds of saturated fats.

8. **The correct answer is (D).** Macromolecules and fluid cross cellular membranes by bulk transport, in which the transported materials are contained within vesicles and do not mix with other materials of the cytoplasm. There are two forms of bulk transport: endocytosis and exocytosis. Endocytosis of a solid is known as phagocytosis.

9. **The correct answer is (D).** In active transport, energy (ATP) is needed. Mitochondria is the main organelle for ATP synthesis.

10. **The correct answer is (C).** Red blood cells have 0.9% salt solution whereas sea water has more solute than red blood cells, so it is a hypertonic solution compared to red blood cells.

11. **The correct answer is (C).** If any cell is placed in a hypertonic solution, the cell loses its water, dehydrates and dies because the cell is hypotonic (more water) compared to outside solutions.

12. **The correct answer is (C).** The movement of materials against a concentration gradient need energy. (See answer 3.)

13. **The correct answer is (D).** Every living organism is covered by a cell membrane.

14. **The correct answer is (A).** Water

15. **The correct answer is (B).** Prokaryote cells do not have membrane-bound organelles.

16. **The correct answer is (B).** The half-life indicates that 100 years are required for ½ of the sample to decay. Therefore, the 31.5 kg should be doubled 4 times.

17. **The correct answer is (B).** Water is a polar molecule whereas oil is a nonpolar molecule. Water molecules have a slightly negative charge in one side and slightly positive charge in the other side, but lipid molecules do not have any charges.

18. **The correct answer is (B).** All plant cells have an outer rigid covering called a cell wall made up of polysaccharide cellulose; animals do not have cell walls, only cell membranes.

19. **The correct answer is (D).** Prokaryote cells (example bacteria and blue-green algae) do not have a membrane-bound nucleus, but they have naked DNA in the cytoplasm.

20. **The correct answer is (D).** The cytoskeleton is a web of fibrous protein that extends throughout the cell. It alters the shape of a cell, moves the whole cell from one place to another, and pushes or pulls organelles.

21. **The correct answer is (B).** Lysosomes are essentially membrane bags that enclose hydrolytic enzymes, which are involved in breaking down proteins, polysaccharides, and lipids. If the lysosomes break open, the cell itself will be destroyed, because the enzymes they carry are capable of hydrolyzing all the major types of molecules found in a living cell.

22. **The correct answer is (A).** Note the $R-COOH$ group, which makes the compound an acid, with the $R-NH_2$ (amino group) in the alpha position.

23. **The correct answer is (C).** Proteins are composed of chains of amino acids linked by peptide bonds, with primary, secondary, and tertiary structure.

24. **The correct answer is (D).** A virus is not a living cell; it is a submicroscopic, non-cellular particle composed of a nucleic acid core and a protein coat, reproducing only within a host. Therefore, it does not belong to any living kingdom.

25. **The correct answer is (D).** Some bacteria and fungi feed on dead organic matter to get their energy (*saphros* means rotten, putrid).

26. **The correct answer is (C).** Parallel circuits enable electrical currents to take separate paths through individual resistors as in circuit II.

27. **The correct answer is (B).** All circuits in a series circuit, as in I, must travel through all resistors.

28. **The correct answer is (B).** There are two forms of endocytosis, depending on the kind of material brought into the cell. Endocytosis of fluid is known as pinocytosis.

29. **The correct answer is (D).** All cells can exist as distinct entities because of the cell membrane, which regulates the passage of materials into and out of the cell. Latex membrane does not allow the HIV virus to pass through the membrane, preventing HIV infection.

30. **The correct answer is (B).** Membranes control the types of molecules that can pass in and out of the cell and organelles. Cell membranes are permeable to certain molecules and impermeable to others—a phenomenon known as selectively permeable.

31. **The correct answer is (A).** Three different types of filaments have been identified as major participants in the cytoskeletons: microtubules, microfilaments, and intermediate filaments. They maintain the shape of the cell, enable it to move, anchor its organelles, and direct its traffic.

32. **The correct answer is (B).** Both mitochondria and chloroplasts are energy-producing organelles. Mitochondria release the energy from food as a form of ATP, and the chloroplasts pick up the solar energy and convert it to chemical energy (ATP).

33. **The correct answer is (B).** The slope (m) is 10.

34. **The correct answer is (C).** In enzyme-catalyzed reactions, substrate molecules generally outnumber enzyme molecules, which allow the enzyme to become saturated and the reaction to proceed at maximum velocity.

35. **The correct answer is (A).** Autotrophic organisms, such as plants, all algae, and some bacteria, are able to synthesize their own organic food by using CO_2, H_2O, and sunlight.

36. **The correct answer is (B).** The liquid part of the solution is called solvent.

37. **The correct answer is (C).** With limited resources, as the numbers of individuals produced approach the environmental capacity, reproduction declines and eventually stops.

38. **The correct answer is (A).** The assumption of unlimited resources suggests the absence of a K value.

39. **The correct answer is (C).** Mitochondrion is the powerhouse of the cell. It produces maximum amounts of chemical energy (ATP) for sustaining life.

40. **The correct answer is (A).** Membranes are composed of a phospholipid bilayer of molecules interspersed with protein molecules. Any kind of nonpolar molecule, such as lipids or some other organic solvents (ether, acetone, etc.), can easily pass through the lipid layer of membrane.

BIOLOGY

TEST 2

1. **The correct answer is (C).** This is the process by which a glucose molecule is changed to two molecules of pyruvic acid with the liberation of a small amount of energy. In the absence of oxygen, pyruvic acid can be converted to ethanol or to one of several organic acids, of which lactic is the most common. This process is called fermentation.

2. **The correct answer is (D).** In the first stage, aerobic respiration (glycolysis) produces 2 ATP. In the second stage (Krebs cycle), it produces 2 ATP. During the final stage (electron transport chain), it produces 32 ATP.

3. **The correct answer is (D).** Reaction I is an uphill process that takes in radiant energy from the sun and converts it to chemical energy to combine CO_2 and H_2O to produce $C_6H_{12}O_6$ and O_2—which have additional energy.

4. **The correct answer is (C).** The reaction in II is downhill, with energy being released from $C_6H_{12}O_6$, generating CO_2 and H_2O with less energy.

5. **The correct answer is (C).** The reactants of some reactions have more energy than the products. Many such reactions release energy that cells can use, which is what happens during aerobic respiration.

6. **The correct answer is (C).** Each type of enzyme functions best within a certain temperature range. The chemical reaction rates decrease sharply when the temperature becomes too high. Humans usually die when their internal body temperature reaches 44°C (112°F) because it destroys the shape of the enzyme and thereby stops the metabolism.

7. **The correct answer is (C).** The enzyme helpers called coenzymes are complex organic molecules, many of which are derived from vitamins. These coenzymes can pick up hydrogen atoms that are liberated during glucose breakdown.

8. **The correct answer is (C).** The stored form of energy is called potential energy. An example is the glucose molecule; when it breaks down, it releases a large quantity of chemical energy to do work.

9. **The correct answer is (C).** All the pigments are present inside the thylakoids; therefore, the chlorophyll molecules and other pigments pick up the solar energy, convert it to chemical energy as a form of ATP and NADPH, and release oxygen during the non-cyclic light reaction.

10. **The correct answer is (B).** During non-cyclic light reactions, energy from the sun drives the formation of ATP (which carries energy) and NADPH (which carries hydrogen and electrons). Oxygen is a by-product of photosynthesis.

11. **The correct answer is (C).** The light independent reactions are the "synthesis" part of photosynthesis. ATP molecules deliver the required energy for the reaction. NADPH molecules deliver the required hydrogen and electrons, and carbon dioxide diffuses inside the stronin. It then forms the energy-rich molecule glucose (the process is called dark reaction).

12. **The correct answer is (C).** Reduction in the hawk population reduced the pressure on the mouse population, which increased and suppressed the grasshopper numbers, and allowed the sunflower population to increase.

13. **The correct answer is (B).** The highest concentration of energy in a ecological pyramid is at the base (producers). Energy is lost as heat at the successive trophic levels.

14. **The correct answer is (C).** Aerobic cellular respiration is more important to sustaining life because it produces 36 ATP compared to anaerobic, which only releases 2 ATP.

15. **The correct answer is (D).** The organelle chloroplast is responsible for photosynthesis, which produces O_2 and the energy-rich molecule carbohydrate.

16. **The correct answer is (D).** All enzymes are protein molecules, and protein is one of the organic molecules necessary for sustaining life.

17. **The correct answer is (C).** Glycolysis is the first stage of cellular respiration in which glucose is broken down step by step to form 2 pyruvic acid inside the cytoplasm.

18. **The correct answer is (D).** The first stage of respiration, the breaking down of the glucose molecules, always takes place inside the cytoplasm because all the enzymes are there for the reaction.

19. **The correct answer is (D).** Electron transport systems and neighboring channel proteins are the machinery embedded in the inner membrane that divides mitochondrion into two compartments.

TEST 3

1. **The correct answer is (B).** The adult bodies of most plants and animals consist of diploid (2n) rather than haploid (n) cells. A gamete (male sperm and female egg) is always a haploid cell, which means it has one set of chromosomes formed by meiosis of germ cells (2n). So if the germ cell is 40, the gamete will be 20.

2. **The correct answer is (A).** When two alternative alleles are fully apparent in a hybrid, with both phenotypes showing in the organism, we say that the hybrids exhibit codominance. Blood typing of humans provides an excellent example of codominance. The AB blood type inherits an A allele and a B allele. Neither allele is dominant over the other; therefore, codominance causes a new blood type, AB.

3. **The correct answer is (A).** The blood cells of humans divide by mitosis. In mitosis, the diploid number of chromosomes is maintained and the resulting daughter cells are identical to the parent cell.

4. **The correct answer is (D).** Meiosis is the nuclear division that reduces the number of chromosomes in the resulting cells by half. Meiosis is necessary for the production of gametes or sex cells and results in 4 non-identical haploid cells (sperms and eggs).

5. **The correct answer is (C).** The first part of sexual reproduction is meiosis, where the germ cells divide and produce four haploid gametes.

6. **The correct answer is (B).** Asexual reproduction occurs without sex and transfers the genes of just one parent to each offspring; it produces offspring that are genetically identical to one another and to their single parent by the process of mitosis.

7. **The correct answer is (C).** The first pattern of inheritance discovered by Mendel was the Law of Segregation. This law describes how the two copies of each gene segregate (separate) during meiosis so that just one copy ends up in each gamete (sperm and egg).

8. **The correct answer is (D).** The dominant will always show the dominant characteristic in their phenotype.

9. **The correct answer is (B).** The sex chromosome of a mother is always XX and the father XY. So, the sex of the child depends on whether he or she gets X or Y from the father. If the child gets X from the father and X from the mother, the child will be a female. If the child gets Y from the father and X from the mother, the child will be a male.

10. **The correct answer is (D).** In normal cells, the cell division is controlled by two sets of genes: one set stimulates and the other set suppresses. In cancer, defective genes may overstimulate cell division or fail to halt cell division.

11. **The correct answer is (B).** Sperm cells are haploid (N), which are formed by meiosis of germ cells (2N); therefore, if the haploid is 30, then germ cells should be 60.

12. **The correct answer is (D).** A person with Down Syndrome has three copies in chromosome 21 rather than two copies. The extra chromosome affects practically every part of the body.

13. **The correct answer is (D).** If we do the Punnet square for a woman who is a heterozygous carrier for sex-linked recessive gene and married to a normal man, half of her sons and half of her daughters will receive this gene.

    $X^C X$—girl with recessive gene
    $X^C Y$—boy with recessive gene
    XY—normal boy
    XX—normal girl

14. **The correct answer is (C).** Hemophilia is one of the disorders caused by a Y-linked recessive allele. Many genes in many chromosomes contribute to normal blood clotting, but two gene loci in the Y chromosome are responsible for the two most common clotting disorders—hemophilia A and hemophilia B.

15. **The correct answer is (D).** Hemophilia is a sex-linked disorder because the defective gene is present in the Y sex chromosome.

16. **The correct answer is (C).** The sex-linked trait is present in the X chromosome; therefore, the father cannot pass the gene to his son because the son always receives the Y chromosome, not the X chromosome, from his father.

17. **The correct answer is (C).** The blue gene is the autosomal recessive trait, whereas hemophilia is the sex-linked recessive trait. To get the blue eyes, the person should have two blue-eyes recessive genes. If the person is male, he needs only one recessive gene for hemophilia.

18. **The correct answer is (C).** If both parents are AB, they can only produce two different kinds of gametes (sperm and eggs), A and B. So the blood types of children will be A, AB, and B.

19. **The correct answer is (D).** Blood type O has neither A nor B polysaccharides (antigen) for antibodies to attack.

20. **The correct answer is (C).** Non-disjunction of sex chromosomes (XY) in a man produces four types of abnormal sperms. When these abnormal sperm (YY) fertilize normal X carrying chromosomes, they produce abnormal genotypes (XYY).

Test 4: Human Anatomy and Physiology

1. **The correct answer is (D).** Only the lymphatic system is involved in all three of these processes, although the urinary system does receive fluid from blood vessels.

2. **The correct answer is (A).** Internal and abdominal muscles aid expiration. The external intercostal aid inspiration, but the diaphragm is the major muscle.

3. **The correct answer is (A).** The integument is comprised of skin, hair, nails, and associated structures, such as sweat and sebaceous glands.

4. **The correct answer is (B).** Oxytocin and antidiuretic hormone (ADH) are both products of the posterior pituitary. Oxytocin acts on uterine smooth muscle and mammary tissue, whereas ADH acts within the kidneys to promote water reabsorption. ADH is also a vasoconstriction, and these two actions combine to elevate blood pressure.

5. **The correct answer is (B).** Homeostasis, the tendency to maintain a constant internal environment, most commonly depends upon negative feedback processes, which tend to counter the effects of change. Positive feedback mechanisms enhance the effects of change, and they generally have a beneficial effect on homeostasis.

6. **The correct answer is (D).** Central chemoreceptors respond to changes in CO_2, which is the most important factor in the control of minute-to-minute respiration.

7. **The correct answer is (C).** Sagittal planes divide the body into left and right parts. Frontal (coronal) planes vertically divide the body into anterior and posterior segments. A transverse section divides the body into superior and inferior parts.

8. **The correct answer is (C).** Cardiac output, the volume of blood by the heart per minute, is equal to the product of stroke volume (L./beat) and heart rate (beats/minute).

9. **The correct answer is (B).** Diffusion is the process by which solutes move from an area of high concentration to an area of low concentration. Osmosis is the movement of water down a concentration gradient. Movement of solute against a concentration gradient requires active transport processes and energy.

10. **The correct answer is (D).** Blood exits the right ventricle through the pulmonary semilunar (pulmonic) valve and enters the pulmonary arteries, which lead to the lungs. Atrioventricular valves (bicuspid and tricuspid) are situated between atria and ventricles. Pulmonary veins come from the lungs back to the heart.

11. **The correct answer is (B).** While both norepinephrine and epinephrine act at Alpha and Beta-1 receptors, epinephrine is the primary agonist at the Beta-2 sites, where it leads to pronounced bronchodilation. Acetylcholine and nicotine are not catechol amines.

12. **The correct answer is (B).** The resting membrane is relatively impermeable to sodium, which is in a high concentration in the extracellular space relative to the intracellular space. An action potential results from the opening of sodium channels, allowing sodium to diffuse into the intracellular space and making that region positive relative to the outside of the cell.

13. **The correct answer is (D).** During swallowing, the epiglottis covers the trachea to prevent ingested material from entering the respiratory tract.

14. **The correct answer is (B).** The amount of dissolved oxygen in blood is minimal compared to the amount carried as oxyhemoglobin. Carbon dioxide and bicarbonate are not physiologic oxygen transporters.

15. **The correct answer is (A).** Pyramidal tract fibers are motor in function and originate in the primary motor cortex, which is directly anterior to the central sulcus, the pre-central gyrus. The postcentral gyms is part of the somatosensory system.

16. **The correct answer is (C).** Epinephrine and norepinephrine are catechol amine transmitters in the autonomic and central nervous systems. Acetylcholinesterase is the enzyme that metabolizes acetylcholine at autonomic and neuromuscular sites.

17. **The correct answer is (B).** Arterioles are located between arteries and capillaries. Dilation or constriction of arterioles regulates the flow of blood into capillary beds and provides adjustment of arterial blood pressure.

18. **The correct answer is (C).** Exocytosis moves substances from the intracellular space into extracellular fluid. Endocytosis is a mechanism for moving large particles into cells. Phagocytosis is a type of endocytosis by which solid particles are engulfed. Pinocytosis is endocytosis of fluids.

19. **The correct answer is (B).** Dermatomes are body regions innervated by individual dorsal roots and can be related to segmental spinal levels. Receptive fields, sensory units, and motor units related to innervation are characteristics of individual neurons rather than nerve trunks.

20. **The correct answer is (D).** Epithelial tissue is characterized by cell shape (squamous, cuboidal, columnar) and cell layering (simple or compound).

21. **The correct answer is (D).** Cartilage forms the skeleton of the embryo and is subsequently converted to bone. Cartilage also forms the nasal septum and the rings of the trachea. Its flexibility makes it an appropriate material to join the ribs to the sternum.

22. **The correct answer is (A).** Keratin is a protein that waterproofs and adds structural strength to skin. It is formed in the deepest layer of the epidermis and migrates to the surface with time. Melanin, carotene, and hemoglobin are pigments in the skin.

23. **The correct answer is (D).** Sharp "pricking" pain information is carried over the small, slowly conducting myelinated A delta fibers, while burning and aching pain information is transmitted over the even more slowly conducted unmyelinated C fibers. A alpha fibers, with their high conduction velocity, are involved in other areas, such as proprioception.

24. **The correct answer is (D).** Activation of the parasympathetic division will lead directly to a slowing of the heart through activity of the vagus nerve. Vasoconstriction, increased heart rate and cardiac output, and inhibition of digestion are within the domain of the sympathetic division.

25. **The correct answer is (D).** Muscle spindles respond to moderate muscle stretch. The Gogli tendon organ is the receptor for the inverse stretch reflex, free nerve endings are involved in pain reception, and hair cells are receptors within the auditory and vestibular systems.

26. **The correct answer is (A).** Although the glomerulus is more permeable than most membranes, it still restricts the passage of proteins, blood cells, and other large particles. Damage to the glomerulus can produce filtration disorders such as glomerulonephritis, and substances such as blood and protein may appear in the urine.

27. **The correct answer is (B).** Some CO_2 is carried in a dissolved form obeying Henry's Law, and some is carried by hemoglobin. Most CO_2, however, is carried as bicarbonate.

28. **The correct answer is (B).** Tubular reabsorption is the process by which the kidneys return water and solutes, including glucose, vitamins, and amino acids, to blood. Filtration and secretion involve movement of substances from blood into urine. Glucose is not reabsorbed from the collecting duct.

29. **The correct answer is (D).** Periosteum covers the outer surface of long bones. It contains osteoblasts, cells that form new bone cells. Endosteum lines the hollow inner surface of a long bone. Osteoclasts break down bone cells.

30. **The correct answer is (C).** Activity in the sinoatrial node is responsible for initiating the cardiac cycle, beginning with atrial depolarization and contraction. In a resting subject, the contribution of atrial contraction to ventricular filling is relatively minimal. The AV node is below the atria.

31. **The correct answer is (B).** The first heart sound ("lub") is the atrioventricular valves (tricuspid and bicuspid) closing in response to the ventricles contracting and increasing intraventricular pressure.

32. **The correct answer is (C).** Visual processing occurs within the occipital lobe of the cerebral cortex, which is protected by the occipital bone. Frontal bone covers the frontal cortex, which is involved in, among other things, behavioral and motor events. Parietal bone covers the parietal cortex, which is involved in sensory integration processes, while temporal bone protects the temporal lobe, which is involved in audition.

33. **The correct answer is (A).** Veins have large lumens and thin, distensible walls; they contain up to 65 percent of the body's total blood supply at any time.

34. **The correct answer is (B).** The patella is a sesamoid bone, a special type of short bone.

35. **The correct answer is (A).** The automaticity of the heart is normally a function of the sinoatrial (SA) node, which leads to atrial depolarization. The atrioventricular (AV) node may become a pacemaker under certain pathological conditions.

36. **The correct answer is (A).** Arteries are under the greatest pressure due to the force from the contraction of the heart and the elastic properties of arterial walls.

37. **The correct answer is (D).** Ninety-nine percent of the water filtered at the glomerulus is returned by osmosis, most of which occurs within the proximal convoluted tubule.

38. **The correct answer is (B).** Small, uncharged lipid soluble molecules cross biological membranes more readily than other species. Water-soluble molecules cross if they are sufficiently small.

39. **The correct answer is (A).** The sympathetic division of the autonomic nervous system is involved in dealing with emergencies and stress. Parasympathetic (craniosacral) activity is primarily involved with energy conservation and "vegetative" functions.

40. **The correct answer is (B).** The sympathetic division of the autonomic nervous system is anatomically the thoricolumbar division because of its spinal levels of origin. The parasympathetic division is, anatomically, the craniosacral division.

41. **The correct answer is (C).** Cellular respiration, the utilization of oxygen and glucose, occurs within mitochondria. Rough endoplasmic reticulum is involved in protein synthesis and smooth endoplasmic reticulum is involved in synthesis of lipid materials. Golgi apparatus are involved in cellular packaging and delivery.

42. **The correct answer is (B).** Flexion decreases the angle of a joint, bringing the two bones closer together. Extension increases the angle of a joint, moving the bones farther apart. Retraction and rotation are not joint "bending" in nature.

43. **The correct answer is (A).** Mitosis leading to the formation of new epidermal cells occurs within the stratum germinativum basale, the deepest layer of the epidermis, which has the advantage of being near the blood supply of the underlying dermis.

44. **The correct answer is (C).** Compared to males, females have a larger percentage of fat (and a lower content of water), which is deposited within the subcutaneous layer under the influence of estrogen.

45. **The correct answer is (A).** Mucosal membranes line structures such as components of the digestive, respiratory, and reproductive tracts, which access the outside world. Serous membranes line cavities that do not access the external environment, such as the pleural cavities. Synovial membranes line joint cavities, and cutaneous membranes comprise the skin.

46. **The correct answer is (B).** The epidermis does not contain blood vessels and depends upon the vascular supply of the underlying dermis for its needs.

47. **The correct answer is (B).** Smooth muscle is found within visceral structures (e.g., digestive, reproductive), does not have a striated histological appearance, and is generally under autonomic (involuntary) control. Skeletal muscle is striated and voluntary. Cardiac muscle is striated but involuntary. Postural muscles are skeletal muscles.

48. **The correct answer is (B).** Although carried by the circulatory system and influenced by the endocrine systems, blood cell formation is largely a function of spongy bone within the skeletal system.

49. **The correct answer is (B).** Parathyroid hormone elevates serum calcium levels by initiating mobilization of calcium from the digestive system. Calcitonin lowers blood calcium and leads to deposition of calcium within bone.

50. **The correct answer is (A).** Eccrine sweat glands of the face, palms, and soles are active in children. Apocrine sweat glands become active at puberty. Sebaceous glands produce sebum and are not found on the soles or palms. Ceruminous glands are found within the external auditory meatus.

51. **The correct answer is (B).** The biceps brachii is a flexor of the elbow, and the triceps femoris is a flexor of the knee.

52. **The correct answer is (A).** Apocrine sweat glands become active at puberty under the influence of sex hormones. Eccrine, sebaceous, and ceruminous glands are active in children.

53. **The correct answer is (B).** Calcitonin is responsible for lowering an elevated serum calcium, partially by depositing the excess mineral in bone. Parathormone will elevate serum calcium levels.

54. **The correct answer is (B).** Although hormones are produced by endocrine glands, their delivery to target organs is primarily via the cardiovascular system.

55. **The correct answer is (D).** Myelin, an "insulating" substance, is responsible for saltatory conduction in which the impulse "skips" from one Node of Ranvier to the next and is rapidly conducted to the end of the cell. The larger the diameter of an axon, the less resistance present and the faster the axon can conduct. Myelinated, large diameter axons comprise the axons with the fastest conduction velocities.

56. **The correct answer is (B).** The nephron is the basic functional unit of kidneys. Nephrons include Bowman's capsule, the proximal convoluted tubule, the loop of Henle, the distal convoluted tubule, and the collecting duct. The glomerulus is part of the circulatory system, the ureters convey urine from the kidneys to the bladder, and the urethra carries urine out from the bladder.

57. **The correct answer is (B).** The esophagus enters the stomach below the fundus at the cardiac region, which contains the cardiac sphincter. The body of the stomach is below and the pyloric region marks the most distal portion of the stomach adjacent to the duodenum of the small intestine.

58. **The correct answer is (C).** Oxytocin, produced by the hypothalamus and released by the posterior pituitary, causes contraction of uterine smooth muscle and plays a role in labor and delivery. ADH is also released by the posterior pituitary, but its role is in water conservation within the kidneys.

59. **The correct answer is (B).** ADH, antidiuretic hormone, when released from the posterior pituitary, causes an increased permeability of the collecting duct of the kidneys to water and leads to water reabsorption and conservation. Inhibition of ADH release, produced for example by the ingestion of alcohol, leads to an increase in urine output.

60. **The correct answer is (D).** FSH begins the maturation process of follicles, but it is the elevation of LH levels that leads to the release of mature egg cells (ovulation). ADH and prolactin do not participate in the process.

61. **The correct answer is (B).** The cardiac sphincter is located at the junction of the esophagus and the stomach and is responsible for preventing gastric reflux. The pyloric sphincter is at the junction of the stomach and the small intestine, the ileocecal valve is at the junction of the small and large intestines, and the epiglottis prevents solids and liquids from entering the trachea.

62. **The correct answer is (C).** Bile, produced in the liver and released from the gall bladder, is involved in fat metabolism in the small intestine. Lipase is also involved in fat metabolism, but it is from the pancreas.

63. **The correct answer is (B).** Although some digestion takes place within all of the structures listed, the majority of digestive processes take place within the duodenum.

64. **The correct answer is (C).** Visual receptors, rods and cones, are located at the back of the eye on the retina. The lens and cornea are involved in transmission of light rays from the environment on to the retina; the optic tract is part of the optic neural pathway.

65. **The correct answer is (C).** Food absorption takes place primarily within the ileum and jejunum. Functions of the stomach and duodenum are primarily digestive, while the colon is principally involved in water reabsorption, some digestion, and vitamin synthesis.

66. **The correct answer is (C).** The medulla begins at, and is indistinguishable from, the rostral end of the spinal cord, forming the lowest portion of the brain stem, which also includes the pons and the midbrain, both superior. The thalamus, part of the diencephalon, is yet further rostral.

67. **The correct answer is (B).** Although stored and delivered by the gall bladder, bile is manufactured within the liver. The duodenum is the major site of digestion, where it receives digestive materials from the pancreas.

68. **The correct answer is (B).** Thyroid hormone contributes to growth and maturation of the nervous system. A hypothyroid infant will show both physical and mental deficits not seen in the adult, since skeletal and brain development have been completed.

69. **The correct answer is (C).** Rods, which provide vision in black and white, and cones, which provide color vision, are located on the retina at the back of the eye. Hair cells are receptors within the auditory and vestibular systems.

70. **The correct answer is (A).** Lining the inside of the digestive system is the epithelial mucosal layer, which provides an appropriate setting for absorption of materials into the submucosal layer that contains blood vessels, lymphatics, and nerves. Serosal membranes surround the digestive tract to form a protective layer.

71. **The correct answer is (B).** The pancreas is classed as an endocrine gland because of its production of insulin and glucagon, which are secreted directly into blood. As an exocrine gland, the pancreas produces a series of enzymes contained in pancreatic juice, carried by the pancreatic duct.

72. **The correct answer is (C).** Lacrimation is the activity of the lacrimal glands, which produce lacrimal fluid or tears.

73. **The correct answer is (A).** Olfaction, the sense of smell, is the domain of the first cranial nerve, the olfactory nerve. Nerves II, III, and IV are involved in the sensory and motor functions of the head and face but not the sense of smell.

74. **The correct answer is (D).** Immediately distal to the neck of the bladder is the prostate gland. Its enlargement, common in males beginning at about the age of 40, interferes with urine outflow. Benign hyperplasia prostate (BHP) is a non-malignant enlargement of the gland, which is also a common site for cancer in males. Although located in the same general area, the seminal vesicles and bulbourethral (Cowper's) glands do not normally hypertrophy with aging.

75. **The correct answer is (B).** Linear (vertical and horizontal) acceleration is sensed by receptors within the utricles and saccules; the semicircular canals contain receptors activated by rotational movement. Receptors within the cochlea detect sound, and the middle ear does not contain auditory or vestibular receptor devices.

76. **The correct answer is (B).** Although the globulins and fibrin are blood proteins, albumin is the protein in the highest plasma concentration.

77. **The correct answer is (A).** Union of sperm and egg normally occurs within the fallopian (uterine) tubes prior to implantation within the uterus. Implantation at non-uterine sites is termed an ectopic pregnancy.

78. **The correct answer is (B).** Depression may result from low levels of serotonin or decreased responsiveness of sertotonergic receptors in the brain, and this is the basis for the use of serotonin reuptake inhibitors in the treatment of clinical depression. High levels of catechol amines may contribute to clinical anxiety.

79. **The correct answer is (B).** Lymphatic vessels begin as lymphatic capillaries, blind pouches found in peripheral tissue. Lymph nodes are more proximal structures, and lymphocytes are forms of white blood cells.

80. **The correct answer is (A).** HCG rises to detectable levels following egg fertilization, and its presence in blood and urine forms the basis of pregnancy testing. The function of HCG is to maintain the corpus luteum, which is responsible for maintaining estrogen and progesterone levels, and their effects on the endometrium, during early and middle pregnancy.

81. **The correct answer is (C).** Sweet, sour, and salty taste sensations result from activity in the facial nerve, the seventh cranial nerve. The first cranial nerve is involved in olfaction; the fifth is involved in motor and sensory mechanisms of the head and face. Nerve x, the vagus, is not involved in taste from the tongue.

82. **The correct answer is (B).** The parasympathetic division of the autonomic nervous system is primarily involved with energy production and conservation. Its outward effects can be remembered by the acronym, SLUD, salivation, lacrimation, urination, and defecation.

83. **The correct answer is (A).** After their formation within the seminiferous tubules, sperm are stored within the epididymis lying alongside the testes. The epididymis leads to the vas deferens, which ultimately empties into the urethra, which receives material from the seminal vesicles.

84. **The correct answer is (B).** Glucagon elevates blood glucose by (1) promoting the breakdown of glycogen to glucose (glycogenolysis), (2) promoting glucose synthesis (gluconeogenesis), and (3) promoting the release of glucose from liver.

85. **The correct answer is (B).** Erythrocytes (red blood cells) are much more numerous than white cells in blood. Globulins and albumin are proteins, not formed elements.

86. **The correct answer is (A).** Although not as powerful as pH regulating mechanisms in the respiratory or renal systems, buffer systems essentially act at the rate of chemical reactions. The liver is not involved in the normal control of blood pH.

87. **The correct answer is (B).** Arterial blood pH is critically maintained between 7.35 and 7.45. Either a decline of pH (acidosis) to a level of 7.0 or an increase in pH (alkalosis) to 8.0 is potentially fatal.

88. **The correct answer is (B).** While the hematocrit reveals the level of plasma, it is intended to evaluate the percentage of erythrocytes (red blood cells) in whole blood and subsequently the oxygen carrying capacity of blood. Normal hematocrit values for females are 37–47 percent, 42–54 percent for males. Platelet and white cell enumerations are also useful diagnostics but do not involve the hematocrit.

89. **The correct answer is (A).** Although about 5 liters of blood are pumped through the heart per minute, the myocardial muscle is dependent upon the coronary arteries for delivery of oxygen.

90. **The correct answer is (B).** The term hair cell is applied to receptors within the auditory and vestibular systems. Rods and cones are visual receptors, and muscle spindles are the receptors for stretch reflexes.

91. **The correct answer is (A).** Blood typing is based on determining the antigen(s) located on the surfaces of erythrocytes; the "opposite" antibody is located within the individual's plasma. A type A patient therefore has the A antigen and the anti-B antibody. Rh antigens are also located on erythrocyte surfaces leading to an individual being typed as Rh positive (antibody present) or Rh negative (no Rh antigen).

92. **The correct answer is (D).** Sickle cell anemia develops when hemoglobin forms long crystalline chains within erythrocytes, forcing the cells into their bizarre shapes. Pernicious anemia refers to abnormal destruction of red blood cells; iron-deficiency and aplastic anemias involve abnormal blood cell formation.

93. **The correct answer is (D).** Hair cells are the auditory receptors located within the cochlea, part of the inner ear. Auditory ossicles are small bones involved in conduction of vibration through the middle ear.

94. **The correct answer is (D).** Female menopause follows aging of the ovaries and is characterized by low estrogen levels, which, in turn, result in high levels of GnRH, FSH, and LH. The latter two appear to be correlated with the "hot flashes" of menopause.

95. **The correct answer is (B).** Hyperventilation can lead to a decreased arterial CO_2 level, which may result in alkalosis of respiratory origin. Extreme alkalosis may lead to convulsions and may produce seizure activity in epileptic patients.

96. **The correct answer is (C).** Plasma is approximately 90 percent water, with the rest being comprised of numerous solutes, including proteins, nutrients, gases, hormones, ions, and products of cell activity.

97. **The correct answer is (B).** Estrogen is involved in a feedback loop to the hypothalamus such that high levels of estrogen inhibit the release of GnRH, which reduces levels of LH and prevents ovulation.

98. **The correct answer is (D).** Heparin is an endogenous anticoagulant produced by basophils. Fibrin, calcium, and thrombin are all promoters of the coagulation process.

99. **The correct answer is (B).** GnRH from the hypothalamus controls the release of FSH and LH from the anterior pituitary. FSH initiates follicle development, and LH leads directly to ovulation, the release of a mature egg.

100. **The correct answer is (D).** Testosterone is produced by interstitial (Leydig) cells under the influence of ICSH, interstitial cell stimulating hormone. The epididymis and prostate gland are not involved in testosterone synthesis.

TEST 5: CHEMISTRY

1. **The correct answer is (B).** Acidic solutions contain hydrogen (H^+) ions, while basic (or alkaline) solution contain a basic ion, such as the hydroxyl ion (OH^-).

2. **The correct answer is (D).** Carbohydrates consist of molecules made up of C, H, and O in a ratio of 1:2:1 (e.g., glucose is $C_6H_{12}O_6$). Polysaccharides are chains of three or more simple sugars (e.g., glucose).

3. **The correct answer is (D).** Whether a watery solution is acidic or alkaline depends on its concentration of hydrogen ions (H^+) in relation to hydroxyl ions (OH^-). The ratio is expressed as the solution pH (the letters stand for potential of hydrogen). The pH scale ranges from O (most acidic) to 14 (most alkaline). Pure water is neutral with a pH of 7 because it has equal amounts of hydrogen and hydroxyl ions.

4. **The correct answer is (D).** Carbohydrates consist of molecules made up of C, H, and O in a ratio of 1:2:1, whereas cholesterol is a lipid (steroid) formed of four carbon rings.

5. **The correct answer is (D).** Organic molecules are molecules that contain carbon; they are found in living things.

6. **The correct answer is (B).** Covalence is the mutual attraction between two atoms that share a pair of electrons. It is the strongest type of chemical bond.

$$H^+ = H^+ \rightarrow H^2$$

7. **The correct answer is (B).** For many atoms, the simplest way to attain a completely filled outer energy level is either to gain or to lose one or two electrons.

8. **The correct answer is (B).** Dissaccharides are double sugars and are formed by linking two simple sugars. For example, glucose and fructose form sucrose, a disaccharide (table sugar).

9. **The correct answer is (D).** Wax is made of glycerol and fatty acids. It is nonpolar and insoluble in water. It is a lipid molecule.

10. **The correct answer is (C).** Proteins are made up of units called amino acids. Amino acids join together by a covalent bond and form polypeptide chains (the primary structure of proteins).

11. **The correct answer is (D).** The nucleus of an atom consists of protons and neutrons. A proton is a subatomic particle with positive electric charge. The number of protons in the nucleus of an atom is equal to the atomic number.

12. **The correct answer is (B).** The chemical activity of an atom is how it reacts with other atoms. Atoms are governed by the number of electrons in their outermost shell. Helium, neon, and other atoms with no electron vacancies in their outermost shell are inert; they tend not to enter into chemical reactions. Hydrogen, oxygen, and other atoms with electron vacancies in their outermost shell tend to interact with other atoms.

13. **The correct answer is (C).** Regardless of the element, atoms have just as many electrons as protons. This means that they carry no net charge, overall. A proton is always positively charged, and an electron is negatively charged.

14. **The correct answer is (C).** Basic or alkaline solutions have fewer H^+ than OH^- ions; their pH is above 7.

15. **The correct answer is (C).** Alkaline solutions always have a higher pH and more OH^- ions.

16. **The correct answer is (D).** Glucose is a 6-carbon simple sugar and serves as a precursor of many complex compounds and as a building block for larger carbohydrates.

17. **The correct answer is (A).** The basic building block of protein is the amino acid. Each amino acid is a small organic compound with an amino group, a carboxyl group (an acid), a hydrogen atom, and one or more atoms, called its R group. Total amino acids are 20. Examples of amino acids are tryptophane, alanine, glycine, aspartic acid, lysine, proline, etc.

18. **The correct answer is (B).** The small organic compounds called nucleotides have three components: a 5-carbon sugar, a phosphate group, and a nitrogen-containing base. Nucleotides are the basic building blocks of DNA and RNA.

19. **The correct answer is (A).** In polar covalent bonds, atoms of different elements, which have a different number of protons, do not exert the same pull in shared electrons. The more attractive atom ends up with a slight negative charge; the atom is "electronegative." Its effect is balanced out by the other atoms, resulting in a slight positive charge. In simple words, a polar covalent bond has no net charge—but the charge is distributed unevenly between the bond's two ends.

20. **The correct answer is (B).** In a hydrogen bond, a small, highly electronegative atom of a molecule interacts weakly with a hydrogen atom that is already participating in a polar covalent bond.

21. **The correct answer is (B).** Genetic information is encoded in the particular order of nucleotides bases, which follow one another in DNA. RNA molecules function in the processes by which the genetic information in DNA is used to build proteins.

TEST 6: CHEMISTRY AND PHYSICAL SCIENCE

1. **The correct answer is (D).** Polarity is determined by differences in electronegativities between atoms involved in a bond. The difference in electronegativities between hydrogen and oxygen on a scale devised by Linus Pauling is 1.4, and between carbon and oxygen, it is 1.0. Carbon and hydrogen differ by only 0.4 and consequently form nonpolar bonds.

2. **The correct answer is (A).** Hydrochloric acid has the weakest conjugate base (Cl) and therefore dissociates most thoroughly (virtually completely in water) and yields hydrogen ions in high concentration. The other compounds shown dissociate less completely because of their stronger conjugate bases.

3. **The correct answer is (B).** Sucrose is a disaccharide that has nearly twice the molar mass of the other two sugars, which are monosaccharides.

4. **The correct answer is (C).** A hydrogen atom must accept an electron in order to form a hydride ion. No other changes occur. The hydride therefore has a single negative charge, whereas the hydrogen atom is neutral. An extra negative charge with no change in positive charge expands the radius.

5. **The correct answer is (D).** The functional group contains carbonyl plus a hydrogen linked to the carbon (—C—H). The other connection of the carbonyl group is to another carbon atom. The groups COOH, —OH, and —COOR are found in carboxylic acids, alcohols, and esters, respectively.

6. **The correct answer is (C).** Calcium oxide is the only compound in the four that is a metal oxide. Metal oxides form hydroxides (bases) when dissolved in water, but non-metal oxides form acids.

7. **The correct answer is (D).** The statement given is the definition of isotope, a form of atom of an element that differs from other atoms of the same element by the number of neutrons.

8. **The correct answer is (A).** Oxidation, the loss of electrons, occurs at the anode. Molten sodium chloride has only sodium ($Na+$) and chloride ($Cl-$) ions, the latter of which each have a single electron to donate to achieve neutrality. Loss of one electron each yields chlorine atoms, which stabilize by forming diatomic molecules of chlorine gas.

9. **The correct answer is (D).** Sugar alone is the only molecular compound of this group. The others readily dissociate as ions in polar solvents, such as water.

10. **The correct answer is (D).** Isopropyl alcohol has a low enough molecular weight to make it volatile and thus capable of giving a noticeable cooling effect during evaporation. It is unsuitable for internal consumption, but it is relatively inexpensive. There are disadvantages for the use of any of the others as rubbing alcohol. Methyl alcohol is toxic, phenol causes skin burns, and ethyl alcohol is too valuable for internal consumption and other commercial purposes.

11. **The correct answer is (B).** Argon, barium, and aluminum are in groups VIIIA, IIA, and IIIA, respectively. Copper is the only element that is in the transition area of the periodic table (group IB).

12. **The correct answer is (C).** Calcium and the other metals of the group IIA ionize by losing two electrons. It achieves the stable electron structure of argon, with eight electrons in the outer shell.

13. **The correct answer is (D).** In the series for the oxyhalogen ions (e.g., ClO_4^-, ClO_3^-, ClO^-), the one with the least amount of oxygen is designated hypochlorite.

14. **The correct answer is (B).** Chemical kinetics is the study of reaction rates and how these change with variation of conditions along with the various molecular events that transpire during the overall reaction.

15. **The correct answer is (C).** There is one phosphorus in the formula, but there are three potassiums and four oxygens. The number of atoms or ions present per formula unit equals the corresponding number of moles of each type in one molecule of the compound (the amount present in a liter of a 1 molar solution). In solution, potassium phosphate would separate as potassium ions and phosphate ions.

16. **The correct answer is (D).** Single bonds between carbon atoms are longer but weaker than double bonds between carbon atoms.

17. **The correct answer is (B).** The rare gases have stable electronic structures with eight outer "valence" electrons (2 S and 6 P) and therefore have no compulsion to seek means of donating, accepting, or sharing electrons. The halogens need an electron to achieve stability, whereas group IIA need to donate two electrons to form stable ions with eight electrons on the outermost shell. Group IB metals react but show a high resistance to oxidation.

18. **The correct answer is (C).** A molar solution contains one mole of solute per liter of solution. Therefore, one mole of solute is combined with less than one kilogram (one liter) of water. In a one molal solution, which contains one mole of solute per kilogram of water, the total volume for a solution of one mole exceeds one liter. Therefore, one liter of a one molal solution contains less than one mole.

19. **The correct answer is (D).** For a molecular compound, the gram formula weight is the same as the gram molecular weight. The empirical formula represents the smallest ratio of the different atoms possible in the compound. The molecular formula may be a multiple of the empirical formulas (e.g., twice).

20. **The correct answer is (D).** The ratio of the rates of effusion of two gases (proportional to the speeds of the gas molecules) is inversely proportional to the square roots of their molecular weights; consequently, rate of effusion of A/rate of effusion of $B = \sqrt{\dfrac{1}{4}} = \dfrac{1}{2}$.

21. **The correct answer is (B).** The greater the concentration of soluble particles, the greater the lowering of the freezing point of the solvent. A mole of calcium chloride contains one mole of calcium ions and two moles of chloride ions. A mole of sodium chloride contains only two moles of ions, and sucrose and methanol have only one mole of particles each per liter of one molar solution.

22. **The correct answer is (B).** If the atomic mass of an isotope is unknown, the number of neutrons cannot be determined. However, if the atomic number is known, the number of protons is known. In an atom, there is no charge, so the number of electrons must equal the number of protons and the atomic number.

23. **The correct answer is (D).** Nitrogen makes up about 80 percent of the air and therefore contributes about 80 percent of the total atmospheric pressure— $0.80 \times 760mm = 608mm$.

24. **The correct answer is (D).** A supersaturated solution contains more dissolved solute than is normal at a given temperature. A disturbance will cause the solution to adjust to the normal concentration with the concurrent expulsion of the excess solute. A saturated solution will remain stable.

25. **The correct answer is (A).** A first order reaction has a rate that is proportional to the concentration of only one reactant.

26. **The correct answer is (A).** The loss of an alpha particle reduces the number of positive charges by two and the atomic mass by four.

27. **The correct answer is (D).** Positron (with the mass of an electron) emission can occur, but protons are never expelled from the nucleus during radioactive decay.

28. **The correct answer is (A).** Fat yields the highest amount of energy per gram of any of the foods consumed.

29. **The correct answer is (C).** The total number of moles of reactants and products are equal; therefore, a change of pressure has no effect in the equilibrium. Increasing hydrogen or reducing hydrogen bromide drives the reaction to the right. Only increasing hydrogen bromide shifts the equilibrium to the left.

30. **The correct answer is (C).** One gram of carbon-14 must go through four half lives to be reduced to 0.0625 grams. Four $\times$ 5.73 $\times$ 10 years equal 22.92 $\times$ 10 years.

31. **The correct answer is (D).** Since the oxidation number of a compound is O, the total positive values must equal the total negative values. Consequently, four times the value for oxygen (-2) must equal the positive values due to potassium ($+1$ each) and manganese (Mn).

   1 (Oxidation number of Mn) +
   2 (Oxidation number of K) +
   4 (Oxidation number of 0) = 0

   Oxidation number of Mn + 2($+1$) + 4(-2) = 0
   Oxidation number of Mn = $+8 - 2 = +6$

32. **The correct answer is (A).** Within a group, the element with the lowest atomic number has the highest ionization energy.

33. **The correct answer is (D).** Within a group of nonmetals such as the halogens, the one with the highest atomic number has the least electronegative value.

34. **The correct answer is (B).** The atomic radii of a group of metals increase as the atomic number increases. Therefore, the element with the lowest atomic number has the smallest atomic radius.

35. **The correct answer is (B).** The salt that would yield a weak acid when mixed with acid would dissolve most readily. Calcium carbonate yields carbonic acid (H_2CO_3) when it is acidified. The other salts yield hydrochloric acid (HC1), nitric acid (HNO_3), or phosphoric acid (H_3PO_4), which are both strong acids.

36. **The correct answer is (B).** The conjugate base is obtained when the acid loses a hydrogen ion. Therefore, the conjugate base of carbonic acid, H_2CO_3, is the hydrogen carbonate ion (HCO^-_3).

37. **The correct answer is (D).** The number of moles of HCl required for the titration must equal the number of moles of NaOH (40 ml $\times$ 0.2 m = 8 moles). Therefore 20 ml of 0.4 ml Cl is required. After titration, the total volume of the mixture is 40 + 20 = 60 ml.

38. **The correct answer is (D).** The salt of a weak acid would hydrolyze in solution to remove hydrogen ions from water and leave an excess of hydroxide ions. $H_2O + A \rightarrow HA + OH$. The salt of a strong acid would hydrolyze by removing hydroxide ions from water. $NH_4 + H_2O \rightarrow NH_4OH + H^+$.

39. **The correct answer is (A).** Heat is produced by the reaction, and, according to Le Chatalier's Principle, the system will adjust to maintain equilibrium. Heating would force the reaction to the left. A pressure increase shifts the reaction in the direction of smaller volumes (right), and addition of more reactant (N_2 or H_2) also pushes the reaction to the right.

40. **The correct answer is (C).** Colligative properties are based on the number of particles. Vapor pressure, osmotic pressure, boiling point elevation, and freezing point lowering all are colligative properties. Density is not.

41. **The correct answer is (C).** Molecular solids are held together by rather weak London forces, which increase with molecular weight. The melting points of molecular substances are relatively low since there are no strong forces, such as ionic forces, to overcome.

42. **The correct answer is (D).** Ionic compounds form readily between non-metals and metals. The only set that has no such combination is CH_2O, H_2S, and NH_3.

43. **The correct answer is (C).** An atom lying at the corner of a unit cell will touch four corners of cubes below and four corners of cubes above.

44. **The correct answer is (A).** A higher boiling point for a liquid is seen when more energy is needed to separate the gaseous molecules from the liquid. It shows that for the same amount of energy, a higher boiling liquid would expel fewer molecules as vapor at any temperature, resulting in a lower vapor pressure. The lowest boiling substance vaporizes most easily and therefore would have the highest vapor pressure at a specific temperature.

45. **The correct answer is (A).** The mass number of an isotope is the sum of the protons and neutrons in an atom. Seventeen protons and seventeen neutrons are necessary to give a mass number of thirty-four. The number of electrons equals the number of protons in an atom.

46. **The correct answer is (A).** Electronegativism decreases within a group in the periodic table as the atomic number increases. The example shown here is the progression from fluorine to iodine.

47. **The correct answer is (D).** Phosphorus has fifteen electrons, all of which are paired except one.

48. **The correct answer is (C).** Chlorine is in the third period and has seven electrons in its outermost shell. Two electrons are in an S orbital, leaving five electrons for the P orbitals.

49. **The correct answer is (B).** Sulfur in group VIA needs two electrons added to its six to achieve a stable outer shell of eight electrons.

50. **The correct answer is (B).** Since all three gases are in equal size flasks with the same temperature and pressure, the total number of moles (hence, the total number of molecules) is equal in each case. However, a molecule of NH_3 contains four atoms, a molecule of NO contains two atoms, and a molecule of N_2 contains two atoms.

READING COMPREHENSION

ANSWER SHEET

READING PASSAGE 1

1. Ⓐ Ⓑ Ⓒ Ⓓ
2. Ⓐ Ⓑ Ⓒ Ⓓ
3. Ⓐ Ⓑ Ⓒ Ⓓ
4. Ⓐ Ⓑ Ⓒ Ⓓ

READING PASSAGE 2

1. Ⓐ Ⓑ Ⓒ Ⓓ
2. Ⓐ Ⓑ Ⓒ Ⓓ
3. Ⓐ Ⓑ Ⓒ Ⓓ
4. Ⓐ Ⓑ Ⓒ Ⓓ

READING PASSAGE 3

1. Ⓐ Ⓑ Ⓒ Ⓓ   5. Ⓐ Ⓑ Ⓒ Ⓓ
2. Ⓐ Ⓑ Ⓒ Ⓓ   6. Ⓐ Ⓑ Ⓒ Ⓓ
3. Ⓐ Ⓑ Ⓒ Ⓓ   7. Ⓐ Ⓑ Ⓒ Ⓓ
4. Ⓐ Ⓑ Ⓒ Ⓓ   8. Ⓐ Ⓑ Ⓒ Ⓓ

READING PASSAGE 4

1. Ⓐ Ⓑ Ⓒ Ⓓ   4. Ⓐ Ⓑ Ⓒ Ⓓ   7. Ⓐ Ⓑ Ⓒ Ⓓ
2. Ⓐ Ⓑ Ⓒ Ⓓ   5. Ⓐ Ⓑ Ⓒ Ⓓ   8. Ⓐ Ⓑ Ⓒ Ⓓ
3. Ⓐ Ⓑ Ⓒ Ⓓ   6. Ⓐ Ⓑ Ⓒ Ⓓ   9. Ⓐ Ⓑ Ⓒ Ⓓ

READING PASSAGE 1

4 QUESTIONS ◼ TIME—9 MINUTES

Directions: Carefully read the following passage and then answer the accompanying questions, basing your answers on what is stated or implied in the passage. When you have decided which choice is best, fill in the corresponding space on your answer sheet. There is only one best answer for each question.

Communicable means "capable of being transmitted or passed through a medium." A communicable disease is an infection that may be transmitted directly or indirectly from one individual to another. The primary objective of programs for the prevention and control of communicable diseases is to prevent the transmission or spreading of the disease by eliminating conditions supportive to infection. Since communicable diseases are caused by microorganisms, the process of infection can be avoided or reversed by eliminating microbial sources, destroying the infectious organisms, creating conditions unfavorable to the growth of infectious microorganisms, and building up the body defenses against microbial attack.

Any measure designed to control or protect anyone from the hazards of the infectious microbes in the environment is called a barrier. The use of barriers is based upon three factors: time, distance, and shielding. "Time" refers to avoiding prolonged exposure; "distance" refers to keeping away from the infectious source; and "shielding" refers to avoiding bodily contact when exposure cannot be avoided (e.g., wearing a mask). The specific plan for selecting barriers in cases where infection exists and for preventing the occurrence of infection is dependent upon the characteristics of the causative microorganism(s). All of these microbes have a certain structure, a specific way of digesting foods, a system for utilizing oxygen or the oxidation-reduction processes, and a technique for reproducing. These microbes are classified by similarities in life characteristics. Therefore, the approach to prevention and control of communicable disease is to eliminate environmental sources or to identify the kind of organisms (by characteristics) and alter their life processes, in order to protect human beings from attack.

1. Infectious diseases are "communicable" because they
   (A) attack human beings.
   (B) spread from one source to another.
   (C) cannot be controlled by barriers.
   (D) can cause disease.

2. The approach to *controlling* communicable diseases differs from the approach to *prevention* of disease in that
   (A) an infectious source exists and could be spread.
   (B) infection has not occurred, and sources are being eliminated.
   (C) transmission has occurred, but there is no infection.
   (D) transmission cannot occur because there is no medium.

3. A barrier that represents "shielding" would be
   (A) isolating a child with a cold.
   (B) using a stick to pick up infected material.
   (C) short visits with a friend who has pneumonia.
   (D) looking at a baby through a nursery window.

4. Having knowledge of the characteristics of an infectious microorganism helps in the prevention and control of communicable disease in that it
   (A) determines how long the infection will last.
   (B) identifies which methods should be used to counteract the infection.
   (C) establishes whether or not the organism is a hazard.
   (D) relates to the severity of the infection.

STOP If you finish before time is called, you may check your work on this section only. Do not turn to any other section in the test.

READING PASSAGE 2

4 QUESTIONS ▪▭ TIME—9 MINUTES

Directions: Carefully read the following passage and then answer the accompanying questions, basing your answers on what is stated or implied in the passage. When you have decided which choice is best, fill in the corresponding space on your answer sheet. There is only one best answer for each question.

The "liberated woman" is a phrase that most of us associate with the sixties and seventies. The ERA and NOW's consciousness-raising and bra-burning blitzed the media with a fury. In reality, the American woman had begun to cast off the restraints of feminine suppression long before the seventies, by snipping the strings of her proverbial apron, if not the straps of her bra. We are referring to both the 1920s and the postwar era.

The flood of labor-saving and timesaving devices pouring from the factories freed women of much of the never-ending drudgery that had been the plight of housewives since the beginning of time.

Women also found new freedom outside the home. The vote was finally rendered to women via the Nineteenth Amendment to the Constitution, and the long awaited dream of political equality between the sexes was fulfilled. Members of what was once known as the "gentle sex" cast down their brooms, cast forth their ballots, and fled their kitchens to take part in a social freedom that catapulted their grandmothers right out of their rocking chairs. Chaperones no longer made the scene at young people's parties. Fashion editors reported "the American woman has lifted her skirt far beyond any modest limitation." The hemline was being hoisted nine inches from the ground and was heading for the knee.

The boyish look was in, and women everywhere invaded the strictly male territory known as the barbershop to have their beautiful and once-treasured tresses "bobbed." Breast implants, no way! Damsels of every social station were binding their chests to acquire that fashionable look of masculinity. In contrast to this trend of fashion, beautiful debutantes took heed to the cliche "powder and paint will make you what you ain't" and plastered their faces doll-style with rouge and lipstick.

Young ladies no longer puffed secretly into the fireplaces of their homes to conceal the damnable sin of which they were partaking. Women were smoking in public for the first time.

Extensive vicissitudes in lifestyle and values placed women in the workplace. The "roaring twenties" were characterized by women finding new opportunities for employment in the booming cities. Though they were limited to a few low-paying jobs hastily labeled "women's work," such as retail clerking and office typing, they were making an impact on the post-war era. A feisty feminist, Margaret Sanger, led a birth-control movement and openly defended the use of contraceptives. To add insult to injury, the women of the twenties deflated many a male ego with the organization of the National Women's Party in 1923.

"You've Come A Long Way Baby" was putting it mildly in the twenties. In all probability, the women of the 1990s can anticipate recoining the phrase ". . . and you ain't seen nothin' yet!"

1. This passage would suggest that women of the 1920s were
   (A) docile in their attitudes regarding social change.
   (B) assertive in their views on women's social and political status.
   (C) willing to compromise on political issues concerning women.
   (D) eager to return to life in the kitchen.

2. A fitting title for this passage would be
   (A) "You've Come a Long Way Baby—Twenties Style."
   (B) "Women in the Workplace."
   (C) "Women's Political Advancements in the Twenties."
   (D) "Male Bashing in the Twenties."

3. The tone of this passage would suggest that the author is
   (A) a male chauvinist.
   (B) a product of the seventies.
   (C) a trendy individual.
   (D) an advocate of women's lib.

4. This passage reflects that the era known as the "Roaring Twenties" was characterized by
   (A) an increase in women's unemployment.
   (B) marked social change.
   (C) an industrial slump.
   (D) an indifference to fashion and style.

STOP   If you finish before time is called, you may check your work on this section only. Do not turn to any other section in the test.

READING PASSAGE 3

8 QUESTIONS ▪ TIME—10 MINUTES

Directions: Carefully read the following passage and then answer the accompanying questions, basing your answers on what is stated or implied in the passage. When you have decided which choice is best, fill in the corresponding space on your answer sheet. There is only one best answer for each question.

Every cell in the body is bathed in water. The substances dissolved in the water provide the immediate environment for the cells' existence, that is, for their respiration, digestion, excretion, and reproduction. This water—70% of our body weight and originally from our food and drink—is carried in the blood and is distributed in three places in the body. In terms of body weight:

5% remains in blood
15% goes to tissue spaces
50% goes inside the cell

Of course, more water is needed in the cell than elsewhere in the body because there are more solutes to be dissolved and because ionization must take place for anabolism and catabolism.

All of the substances inside the cell and outside the cell in the tissue spaces were at one time a part of the blood. The blood is the transportation system of the body and, therefore, is the recipient of all substances. Substances are "unloaded" by pushing out those that can filter through the tiny openings of the semipermeable membranes of the capillaries into the tissue spaces. These substances, along with water, are then sucked into the semipermeable membranes of the cells. At the same time, the cell has produced waste substances; it now pushes those out into the tissue fluid so that they can be pushed into the capillaries and thereby excreted by the kidneys, skin, respiratory system, etc.

The pushing and sucking forces are regulated by concentrations. The more concentrated a substance is, the more force it has. What determines whether that force will push or suck is whether the substance is primarily water (solvent) or particles dissolved in water (solute). If water is the primary component of a substance, it will be sucked; that is, it will pass from a lesser to a greater concentration. This is called osmosis. The substance that is sucking in the water has the greater force or pull, called osmotic pressure, because it has the greater concentration. If solutes are the primary component, they can be pushed only by diffusion from a greater to a lesser concentration. The sucking and pushing processes go on simultaneously, and that is why we identify this mechanism as being dynamic. The "equilibrium" of body fluids is explained in terms of a balance of forces. This dynamic factor is controlled by three things:

1. How much of the substance is present (solute/solvent)

2. What kind of substance is present (electrolytes/non-electrolytes)

3. The placement and distribution of the substance (cell/tissue space/blood)

The concentration of a solution is determined by the relationship between the solutes and water. "Solutes" may be electrolytes or non-electrolytes. Non-electrolytes do not ionize and, therefore, they affect the concentration of a solution and its diffusion processes, but they do not affect the osmolarity of a solution. Osmotic pressure is determined by "tonic" relationships. "Tonic" refers to the comparison of the number of specific ions per unit volume in two given solutions—iso being "the same as," hypo being "less than," and hyper being "more than."

Given two solutions of the same solute, the more concentrated solution contains more solute particles, has a higher potential osmotic pressure, and is hypertonic as compared with the less concentrated solution. Given two solutions of different solutes, the solution containing more particles has the greater concentration, but there are no "tonic" relationships.

1. Why is an adequate intake of water essential to life?

   (A) Solutes will dissolve only in water.
   (B) Water is the medium for exchange of solutes.
   (C) Osmosis will take place only in water.
   (D) Water is necessary for metabolism.

2. The blood is described as "the transportation system of the body" because

   (A) blood has the capacity for osmosis and diffusion.
   (B) all nutrients and wastes are received by the blood.
   (C) blood has a higher concentration than any other body fluid.
   (D) all metabolic processes are controlled by the blood.

3. The concentration of a solution is directly determined by

   (A) placement of solutes.
   (B) distribution of water.
   (C) percentage of solute to solvent.
   (D) percentage of electrolytes to non-electrolytes.

4. The largest percentage of H_2O in the body is found

   (A) intracellularly.
   (B) extracelluarly.
   (C) intravascularly.
   (D) interstitially.

5. In the process of osmosis (sucking), the primary factor is

   (A) water.
   (B) solute.
   (C) ionization.
   (D) force.

6. If blood cells were placed in a hypertonic solution of salt, which one of the following blood cell reactions would take place?

   (A) Swelling
   (B) Shrinkage
   (C) Destruction
   (D) No change

7. The primary factor in diffusion (pushing) is

   (A) water.
   (B) solute.
   (C) ionization.
   (D) force.

8. If there are two solutions of sodium chloride, which of the following factors will determine which solution has the highest potential for osmosis?

   (A) Isotonicity
   (B) Hypotonicity
   (C) Hypertonicity
   (D) All of the above

STOP   If you finish before time is called, you may check your work on this section only. Do not turn to any other section in the test.

READING PASSAGE 4

9 QUESTIONS ▪ TIME—17 MINUTES

Directions: Carefully read the following passage and then answer the accompanying questions, basing your answers on what is stated or implied in the passage. When you have decided which choice is best, fill in the corresponding space on your answer sheet. There is only one best answer for each question.

As the world's population grows, the part played by humans in influencing plant life becomes increasingly great. In old and densely populated countries, as in western Europe, humans determine almost wholly what shall grow and what shall not grow. In such regions, the influence of humans on plant life is in large measure a beneficial one. Laws, often centuries old, protect plants of economic value and preserve soil fertility. In newly settled countries the situation is, unfortunately, quite the reverse. The pioneer's life is too strenuous for him to think of posterity.

Some years ago Mt. Mitchell, the highest summit east of the Mississippi, was covered with a magnificent forest. A lumber company was given full rights to fell the trees. Those not cut down were crushed. The mountain was left a waste area where fire would rage and erosion complete the destruction. There was no stopping the devastating foresting of the company, for the contract had been given. Under a more enlightened civilization, this could not have happened. The denuding of Mt. Mitchell is a minor chapter in the destruction of lands in the United States; and this country is by no means the only sufferer. China, India, Egypt, and East Africa all have their thousands of square miles of wasteland, the result of human indifference to the future.

Deforestation, grazing, and poor farming techniques are the chief causes of the destruction of land fertility. Wasteful cutting of timber is the first step. Grazing follows lumbering, often bringing about ruin. The Caribbean slopes of northern Venezuela are barren wastes, owing first to ruthless cutting of forests and then to destructive grazing. Hordes of goats roamed these slopes until only a few thorny acacias and cacti remained. Erosion completed the devastation. What is illustrated there on a small scale is the story of vast areas in China and India, countries where famines occur regularly.

Humans are not wholly to blame, for nature is often merciless. In parts of India and China, plant life, even when left undisturbed, cannot cope with either the disastrous floods of wet seasons or the destructive winds of the dry season. Humans have learned much; prudent land management has been the policy of the Chinese people since 2700 B.C.E., but even they have not learned enough.

When the American forestry service was in its infancy, it met with much opposition from legislators, who loudly claimed that the protected land would in one season yield a crop of cabbages of more value than all the timber on it. Herein lay the fallacy: that one season's crop is all that need be thought of. Nature, through the years, adjusts crops to the soil and to the climate. Forests usually occur where precipitation exceeds evaporation. If the reverse is true, grasslands are found; where evaporation is still greater, desert or scrub vegetation alone survives. The phytogeographic map of a country is very similar to the climatic map based on rainfall, evaporation, and temperature. Humans ignore this natural adjustment of crops and strive for one "bumper" crop in a single season; it may be produced, but "year in and year out, the yield of the grassland is certain; that of the planted fields, never."

Humans are learning; we spray trees with insecticides and fungicides; import ladybugs to destroy aphids; irrigate, fertilize, and rotate crops; but we are still indifferent to many of the consequences of short-sighted policies.

In spite of the evidence from the experience of this country, the people of other countries still in the pioneer stage farm as wastefully as did our own pioneers. In the interiors of Central and South

America, natives fell superb forest trees and leave them to rot in order to obtain virgin soil for cultivation. Where the land is hilly, it readily washes, and after one or two seasons, it is unfit for crops. So the frontier farmer pushes back into the primeval forest, moving his hut as he goes, and fells more monarchs to lay bare another patch of ground for his plantings to support his family. Valuable timber that will require a century to replace is destroyed and the land laid waste to produce what could be supplied for a pittance.

How badly humans can err in the handling of land is shown by the draining of extensive swamp areas, which to the uninformed would seem to be a very good thing to do. One of the first effects of the drainage is the lowering of the water table, which may bring about the death of the dominant species and leave to another species the possession of the soil, even when the difference in water level is little more than an inch. Bog country will frequently yield marketable crops of cranberries and blueberries, but, if drained, will grow neither these nor any other economically useful plant on the fallow soil. Swamps and marshes may have their drawbacks, but humans should beware of disturbing the ecosphere. When drained, wetlands may leave waste land, the surface of which can erode rapidly and be blown away in dust blizzards disastrous to both humans and wild beasts.

1. The best title for this passage might be
   (A) "How to Increase Soil Productivity."
   (B) "Conservation of Natural Resources."
   (C) "Humans' Effect on Soil."
   (D) "Soil Conditions and Plant Growth."

2. A policy of good management is sometimes upset by
   (A) the indifference of humans.
   (B) centuries-old laws.
   (C) floods and winds.
   (D) grazing animals.

3. Areas in which the total amounts of rain and snow falling on the ground are greater than the moisture evaporated will support
   (A) forests.
   (B) grasslands.
   (C) scrub vegetation.
   (D) no plants.

4. Pioneers usually do not have a long range view on soil problems since they   .
   (A) are not protected by laws.
   (B) live under adverse conditions.
   (C) use poor methods of farming.
   (D) must protect themselves from famine.

5. *Phytogeographic* maps are those that show
   (A) areas of grassland.
   (B) areas of bumper crops.
   (C) areas of similar climate.
   (D) areas of similar plants.

6. What is meant by, "the yield of the grasslands is certain; that of the planted field, never"?
   (A) It is impossible to get more than one bumper crop from any one cultivated area.
   (B) Crops planted in former grasslands will not give good yields.
   (C) Through the indifference of humans, dust blizzards have occurred in former grasslands.
   (D) If humans do not interfere, plants will grow in the most suitable environment.

7. The first act of prudent land management might be to
   (A) prohibit drainage of swamps.
   (B) use irrigation and crop rotation in planted areas.
   (C) increase use of fertilizers.
   (D) prohibit excessive forest lumbering.

GO ON TO THE NEXT PAGE

8. The results of effective land management may usually be found in

(A) heavily populated areas.
(B) areas not given over to grazing.
(C) underdeveloped areas.
(D) ancient civilizations.

9. Long-range programs of soil management are possible only in

(A) young nations.
(B) ancient civilizations.
(C) those nations with an agricultural economy.
(D) those nations that want it.

STOP If you finish before time is called, you may check your work on this section only. Do not turn to any other section in the test.

ANSWER KEY

Reading Passage 1

1. **B**
2. **A**
3. **D**
4. **B**

Reading Passage 2

1. **B**
2. **A**
3. **D**
4. **B**

Reading Passage 3

1. **D**   5. **A**
2. **B**   6. **A**
3. **C**   7. **B**
4. **A**   8. **C**

Reading Passage 4

1. **C**   4. **B**   7. **D**
2. **C**   5. **D**   8. **A**
3. **A**   6. **D**   9. **C**

PART IV

PRACTICE FOR PRACTICAL/VOCATIONAL NURSING SCHOOL ENTRANCE EXAMINATIONS

Introduction

Modern nursing is complex and multifaceted. Nurses practice in a variety of settings that emphasize different roles. Various educational programs are available to provide opportunities for nurses to enter different careers within the same profession of nursing. Nursing has experienced many changes throughout its history, and the changes are not over yet. A major change that has occurred in practical/vocational nursing history is a gradual increase in the required formal knowledge base.

Prior to the Civil War, untrained compassionate women cared for sick relatives and friends using skills that they had learned from their mothers and friends. The practical/vocational nurse became a permanent member of the health team when society needed a trained individual who could render competent and intelligent bedside care to patients. The need for an educational program for practical/vocational nurses was recognized, and in 1893, the first school for practical nurses in the United States was founded in New York. This was the Ballard School, which consisted of a three-month educational program.

Today's practical/vocational nurses are educationally prepared and technically skilled individuals capable of rendering competent, scientific, and personal care to patients. The educational program is approximately one year in length. The emphasis in practical/vocational nursing education is on learning basic skills that can be used in a variety of clinical settings. Care is rendered to patients in hospitals, physicians' offices, extended-care facilities, community health centers, private homes, day camps, industries, nursing homes, hospice facilities, and the armed forces. Men as well as women find practical/vocational nursing a rewarding vocation.

The practical/vocational nurse works under the supervision and direction of the registered nurse, physician, or other person(s) authorized by law. The practical/vocational nurse participates in assessing the patient's physical and mental health; records and reports; participates in implementing health-care plans designed by the registered nurse or other authorized persons; reinforces teaching; and documents the patient's response to nursing care.

The practical/vocational nurse is a graduate of a state-approved school and is licensed to practice after passing the National Council Licensure Examination (NCLEX-PN), which is a computerized test. Practical/vocational nursing programs may be administered at technical and vocational schools; community and junior colleges: universities; hospitals; and private or government agencies. Knowledge is basic to all occupations. Because nursing is comprehensive, you will be required to take many courses in theory and practice to provide you with the knowledge and information essential to your vocation. The nursing curriculum is based on scientific theory from the natural, social, and health sciences. Basic principles of selected nursing techniques are also included. Clinical experience is provided in such areas as nursing care of mothers and infants, pediatrics, care of the mentally ill, medical and surgical nursing, and care of the aged and chronically ill. Licensed practical/vocational nurses (LPNs or LVNs) have excellent employment opportunities. Many new positions have been created by population growth and the increase in public-health consciousness. Salaries for practical/vocational nurses have increased proportionately, as they have for registered nurses. The salary for the licensed practical nurse or licensed vocational nurse is usually three-fourths that of the registered nurse.

Any career that you choose entails effort, trials, and preserverance. Your nursing program is no exception and will present many exciting challenges to you. A nursing examination is usually required before admission to a practical/vocational nursing program. This section is designed to help you achieve an acceptable score on the examination.

TEST-TAKING STRATEGIES

An important objective in preparing for admission into nursing school is to develop your test-taking skills. Success in test-taking is very important to the majority of us. We learn early on in life that by obtaining certain test scores, we are permitted or denied certain opportunities. With the importance that our society has placed on passing or failing tests, it is understandable that there will be a certain amount of stress before, during, and after a test. This feeling can be termed "test stress."

Effects of Stress

Stress is a normal part of everyday life, and it is inherent in health-care professions. Stress is the wear and tear put on the body through normal or abnormal events of life. Our reactions to stress may include painful emotions, such as fear, anxiety, confusion, and humiliation. Minimal stress can be helpful and positive because it keeps us alert and "on our toes." Intense stress is negative because it interferes with the learning process by elevating your anxiety level until it causes a blockage. For example, a person under stress may be unable to concentrate, may forget, and may make errors in judgment. All in all, the combined effects of stress can be a deciding factor in whether a test-taker will be successful or unsuccessful in passing tests.

Reducing Test Stress

It has been determined that test-takers who anticipate failure will have an increase in their stress level. You must learn to control this source of stress by focusing on positive events that have occurred in your life and by anticipating future successes. Focus on positive thinking!

Relaxation exercises can be very effective in relieving tension and stress. One technique is to take deep, slow, deliberate breaths. Following this, you should tense each major muscle group for ten seconds, then relax. Once you learn how to perform these exercises, you can use them any time you feel tense or stressed.

Tests are a fact of life for students. You must be prepared to deal with them. Preparation for tests includes planned study or review sessions. This preparation will help to build your self-confidence. If you study effectively, concentrate, and apply what you have learned, you will reduce stress to a minimum.

Many people experience stress when dealing with the unknown. Try to learn as much as you can about the examination and the condition of testing. Sample tests included in this book will help you to prepare for the unknown.

TEST-TAKING TACTICS

In the following paragraphs, ten tactics for test-taking have been identified for you. These tactics provide solutions to the most common problems faced by test-takers.

Many of the tests that you take will be multiple choice. How do you successfully take a multiple-choice test? The answer to this question can be complex, but the more practice you have, the better you will become. Listed below are general tactics for taking multiple-choice tests.

1. Read instructions or directions carefully. Reading directions may seem like a simple matter, but mistakes can be made when the test-taker does not read the information carefully and completely.

2. Manage your time effectively during test-taking. If you are a slow test-taker, practice reading at a faster pace. Do not spend too much time on one question; move on if you have to and return to it later. If you progress in a timely fashion, you will feel confident and maintain composure during the testing situation.

3. Do not change answers without good reason or sound rationale. Usually your first answer is the best, unless you are positive that it is wrong. Your first attempt at answering a test item is usually accomplished by a logical and orderly thinking process. If you are uncertain of an answer and you change it, you are most likely doing it impulsively, not because of logical thinking. Do not change your answer unless you have a SOUND reason to do so.

4. Use a process of elimination to weed out unsound, unreasonable options that do not fit. By reducing your choices on a difficult question, you can sharpen your focus and make the question more manageable.

5. Do not become angry or upset with a question. Put the emotion away until after the test.

6. Maintain a positive attitude. You may not know the answer, but try to figure it out.

7. Don't overlook key words or phrases such as "not," "except," "never," "all," "always," and "only." Words such as these may cause you to give an inaccurate response.

8. Attempt every question. Do not avoid questions that seem complicated. After you read them carefully, they may be easier than you think.

9. Do not jump to conclusions. Read the questions slowly and carefully.

10. Do not read too deeply into questions or answers. Answer only what is being asked, not what you think should be asked.

Will these tactics improve your test-taking skills? When combined with a proper, planned review, these strategies should help you to do better on the admission examination and achieve your goal of becoming a practical/vocational nurse.

VERBAL SKILLS

ANSWER SHEET

ANTONYMS

TEST 1

1. Ⓐ Ⓑ Ⓒ Ⓓ	11. Ⓐ Ⓑ Ⓒ Ⓓ	21. Ⓐ Ⓑ Ⓒ Ⓓ	31. Ⓐ Ⓑ Ⓒ Ⓓ	41. Ⓐ Ⓑ Ⓒ Ⓓ
2. Ⓐ Ⓑ Ⓒ Ⓓ	12. Ⓐ Ⓑ Ⓒ Ⓓ	22. Ⓐ Ⓑ Ⓒ Ⓓ	32. Ⓐ Ⓑ Ⓒ Ⓓ	42. Ⓐ Ⓑ Ⓒ Ⓓ
3. Ⓐ Ⓑ Ⓒ Ⓓ	13. Ⓐ Ⓑ Ⓒ Ⓓ	23. Ⓐ Ⓑ Ⓒ Ⓓ	33. Ⓐ Ⓑ Ⓒ Ⓓ	43. Ⓐ Ⓑ Ⓒ Ⓓ
4. Ⓐ Ⓑ Ⓒ Ⓓ	14. Ⓐ Ⓑ Ⓒ Ⓓ	24. Ⓐ Ⓑ Ⓒ Ⓓ	34. Ⓐ Ⓑ Ⓒ Ⓓ	44. Ⓐ Ⓑ Ⓒ Ⓓ
5. Ⓐ Ⓑ Ⓒ Ⓓ	15. Ⓐ Ⓑ Ⓒ Ⓓ	25. Ⓐ Ⓑ Ⓒ Ⓓ	35. Ⓐ Ⓑ Ⓒ Ⓓ	45. Ⓐ Ⓑ Ⓒ Ⓓ
6. Ⓐ Ⓑ Ⓒ Ⓓ	16. Ⓐ Ⓑ Ⓒ Ⓓ	26. Ⓐ Ⓑ Ⓒ Ⓓ	36. Ⓐ Ⓑ Ⓒ Ⓓ	46. Ⓐ Ⓑ Ⓒ Ⓓ
7. Ⓐ Ⓑ Ⓒ Ⓓ	17. Ⓐ Ⓑ Ⓒ Ⓓ	27. Ⓐ Ⓑ Ⓒ Ⓓ	37. Ⓐ Ⓑ Ⓒ Ⓓ	47. Ⓐ Ⓑ Ⓒ Ⓓ
8. Ⓐ Ⓑ Ⓒ Ⓓ	18. Ⓐ Ⓑ Ⓒ Ⓓ	28. Ⓐ Ⓑ Ⓒ Ⓓ	38. Ⓐ Ⓑ Ⓒ Ⓓ	48. Ⓐ Ⓑ Ⓒ Ⓓ
9. Ⓐ Ⓑ Ⓒ Ⓓ	19. Ⓐ Ⓑ Ⓒ Ⓓ	29. Ⓐ Ⓑ Ⓒ Ⓓ	39. Ⓐ Ⓑ Ⓒ Ⓓ	49. Ⓐ Ⓑ Ⓒ Ⓓ
10. Ⓐ Ⓑ Ⓒ Ⓓ	20. Ⓐ Ⓑ Ⓒ Ⓓ	30. Ⓐ Ⓑ Ⓒ Ⓓ	40. Ⓐ Ⓑ Ⓒ Ⓓ	50. Ⓐ Ⓑ Ⓒ Ⓓ

TEST 2

1. Ⓐ Ⓑ Ⓒ Ⓓ	5. Ⓐ Ⓑ Ⓒ Ⓓ	9. Ⓐ Ⓑ Ⓒ Ⓓ	13. Ⓐ Ⓑ Ⓒ Ⓓ	17. Ⓐ Ⓑ Ⓒ Ⓓ
2. Ⓐ Ⓑ Ⓒ Ⓓ	6. Ⓐ Ⓑ Ⓒ Ⓓ	10. Ⓐ Ⓑ Ⓒ Ⓓ	14. Ⓐ Ⓑ Ⓒ Ⓓ	18. Ⓐ Ⓑ Ⓒ Ⓓ
3. Ⓐ Ⓑ Ⓒ Ⓓ	7. Ⓐ Ⓑ Ⓒ Ⓓ	11. Ⓐ Ⓑ Ⓒ Ⓓ	15. Ⓐ Ⓑ Ⓒ Ⓓ	19. Ⓐ Ⓑ Ⓒ Ⓓ
4. Ⓐ Ⓑ Ⓒ Ⓓ	8. Ⓐ Ⓑ Ⓒ Ⓓ	12. Ⓐ Ⓑ Ⓒ Ⓓ	16. Ⓐ Ⓑ Ⓒ Ⓓ	20. Ⓐ Ⓑ Ⓒ Ⓓ

SYNONYMS

TEST 3

1. Ⓐ Ⓑ Ⓒ Ⓓ
2. Ⓐ Ⓑ Ⓒ Ⓓ
3. Ⓐ Ⓑ Ⓒ Ⓓ
4. Ⓐ Ⓑ Ⓒ Ⓓ
5. Ⓐ Ⓑ Ⓒ Ⓓ
6. Ⓐ Ⓑ Ⓒ Ⓓ
7. Ⓐ Ⓑ Ⓒ Ⓓ
8. Ⓐ Ⓑ Ⓒ Ⓓ
9. Ⓐ Ⓑ Ⓒ Ⓓ
10. Ⓐ Ⓑ Ⓒ Ⓓ

11. Ⓐ Ⓑ Ⓒ Ⓓ
12. Ⓐ Ⓑ Ⓒ Ⓓ
13. Ⓐ Ⓑ Ⓒ Ⓓ
14. Ⓐ Ⓑ Ⓒ Ⓓ
15. Ⓐ Ⓑ Ⓒ Ⓓ
16. Ⓐ Ⓑ Ⓒ Ⓓ
17. Ⓐ Ⓑ Ⓒ Ⓓ
18. Ⓐ Ⓑ Ⓒ Ⓓ
19. Ⓐ Ⓑ Ⓒ Ⓓ
20. Ⓐ Ⓑ Ⓒ Ⓓ

21. Ⓐ Ⓑ Ⓒ Ⓓ
22. Ⓐ Ⓑ Ⓒ Ⓓ
23. Ⓐ Ⓑ Ⓒ Ⓓ
24. Ⓐ Ⓑ Ⓒ Ⓓ
25. Ⓐ Ⓑ Ⓒ Ⓓ
26. Ⓐ Ⓑ Ⓒ Ⓓ
27. Ⓐ Ⓑ Ⓒ Ⓓ
28. Ⓐ Ⓑ Ⓒ Ⓓ
29. Ⓐ Ⓑ Ⓒ Ⓓ
30. Ⓐ Ⓑ Ⓒ Ⓓ

31. Ⓐ Ⓑ Ⓒ Ⓓ
32. Ⓐ Ⓑ Ⓒ Ⓓ
33. Ⓐ Ⓑ Ⓒ Ⓓ
34. Ⓐ Ⓑ Ⓒ Ⓓ
35. Ⓐ Ⓑ Ⓒ Ⓓ
36. Ⓐ Ⓑ Ⓒ Ⓓ
37. Ⓐ Ⓑ Ⓒ Ⓓ
38. Ⓐ Ⓑ Ⓒ Ⓓ
39. Ⓐ Ⓑ Ⓒ Ⓓ
40. Ⓐ Ⓑ Ⓒ Ⓓ

41. Ⓐ Ⓑ Ⓒ Ⓓ
42. Ⓐ Ⓑ Ⓒ Ⓓ
43. Ⓐ Ⓑ Ⓒ Ⓓ
44. Ⓐ Ⓑ Ⓒ Ⓓ
45. Ⓐ Ⓑ Ⓒ Ⓓ
46. Ⓐ Ⓑ Ⓒ Ⓓ
47. Ⓐ Ⓑ Ⓒ Ⓓ
48. Ⓐ Ⓑ Ⓒ Ⓓ
49. Ⓐ Ⓑ Ⓒ Ⓓ
50. Ⓐ Ⓑ Ⓒ Ⓓ

TEST 4

1. Ⓐ Ⓑ Ⓒ Ⓓ
2. Ⓐ Ⓑ Ⓒ Ⓓ
3. Ⓐ Ⓑ Ⓒ Ⓓ
4. Ⓐ Ⓑ Ⓒ Ⓓ

5. Ⓐ Ⓑ Ⓒ Ⓓ
6. Ⓐ Ⓑ Ⓒ Ⓓ
7. Ⓐ Ⓑ Ⓒ Ⓓ
8. Ⓐ Ⓑ Ⓒ Ⓓ

9. Ⓐ Ⓑ Ⓒ Ⓓ
10. Ⓐ Ⓑ Ⓒ Ⓓ
11. Ⓐ Ⓑ Ⓒ Ⓓ
12. Ⓐ Ⓑ Ⓒ Ⓓ

13. Ⓐ Ⓑ Ⓒ Ⓓ
14. Ⓐ Ⓑ Ⓒ Ⓓ
15. Ⓐ Ⓑ Ⓒ Ⓓ
16. Ⓐ Ⓑ Ⓒ Ⓓ

17. Ⓐ Ⓑ Ⓒ Ⓓ
18. Ⓐ Ⓑ Ⓒ Ⓓ
19. Ⓐ Ⓑ Ⓒ Ⓓ
20. Ⓐ Ⓑ Ⓒ Ⓓ

TEST 5: SPELLING USAGE

1. Ⓐ Ⓑ Ⓒ Ⓓ
2. Ⓐ Ⓑ Ⓒ Ⓓ
3. Ⓐ Ⓑ Ⓒ Ⓓ
4. Ⓐ Ⓑ Ⓒ Ⓓ
5. Ⓐ Ⓑ Ⓒ Ⓓ
6. Ⓐ Ⓑ Ⓒ Ⓓ
7. Ⓐ Ⓑ Ⓒ Ⓓ

8. Ⓐ Ⓑ Ⓒ Ⓓ
9. Ⓐ Ⓑ Ⓒ Ⓓ
10. Ⓐ Ⓑ Ⓒ Ⓓ
11. Ⓐ Ⓑ Ⓒ Ⓓ
12. Ⓐ Ⓑ Ⓒ Ⓓ
13. Ⓐ Ⓑ Ⓒ Ⓓ
14. Ⓐ Ⓑ Ⓒ Ⓓ

15. Ⓐ Ⓑ Ⓒ Ⓓ
16. Ⓐ Ⓑ Ⓒ Ⓓ
17. Ⓐ Ⓑ Ⓒ Ⓓ
18. Ⓐ Ⓑ Ⓒ Ⓓ
19. Ⓐ Ⓑ Ⓒ Ⓓ
20. Ⓐ Ⓑ Ⓒ Ⓓ
21. Ⓐ Ⓑ Ⓒ Ⓓ

22. Ⓐ Ⓑ Ⓒ Ⓓ
23. Ⓐ Ⓑ Ⓒ Ⓓ
24. Ⓐ Ⓑ Ⓒ Ⓓ
25. Ⓐ Ⓑ Ⓒ Ⓓ
26. Ⓐ Ⓑ Ⓒ Ⓓ
27. Ⓐ Ⓑ Ⓒ Ⓓ
28. Ⓐ Ⓑ Ⓒ Ⓓ

29. Ⓐ Ⓑ Ⓒ Ⓓ
30. Ⓐ Ⓑ Ⓒ Ⓓ
31. Ⓐ Ⓑ Ⓒ Ⓓ
32. Ⓐ Ⓑ Ⓒ Ⓓ
33. Ⓐ Ⓑ Ⓒ Ⓓ
34. Ⓐ Ⓑ Ⓒ Ⓓ
35. Ⓐ Ⓑ Ⓒ Ⓓ

ANTONYMS
TEST 1

50 QUESTIONS ■□ TIME—30 MINUTES

Please refer to Unit 1 for review before completing this section.

Directions: For each question, select the word that is opposite in meaning to the capitalized word. Fill in the corresponding space on your answer sheet.

1. GARRULOUS
    - (A) talkative
    - (B) reserved
    - (C) unruly
    - (D) fraternal

2. TRANSLUCENT
    - (A) patent
    - (B) transitory
    - (C) transparent
    - (D) opaque

3. BENEVOLENT
    - (A) generous
    - (B) charitable
    - (C) malevolent
    - (D) good

4. LETHARGIC
    - (A) energetic
    - (B) sluggish
    - (C) apathetic
    - (D) fatal

5. AMICABLE
    - (A) lonely
    - (B) reactionary
    - (C) hostile
    - (D) laconic

6. TRANQUILITY
    - (A) complacency
    - (B) tumult
    - (C) plagiarism
    - (D) prophecy

7. PROCRASTINATE
    - (A) elegiac
    - (B) mediate
    - (C) expedite
    - (D) investiture

8. QUIESCENT
    - (A) restless
    - (B) lethargic
    - (C) mendicant
    - (D) malignant

9. DELETERIOUS
    - (A) fractious
    - (B) pathetic
    - (C) salubrious
    - (D) gullible

10. COGNIZANCE
    - (A) ignorance
    - (B) abeyance
    - (C) anecdote
    - (D) idiom

11. CLEMENCY
    - (A) mercy
    - (B) indulgence
    - (C) kindness
    - (D) vindictiveness

GO ON TO THE NEXT PAGE

12. IGNOBLE
    (A) honorable
    (B) shameful
    (C) disgraceful
    (D) humble

13. CURSORY
    (A) hasty
    (B) superficial
    (C) awful
    (D) thorough

14. ADMONISH
    (A) warn
    (B) praise
    (C) advise
    (D) reprove

15. PHLEGMATIC
    (A) energetic
    (B) dull
    (C) extraordinary
    (D) morbid

16. LAMENTABLE
    (A) laughable
    (B) generous
    (C) emotional
    (D) doleful

17. PERILOUS
    (A) vivacious
    (B) fatal
    (C) safe
    (D) hazardous

18. INIQUITOUS
    (A) unequaled
    (B) unfriendly
    (C) righteous
    (D) injurious

19. ASSIDUOUS
    (A) cooperative
    (B) indifferent
    (C) active
    (D) satisfactory

20. CORROBORATE
    (A) fascinate
    (B) corrupt
    (C) confirm
    (D) dispute

21. CONFLUENCE
    (A) convention
    (B) sympathy
    (C) divergence
    (D) concurrence

22. DASTARDLY
    (A) cowardly
    (B) bravely
    (C) friendly
    (D) sinfully

23. ABSTRUSE
    (A) understandable
    (B) hidden
    (C) absurd
    (D) religious

24. ILLUSION
    (A) delusion
    (B) conception
    (C) reality
    (D) dramatization

25. AVARICIOUS
    (A) greedy
    (B) persuasive
    (C) generous
    (D) gracious

26. COERCE
    (A) enforce
    (B) cohere
    (C) forestall
    (D) coax

27. TEMERITY
    (A) recklessness
    (B) prudence
    (C) support
    (D) sanity

28. LACONIC

    (A) verbose
    (B) concise
    (C) serene
    (D) interesting

29. CREDULOUS

    (A) exuberant
    (B) skeptical
    (C) dangerous
    (D) legible

30. INCARCERATE

    (A) immunize
    (B) anesthetize
    (C) transport
    (D) release

31. OBTUSE

    (A) oblique
    (B) obese
    (C) perpendicular
    (D) acute

32. MUNIFICENT

    (A) political
    (B) miserly
    (C) liberal
    (D) educational

33. DERANGED

    (A) unsettled
    (B) paralyzed
    (C) sane
    (D) awkward

34. LEVITY

    (A) flippancy
    (B) peace
    (C) gravity
    (D) trickery

35. EQUANIMITY

    (A) peace
    (B) inflation
    (C) agitation
    (D) tranquility

36. MARAUD

    (A) purchase
    (B) plunder
    (C) masticate
    (D) elevate

37. ENCOMIUM

    (A) immorality
    (B) praise
    (C) egotism
    (D) defamation

38. ABOMINABLE

    (A) delightful
    (B) horrible
    (C) meaningful
    (D) insane

39. ABSTEMIOUS

    (A) frugal
    (B) happy
    (C) greedy
    (D) radiant

40. ADVERTENT

    (A) retentive
    (B) inconsiderate
    (C) empathetic
    (D) abnormal

41. ENIGMATIC

    (A) perplexing
    (B) explicit
    (C) persistent
    (D) officious

42. EXECRABLE

    (A) unusual
    (B) detestable
    (C) fallible
    (D) respectable

43. IGNOMINIOUS

    (A) reputable
    (B) shameful
    (C) intangible
    (D) irascible

GO ON TO THE NEXT PAGE

44. SAGACITY

    (A) sorrowfulness
    (B) support
    (C) satisfaction
    (D) stupidity

45. PROVERBIAL

    (A) innovative
    (B) current
    (C) wise
    (D) cautious

46. ANNIHILATE

    (A) advertise
    (B) destroy
    (C) preserve
    (D) announce

47. AFFABLE

    (A) discourteous
    (B) beloved
    (C) sociable
    (D) debonair

48. CAPRICIOUS

    (A) logical
    (B) agreeable
    (C) awkward
    (D) constant

49. CONTINGENT

    (A) conditional
    (B) independent
    (C) confinable
    (D) familiar

50. OFFICIOUS

    (A) meddling
    (B) modest
    (C) emaciated
    (D) authentic

STOP If you finish before time is called, you may check your work on this section only. Do not turn to any other section in the test.

TEST 2

20 QUESTIONS   TIME—10 MINUTES

Directions: For each question, select the word that is opposite in meaning to the capitalized word. Fill in the corresponding space on your answer sheet.

1. DECEIT
   - (A) fraud
   - (B) truthfulness
   - (C) treachery
   - (D) imposition

2. DOCILE
   - (A) teachable
   - (B) compliant
   - (C) tame
   - (D) inflexible

3. HARMLESS
   - (A) safe
   - (B) hurtful
   - (C) innocent
   - (D) innocuous

4. MELANCHOLY
   - (A) jolly
   - (B) low-spirited
   - (C) dreamy
   - (D) sad

5. IMPETUOUS
   - (A) violent
   - (B) furious
   - (C) calm
   - (D) vehement

6. JOY
   - (A) gladness
   - (B) grief
   - (C) mirth
   - (D) delight

7. LUNACY
   - (A) sanity
   - (B) madness
   - (C) derangement
   - (D) mania

8. MOIST
   - (A) dank
   - (B) dry
   - (C) damp
   - (D) humid

9. PUERILE
   - (A) youthful
   - (B) weak
   - (C) silly
   - (D) mature

10. WEIGHT
    - (A) gravity
    - (B) heaviness
    - (C) lightness
    - (D) burden

11. SUPERFLUOUS
    - (A) necessary
    - (B) excessive
    - (C) unnecessary
    - (D) expanded

12. REFORM
    - (A) amend
    - (B) correct
    - (C) better
    - (D) corrupt

GO ON TO THE NEXT PAGE

13. SCANTY

    (A) bare
    (B) ample
    (C) insufficient
    (D) meager

14. MISERY

    (A) happiness
    (B) woe
    (C) privation
    (D) penury

15. PROPER

    (A) honest
    (B) appropriate
    (C) wrong
    (D) pertinent

16. INCONGRUOUS

    (A) compatible
    (B) absurd
    (C) contrary
    (D) incoherent

17. FATIGUE

    (A) lassitude
    (B) weariness
    (C) malaise
    (D) vigor

18. HASTEN

    (A) delay
    (B) accelerate
    (C) dispatch
    (D) expedite

19. ABSORB

    (A) emit
    (B) engulf
    (C) engross
    (D) consume

20. ABUSE

    (A) ribaldry
    (B) protection
    (C) contumely
    (D) obloquy

S T O P   If you finish before time is called, you may check your work on this section only. Do not turn to any other section in the test.

SYNONYMS
TEST 3

50 QUESTIONS ▪▭ TIME—30 MINUTES

Directions: In each of the following, choose the word that best corresponds in meaning to the italicized word. Fill in the corresponding space on your answer sheet.

1. Her efforts to revive the child were *futile*.
   - (A) strong
   - (B) clumsy
   - (C) useless
   - (D) sincere

2. The supply of pamphlets has been *depleted*.
   - (A) exhausted
   - (B) delivered
   - (C) included
   - (D) rejected

3. The *gist* of his speech was that we should strike.
   - (A) end
   - (B) essence
   - (C) strength
   - (D) spirit

4. The soldier was decorated for his *valor* in battle in Korea.
   - (A) injury
   - (B) ability
   - (C) cooperation
   - (D) courage

5. When Mary arrived in California, her future seemed *auspicious*.
   - (A) bleak
   - (B) uncertain
   - (C) promising
   - (D) somber

6. To our *consternation*, the child's bicycle rolled into the busy street.
   - (A) dismay
   - (B) amazement
   - (C) incompetence
   - (D) annoyance

7. *Indolence* is a habit that cannot be excused.
   - (A) incompetency
   - (B) snoring
   - (C) carelessness
   - (D) idleness

8. The political candidate made *cogent* remarks.
   - (A) pleasing
   - (B) convincing
   - (C) flattering
   - (D) slandering

9. A *prolific* writer is one who is
   - (A) productive.
   - (B) popular.
   - (C) frank.
   - (D) effective.

10. He was *meticulous* when performing his work.
    - (A) careless
    - (B) patient
    - (C) scrupulous
    - (D) nervous

GO ON TO THE NEXT PAGE

11. There were *sporadic* outbreaks of food poisoning at the camp.

    (A) epidemic
    (B) widespread
    (C) serious
    (D) scattered

12. The motion passed even though there were three *dissenting* votes.

    (A) annoying
    (B) disagreeing
    (C) abstaining
    (D) approving

13. It is *traditional* for the bride to wear a white gown.

    (A) normal
    (B) customary
    (C) ordinary
    (D) gracious

14. The company has *rescinded* the order.

    (A) canceled
    (B) revised
    (C) confirmed
    (D) misinterpreted

15. Although the prisoner was released early, he was *vindictive* toward society.

    (A) prejudiced
    (B) impatient
    (C) revengeful
    (D) unreasonable

16. The *sedulous* student worked many hours in the laboratory.

    (A) eager
    (B) persistent
    (C) intelligent
    (D) inexperienced

17. The neighbors were *interrogated* by the police.

    (A) arrested
    (B) detained
    (C) investigated
    (D) questioned

18. The lifeguard *disparaged* his brave rescue of the child.

    (A) explained
    (B) belittled
    (C) demonstrated
    (D) elucidated

19. The water could not *permeate* the rubber apron.

    (A) saturate
    (B) wet
    (C) harm
    (D) discolor

20. The *docile* dog waited at the gate.

    (A) mongrel
    (B) hungry
    (C) intractable
    (D) obedient

21. The two hospitals in our town will *amalgamate* next year.

    (A) close
    (B) expand
    (C) relocate
    (D) merge

22. She wasted her money on *frivolous* things.

    (A) sweet
    (B) expensive
    (C) unimportant
    (D) cheap

23. The teacher *divulged* the test grades.

    (A) whispered
    (B) disregarded
    (C) revealed
    (D) averaged

24. *Remuneration* to the shareholders was 10 percent higher than last year.

    (A) shares
    (B) payment
    (C) liquidation
    (D) speculation

25. The art dealer *scrutinized* the painting to verify its authenticity.

(A) touched
(B) bought
(C) inspected
(D) measured

26. The bridge was closed because it was *decrepit*.

(A) slippery
(B) weak
(C) swaying
(D) flooded

27. The driver *conceded* that he was at fault.

(A) denied
(B) explained
(C) complained
(D) admitted

28. The machinery in the vocational classroom was *obsolete*.

(A) out-of-date
(B) new
(C) reliable
(D) complicated

29. The speaker made *candid* remarks about the candidate's record.

(A) biased
(B) confidential
(C) frank
(D) insulting

30. When the hostage was released, he was speaking *incoherently*.

(A) disconnectedly
(B) cohesively
(C) prolifically
(D) sluggishly

31. The mother tried to *pacify* the child.

(A) detain
(B) restrain
(C) accompany
(D) calm

32. The head nurse on 2 West was young and *vivacious*.

(A) kind
(B) lively
(C) short
(D) talkative

33. The town was *devastated* after the earthquake.

(A) rebuilt
(B) deserted
(C) destroyed
(D) saved

34. The teacher *digressed* from her custom and didn't give any homework.

(A) deviated
(B) reposed
(C) alighted
(D) moored

35.. The Colonel was a *gallant* man.

(A) rude
(B) fastidious
(C) cowardly
(D) chivalrous

36. The family gathering was a *melancholic* scene.

(A) happy
(B) sad
(C) heart-warming
(D) ardent

37. When I visited her in the nursing home, she was *querulous* and unhappy.

(A) satisfied
(B) cheerful
(C) complaining
(D) painful

38. The FBI agent kept a *vigilant* guard on the suspect.

(A) careful
(B) continuous
(C) observant
(D) reciprocal

GO ON TO THE NEXT PAGE

39. The play treated current social issues *satirically*.

(A) frankly
(B) interminably
(C) musically
(D) ironically

40. She felt an *antipathy* for lizards.

(A) aversion
(B) fondness
(C) interest
(D) fear

41. The hiker had a *premonition* of danger.

(A) vision
(B) forewarning
(C) recurrence
(D) apprehension

42. The policeman *confiscated* the illegal drugs.

(A) stored
(B) distributed
(C) destroyed
(D) appropriated

43. John was asked to resign because of his *impropriety*.

(A) age
(B) tardiness
(C) dishonesty
(D) absenteeism

44. There is no *tangible* evidence of damage.

(A) concrete
(B) theoretical
(C) verified
(D) scientific

45. Her *blithe* spirit made her popular.

(A) free
(B) cheerful
(C) kind
(D) insolent

46. The jury *deliberated* for 8 hours.

(A) met
(B) convened
(C) considered
(D) summarized

47. He had a *sinister* motive for entering the building.

(A) practical
(B) wrong
(C) important
(D) honest

48. The requirements for admission to the school were *stringent*.

(A) unusual
(B) numerous
(C) rigid
(D) lax

49. The students refused to give up their *prerogatives*.

(A) demands
(B) rights
(C) ideals
(D) duties

50. The widow and her children were *destitute*.

(A) impoverished
(B) detained
(C) loathed
(D) ill

STOP If you finish before time is called, you may check your work on this section only. Do not turn to any other section in the test.

TEST 4

20 QUESTIONS ▬ TIME—10 MINUTES

Directions: For each question, select the word that corresponds in meaning to the capitalized word. Fill in the corresponding space on your answer sheet.

1. COMPETENT
   - (A) agreeable
   - (B) inept
   - (C) vigorous
   - (D) capable

2. OMNIBUS
   - (A) threatening
   - (B) all-embracing
   - (C) rotund
   - (D) slow-moving

3. INGENUITY
   - (A) deceitfulness
   - (B) appeal
   - (C) cleverness
   - (D) innocence

4. CONCAVE
   - (A) curving inward
   - (B) curving outward
   - (C) oval-shaped
   - (D) rounded

5. CANON
   - (A) barrier
   - (B) noisy place
   - (C) guiding principle
   - (D) vigorous

6. AUSPICIOUS
   - (A) questionable
   - (B) well-known
   - (C) free
   - (D) favorable

7. VACILLATING
   - (A) changeable
   - (B) decisive
   - (C) equalizing
   - (D) progressing

8. FORFEIT
   - (A) exchange
   - (B) relinquish
   - (C) protect
   - (D) withdraw

9. QUERY
   - (A) question
   - (B) look over carefully
   - (C) follow through
   - (D) act peculiarly

10. STEADFAST
    - (A) gradual
    - (B) strong
    - (C) friendly
    - (D) unwavering

11. ACCESS
    - (A) too much
    - (B) extra
    - (C) admittance
    - (D) arrival

12. PERMUTATION
    - (A) alteration
    - (B) permission
    - (C) combination
    - (D) seepage

GO ON TO THE NEXT PAGE

13. SPRITZ

   (A) spray
   (B) bubble
   (C) protrude
   (D) sail

14. PERSONABLE

   (A) intimate
   (B) cheerful
   (C) attractive
   (D) superficial

15. EXPEDITE

   (A) dismiss
   (B) advise
   (C) accelerate
   (D) demolish

16. COMPULSORY

   (A) imperative
   (B) impossible
   (C) imminent
   (D) logical

17. PRACTICABLE

   (A) lenient
   (B) feasible
   (C) simple
   (D) visible

18. AGREE

   (A) inquire
   (B) acquiesce
   (C) discharge
   (D) endeavor

19. FLORID

   (A) overflowing
   (B) ruddy
   (C) seedy
   (D) flowery

20. NEARNESS

   (A) adherence
   (B) declivity
   (C) worldliness
   (D) proximity

STOP   If you finish before time is called, you may check your work on this section only. Do not turn to any other section in the test.

TEST 5: SPELLING USAGE

35 QUESTIONS ▪◻ TIME—20 MINUTES

Directions: Select the letter that belongs in the blank space in the sentence.

1. The demonstrators were _____ from the property.
   - (A) band
   - (B) banned

2. The nurse had to _____ the baby.
   - (A) weigh
   - (B) way

3. She looked on the _____ for the date of the meeting.
   - (A) calendar
   - (B) calender

4. The perfume had a _____ of roses.
   - (A) sent
   - (B) scent

5. The injury caused a _____ on her arm.
   - (A) bruise
   - (B) brews

6. The student received a _____ for passing the test.
   - (A) complement
   - (B) compliment

7. The _____ gave the faculty members their assignments.
   - (A) principal
   - (B) principle

8. The ulcer on the patient's foot did not _____.
   - (A) heel
   - (B) heal

9. A tiny opening in the skin is called a _____.
   - (A) pour
   - (B) pore

10. The _____ after surgery caused the child to cry.
    - (A) pain
    - (B) pane

11. A _____ is a sour berry.
    - (A) current
    - (B) currant

12. It is important to _____ in order to strengthen muscles.
    - (A) exercise
    - (B) exorcise

13. The secretary purchased new _____ on which to type letters.
    - (A) stationery
    - (B) stationary

14. They wanted _____ food right away.
    - (A) there
    - (B) their

15. He was too _____ to climb the stairs.
    - (A) week
    - (B) weak

16. The _____ is a timid animal.
    - (A) dear
    - (B) deer

17. I want to _____ the president.
    - (A) meat
    - (B) meet

18. She wanted a _____ of candy.
    - (A) piece
    - (B) peace

GO ON TO THE NEXT PAGE

19. The child did not _____ the vase.
    (A) brake
    (B) break

20. To _____ means to stop living.
    (A) dye
    (B) die

21. She wanted to purchase two _____ of milk.
    (A) quartz
    (B) quarts

22. He could not _____ his book.
    (A) find
    (B) fined

23. The _____ led to a dead-end street.
    (A) rode
    (B) road

24. The telephone was _____.
    (A) ringing
    (B) wringing

25. The _____ was chocolate cake.
    (A) dessert
    (B) desert

26. The thief was going to _____ the money.
    (A) steel
    (B) steal

27. She placed an _____ in the local newspaper.
    (A) ad
    (B) add

28. He turned _____ because he was so afraid.
    (A) pale
    (B) pail

29. The man wanted the bank to _____ him some money.
    (A) lone
    (B) loan

30. The area around the incision was _____.
    (A) sore
    (B) soar

31. The _____ in the paragraph was not clear.
    (A) clause
    (B) claws

32. The passenger had to pay a _____ to ride the bus.
    (A) fair
    (B) fare

33. When her blood pressure dropped, she started to _____.
    (A) feint
    (B) faint

34. He _____ a loud sound.
    (A) heard
    (B) herd

35. We will go _____ or not it rains.
    (A) weather
    (B) whether

STOP   If you finish before time is called, you may check your work on this section only. Do not turn to any other section in the test.

ANSWER KEY

ANTONYMS

TEST 1

1. **B**	14. **B**	27. **B**	39. **C**
2. **D**	15. **A**	28. **A**	40. **B**
3. **C**	16. **A**	29. **B**	41. **B**
4. **A**	17. **C**	30. **D**	42. **D**
5. **C**	18. **C**	31. **D**	43. **A**
6. **B**	19. **B**	32. **B**	44. **D**
7. **C**	20. **D**	33. **C**	45. **A**
8. **A**	21. **C**	34. **C**	46. **C**
9. **C**	22. **B**	35. **C**	47. **A**
10. **A**	23. **A**	36. **A**	48. **D**
11. **D**	24. **C**	37. **D**	49. **B**
12. **A**	25. **C**	38. **A**	50. **B**
13. **D**	26. **D**		

TEST 2

1. **B**	6. **B**	11. **A**	16. **A**
2. **D**	7. **A**	12. **D**	17. **D**
3. **B**	8. **B**	13. **B**	18. **A**
4. **A**	9. **D**	14. **A**	19. **A**
5. **C**	10. **C**	15. **C**	20. **B**

SYNONYMS

TEST 3

1. C	14. A	27. D	39. D
2. A	15. C	28. A	40. A
3. B	16. B	29. C	41. B
4. D	17. D	30. A	42. D
5. C	18. B	31. D	43. C
6. A	19. A	32. B	44. A
7. D	20. D	33. C	45. B
8. B	21. D	34. A	46. C
9. A	22. C	35. D	47. B
10. C	23. C	36. B	48. C
11. D	24. B	37. C	49. B
12. B	25. C	38. C	50. A
13. B	26. B		

TEST 4

1. D	6. D	11. C	16. A
2. B	7. A	12. A	17. B
3. C	8. B	13. A	18. B
4. A	9. A	14. C	19. B
5. C	10. D	15. C	20. D

TEST 5: SPELLING USAGE

1. B	10. A	19. B	28. A
2. A	11. B	20. B	29. B
3. A	12. A	21. B	30. A
4. B	13. A	22. A	31. A
5. A	14. B	23. B	32. B
6. B	15. B	24. A	33. B
7. A	16. B	25. A	34. A
8. B	17. B	26. B	35. B
9. B	18. A	27. A	

ARITHMETIC AND MATHEMATICS

Arithmetic is an important part of the study of pharmacology and the related sciences. In this section, practice problems on fractions, decimals, ratio, proportion, and percent are included with a review of the appropriate processes. The problem solutions are presented after each set of exercises. If you have made errors, go back to the explanation for that kind of problem. After you have completed all practice tests, take the final test.

REVIEW OF BASIC OPERATIONS

FRACTIONS

Reduction of Fractions

To reduce fractions to lowest terms, divide both the numerator and the denominator by the same number.

Example:

$$\frac{4}{8} = \frac{4 \div 4}{8 \div 4} = \frac{1}{2}$$

Practice Exercise A

Reduce the following fractions to their lowest terms.

1. $\dfrac{8}{16} =$ _____

2. $\dfrac{3}{12} =$ _____

3. $\dfrac{5}{10} =$ _____

4. $\dfrac{25}{100} =$ _____

5. $\dfrac{18}{72} =$ _____

6. $\dfrac{50}{60} =$ _____

7. $\dfrac{27}{54} =$ _____

8. $\dfrac{4}{64} =$ _____

9. $\dfrac{12}{144} =$ _____

10. $\dfrac{25}{150} =$ _____

Improper Fractions

To change an improper fraction to a mixed number, divide the numerator by the denominator and show the remainder, if any, over the denominator. Reduce to the lowest terms.

Example:

$$\frac{21}{7} = 5\overline{)21} \quad \begin{array}{r} 3 \\ \underline{21} \\ 0 \end{array}$$

$$\frac{15}{9} = 1\frac{6}{9} = 1\frac{2}{3}$$

$$9\overline{)15} \quad \begin{array}{r} 1 \\ \underline{9} \\ 6 \end{array}$$

To change a mixed number to an improper fraction, add the numerator of the fraction to the product of the whole number and the denominator of the fraction. Show the total over the denominator of the fraction.

Example:

$$4\frac{3}{8} = \frac{(4 \times 8) + 3}{8} = \frac{32 + 3}{8} = \frac{35}{8}$$

Practice Exercise B
Change the following improper fractions to mixed numbers and vice versa.

1. $\dfrac{15}{4} =$ _____

2. $\dfrac{13}{6} =$ _____

3. $\dfrac{27}{5} =$ _____

4. $\dfrac{17}{3} =$ _____

5. $\dfrac{99}{10} =$ _____

6. $2\dfrac{1}{9} =$ _____

7. $6\dfrac{4}{5} =$ _____

8. $8\dfrac{3}{4} =$ _____

9. $3\dfrac{7}{8} =$ _____

10. $2\dfrac{1}{6} =$ _____

Addition of Fractions
To add two or more fractions, the denominators must be the same. Rewrite each fraction as an equivalent fraction with the Least (smallest) Common Multiple (LCM) as the common denominator. Then add the numerators and reduce the answer to lowest terms.

Example:

Add $\dfrac{2}{3} + \dfrac{3}{4}$

Multiples of 3 = 3, 6, 9, 12, 15, 18, 21, 24, . . .

Multiples of 4 = 4, 8, 12, 16, 20, 24, . . .

Common multiples are 12 and 24

LCM = 12 (the common denominator)

To make an equivalent fraction, divide the common denominator by the original denominator and multiply the original numerator by the result.

$12 \div 3 = 4; 2 \times 4 = 8$

$12 \div 4 = 3; 3 \times 3 = 9$

Add and reduce to lowest terms.

$$\frac{2}{3} + \frac{3}{4} = \frac{8}{12} + \frac{9}{12} = \frac{17}{12} = 1\frac{5}{12}$$

Practice Exercise C

1. $\frac{1}{2}$

    $\frac{1}{3}$

    $\frac{1}{6}$
    _____

2. $\frac{3}{4}$

    $\frac{1}{12}$

    $\frac{2}{3}$
    _____

3. $7\frac{2}{3}$

    $3\frac{5}{24}$

    $5\frac{5}{12}$
    _____

4. $1\frac{1}{4}$

    $5\frac{3}{16}$

    $2\frac{5}{12}$
    _____

5. $26\frac{3}{5}$

    $14\frac{1}{5}$

    $5\frac{7}{8}$
    _____

6. $7\frac{8}{8}$

    $\frac{1}{32}$

    $3\frac{1}{10}$
    _____

7. $4\frac{1}{2}$

    $3\frac{1}{4}$

    $9\frac{3}{8}$
    _____

8. $7\frac{11}{12}$

    $16\frac{3}{4}$

    $2\frac{4}{18}$
    _____

9. $1\frac{3}{24}$

    $8\frac{1}{3}$

    $3\frac{5}{6}$
    _____

10. $5\frac{5}{6}$

    $7\frac{3}{8}$

    $2\frac{3}{10}$
    _____

Subtraction of Fractions

Rewrite each fraction as an equivalent fraction with the LCM as the common denominator, as shown above. If the fraction of the mixed number to be subtracted is larger than the one from which it is to be subtracted, you must borrow 1 from the whole number of the larger mixed number. Add the numerator and denominator of the larger mixed number to make a new numerator. Subtract and reduce to lowest terms.

Example:

$$9\frac{1}{2} = 9\frac{3}{6} = 8\frac{9}{6}$$ Find the common denominator and make equivalent fractions. Borrow from the whole number of the larger mixed number $(9 - 1 = 8)$.

$$1\frac{2}{3} = 1\frac{4}{6} = 1\frac{4}{6}$$ Add the numerator and denominator to make a new numerator $(3 + 6 = 9)$.

$$7\frac{5}{6}$$ Subtract and reduce to lowest terms.

Practice Exercise D

1. $\frac{5}{8}$
    $-\frac{3}{16}$

6. $\frac{17}{20}$
    $-\frac{3}{4}$

2. $7\frac{5}{12}$
    $-3\frac{1}{4}$

7. $5\frac{3}{8}$
    $-1\frac{7}{16}$

3. $\frac{1}{2}$
    $-\frac{1}{8}$

8. $\frac{2}{5}$
    $-\frac{2}{9}$

4. $3\frac{1}{8}$
    $-1\frac{3}{4}$

9. $4\frac{3}{4}$
    $-2\frac{2}{3}$

5. $\frac{7}{9}$
    $-\frac{1}{6}$

10. $11\frac{7}{8}$
    $-1\frac{3}{4}$

Multiplication of Fractions

To multiply fractions, multiply the numerators, then multiply the denominators. You may be able to simplify the fractions before multiplying, which allows you to work with smaller numbers. To simplify, divide the numerator of one fraction and the denominator of another fraction by the same number. Multiply and reduce to lowest terms.

Example:

$$\frac{12}{25} \times \frac{5}{9} = \frac{\overset{4}{\cancel{12}}}{\underset{5}{\cancel{25}}} \times \frac{\overset{1}{\cancel{5}}}{\underset{3}{\cancel{9}}} = \frac{4}{15}$$

To multiply a fraction by a whole number, change the whole number to a fraction by placing the whole number over 1. Multiply, simplify, if possible, and reduce to lowest terms.

Example:

$$4 \times \frac{1}{12} = \frac{4}{1} \times \frac{1}{12} = \frac{\overset{1}{\cancel{4}}}{1} \times \frac{1}{\underset{3}{\cancel{12}}} = \frac{1}{3}$$

To multiply mixed numbers, change the mixed number to an improper fraction. Simplify, if possible, and then multiply as above. Reduce answer to lowest terms.

Example:

$$3\frac{1}{2} \times \frac{6}{21} = \frac{7}{2} \times \frac{6}{21} = \frac{\overset{1}{\cancel{7}}}{\underset{1}{\cancel{2}}} \times \frac{\overset{3}{\cancel{6}}}{\underset{3}{\cancel{21}}} = \frac{3}{3} = 1$$

Practice Exercise E

1. $\frac{2}{3} \times \frac{1}{8} = $ _____

2. $\frac{2}{5} \times \frac{5}{12} = $ _____

3. $\frac{4}{21} \times \frac{7}{8} = $ _____

4. $\frac{15}{16} \times \frac{9}{10} = $ _____

5. $\frac{4}{6} \times \frac{2}{4} = $ _____

6. $3\frac{3}{8} \times \frac{27}{8} = $ _____

7. $\frac{1}{2} \times 8 = $ _____

8. $6\frac{1}{2} \times 5\frac{4}{8} = $ _____

9. $3\frac{2}{3} \times \frac{3}{4} = $ _____

10. $9 \times 3\frac{1}{3} = $ _____

Division of Fractions

To divide fractions, invert the divisor (the second fraction) and change the sign from division ($\div$) to multiplication ($\times$). Then follow the rules for multiplication. Whole numbers are written as fractions with denominator of 1. Mixed numbers are written as improper fractions.

Example:

$$\frac{2}{3} \div \frac{3}{4} = \frac{2}{3} \times \frac{4}{3} = \frac{8}{9}$$

$$5 \div 6\frac{2}{3} = \frac{5}{1} \div \frac{20}{3} = \frac{\overset{1}{\cancel{5}}}{1} \times \frac{3}{\underset{4}{\cancel{20}}} = \frac{3}{4}$$

Practice Exercise F

1. $2\frac{1}{5} \div 11 = $ _____

2. $\frac{1}{50} \div \frac{1}{200} = $ _____

3. $6\frac{3}{5} \div 8\frac{3}{10} = $ _____

4. $\frac{3}{4} \div \frac{1}{8} = $ _____

5. $\frac{5}{12} \div \frac{5}{60} = $ _____

6. $10\frac{1}{2} \div \frac{1}{3} = $ _____

7. $\frac{1}{60} \div \frac{1}{2} = $ _____

8. $8 \div \frac{2}{3} = $ _____

9. $\frac{1}{6} \div \frac{1}{3} = $ _____

10. $\frac{7}{8} \div \frac{3}{4} = $ _____

Decimals, Ratios and Proportions, and Percent Decimals

The decimal system is based on the number 10. All numbers to the right of the decimal point are decimal fractions whose denominator is 10 or a multiple of 10. *Tenths* are directly after the decimal point, *hundredths* two places after, *thousandths* three places after, *ten-thousandths* four places after, etc. Whole numbers are written to the left of the decimal point, and the decimal point is read as "and."

Millions	Hundred-thousands	Ten-thousands	Thousands	Hundreds	Tens	Ones		Tenths	Hundreths	Thousandths	Ten-thousandths	Hundred-thousandths	Millionths

Changing Fractions to Decimals

To change a fraction to a decimal, divide the numerator by the denominator. Write a decimal after the numerator and add as many zeros as needed. The division ends when the remainder is zero.

Example:

$$
\frac{3}{4} = 4\overline{)3.00} \quad
\begin{array}{r}
.75 \\
\hline
28 \\
\hline
20 \\
20 \\
\hline
0
\end{array}
$$

Sometimes the division is not exact and a remainder may repeat itself. Draw a bar over the number in the answer that repeats.

$$
\frac{1}{12} = 12\overline{)1.0000} = .08\overline{3} \quad
\begin{array}{r}
.0833 \\
\hline
96 \\
\hline
40 \\
36 \\
\hline
40 \\
36 \\
\hline
4
\end{array}
$$

Practice Exercise G

Change the following fractions to decimals.

1. $\dfrac{1}{4} =$ _____

2. $\dfrac{7}{8} =$ _____

3. $\dfrac{5}{6} =$ _____

4. $\dfrac{5}{125} =$ _____

5. $\dfrac{5}{16} =$ _____

6. $\dfrac{3}{25} =$ _____

7. $\dfrac{9}{20} =$ _____

8. $\dfrac{1}{75} =$ _____

9. $\dfrac{3}{8} =$ _____

10. $\dfrac{3}{10} =$ _____

Changing Decimals to Fractions

Decimals may be changed to fractions by dropping the decimal point and using the proper denominator. The number of decimal places to the right of the decimal point represents the number of zeros to be used in the denominator preceded by the number 1. Remove the decimal point from the number that you are converting and this becomes the numerator.

Example:

Change 0.025 to a fraction. There are 3 places to the right of the decimal point. Therefore, the denominator is 1 followed by 3 zeros (1,000). Next, remove the decimal point from 0.025; this number (25) becomes the numerator.

$$0.025 = \frac{25}{1000}$$

Practice Exercise H

Change the following decimals to fractions and reduce to lowest terms.

1. 0.16 = _____
2. 0.04 = _____
3. 0.125 = _____
4. 0.06 = _____
5. 0.257 = _____

6. 0.75 = _____
7. 0.250 = _____
8. 0.525 = _____
9. 0.2 = _____
10. 4.75 = _____

Adding Decimals

To add decimals, place the numbers in columns so that the decimal points are directly under one other. Then add in the same manner that you would add columns of whole numbers. Place a decimal point in your answer directly under the others.

Example:

Add 22.05 + 1.375 + 10.2

```
 22.05
  1.375
 10.2
------
 33.625
```

Practice Exercise I

Add the following decimals.

1. 7.2 + 3.57 + 10.8 = _____
2. 48.3 + 18.25 + 4.002 = _____
3. 6.3 + 0.005 + 2.67 = _____
4. 25.4 + 37.06 + 41 = _____
5. 8.50 + 19.625 + 0.17 = _____

6. 29.042 + 2.6 + 3.120 = _____
7. 5.4 + 8.62 + 0.95 = _____
8. 2.246 + 16.8 + 4.26 = _____
9. 16.1 + 1.12 + 3.525 = _____
10. 30.7 + 4.05 + 20.5 = _____

Subtracting Decimals

To subtract decimals, use the same rule as for adding decimals: place decimal points directly under one another. Then subtract in the same manner you would subtract whole numbers, placing the decimal point in your answer directly under the others.

Example:

$$
\begin{array}{r}
50.789 \\
- 24.19 \\
\hline
26.599
\end{array}
$$

Practice Exercise J

Subtract the following decimals.

1. $5.67 - 3.9 =$ _____
2. $37.2 - 25.37 =$ _____
3. $17.4 - 13.262 =$ _____
4. $58.94 - 27.363 =$ _____
5. $2.425 - 0.675 =$ _____

6. $15 - 7.82 =$ _____
7. $205.6 - 105.23 =$ _____
8. $246.52 - 107.988 =$ _____
9. $35.25 - 17.0 =$ _____
10. $1725.5 - 50.6325 =$ _____

Multiplying Decimals

To multiply decimals, multiply the numbers as if they were whole numbers. Then place the decimal point in the answer by counting from the right the number of decimal places in the multiplier and the multiplicand.

Example:

$$
\begin{array}{rl}
2.56 & \text{(2 decimal places)} \\
\times \quad 0.6 & \text{(1 decimal place)} \\
\hline
1.536 & \text{(2 + 1 or 3 decimal places)}
\end{array}
$$

Practice Exercise K

Multiply the following decimals.

1. $5.64 \times 1.2 =$ _____
2. $4.25 \times 12 =$ _____
3. $35.6 \times 2.5 =$ _____
4. $4.92 \times 9.5 =$ _____
5. $51. \times 0.92 =$ _____

6. $28.6 \times 8.16 =$ _____
7. $50.06 \times 2.15 =$ _____
8. $32.2 \times 3.15 =$ _____
9. $21.0 \times 41.6 =$ _____
10. $8.06 \times 3.654 =$ _____

Dividing Decimals

To divide decimals, the divisor must always be a whole number. If the divisor is a decimal, move the decimal to the right as many places as necessary to make the decimal a whole number. Then move the decimal point in the dividend the same number of places to the right to avoid changing the value of the quotient. The decimal point in the quotient is placed directly above the decimal point in the dividend.

Example:

$$
.25\overline{)28} = .25.\overline{)28.00.}
$$

$$
\begin{array}{r}
112 \\
\hline
25 \\
\hline
30 \\
25 \\
\hline
50 \\
50 \\
\hline
0
\end{array}
$$

Practice Exercise L

1. $100 \div 2.5 =$ _____
2. $0.9 \div 0.3 =$ _____
3. $38.6 \div 1.7 =$ _____
4. $115 \div 1.5 =$ _____
5. $5.5 \div 2.5 =$ _____

6. $3.22 \div 0.46 =$ _____
7. $4.65 \div 1.5 =$ _____
8. $15 \div 7.5 =$ _____
9. $0.042 \div 0.3 =$ _____
10. $0.006 \div 0.05 =$ _____

RATIOS AND PROPORTIONS

Ratio

A ratio is the comparison of two numbers by division. A ratio can be written using the symbol (:) or can be written as a fraction. The ratio 1 : 8 shows the relationship between 1 and 8. The ratio 1 : 8 can be written as the fraction $\frac{1}{8}$.

Example:

$$2 : 50 = 1 : 25$$

$$2 : 50 = \frac{2}{50} = \frac{1}{25}$$

$$\therefore 2 : 50 = 1 : 25$$

Practice Exercise M

Write the following fractions as ratios and reduce to lowest terms:

1. $\dfrac{4}{5}$ = _____

2. $\dfrac{1}{3}$ = _____

3. $\dfrac{3}{4}$ = _____

4. $\dfrac{3}{8}$ = _____

5. $\dfrac{1}{10}$ = _____

6. $\dfrac{2}{3}$ = _____

7. $\dfrac{1}{2}$ = _____

8. $\dfrac{25}{50}$ = _____

9. $\dfrac{3}{9}$ = _____

10. $\dfrac{2}{5}$ = _____

Proportion

A proportion states that two ratios are equal. Proportions may be expressed in two ways:

Example:

$$\frac{1}{2} = \frac{50}{100} \text{ or } 1 : 2 :: 50 : 100$$

Both are read: *One is to two as fifty is to one hundred.* The product of the means equals the product of the extremes.

Example:

If one number is not known, substitute an alphabet letter and solve for the unknown number by multiplying the means and the extremes, or multiplying the diagonals.

Example:

$$5 : y = 25 : 125$$
$$\frac{5}{y} = \frac{25}{125}$$

Example:

$$25 \times y = 5 \times 125$$
$$25y = 625$$
$$y = 25$$

Practice Exercise N

Solve for *x* in the following proportions.

1. $8 : 10 = x : 30$ _____

2. $\dfrac{9}{15} = \dfrac{x}{5}$ _____

3. $x : 80 = 3 : 12$ _____

4. $\dfrac{3}{x} = \dfrac{8}{24}$ _____

5. $2 : 3 = x : 63$ _____

6. $5 : 15 = x : 60$ _____

7. $\dfrac{7}{x} = \dfrac{4}{28}$ _____

8. $0.2 : 8 = 25 : x$ _____

9. $\dfrac{5}{7} = \dfrac{x}{28}$ _____

10. $\dfrac{1}{10}x : 2000 = 1 : 100$ _____

PERCENTAGES

To change a decimal to a percent, multiply the decimal by 100 (move the decimal point two places to the right), and then add the percent sign.

Example:

$$0.25 = .25$$

$$= 25\%$$

To find the percent of a number, change the percent to its decimal equivalent, or to a fraction, and multiply.

Example:

Find 7% of 40. (Note: "of" means multiply.)

$$\begin{array}{r} 40 \\ \times\ .07 \\ \hline 2.80 \end{array} \quad \text{or} \quad \frac{7}{\overset{}{\underset{10}{100}}} \times \frac{\overset{4}{\cancel{40}}}{1} = \frac{28}{10} = 2.8$$

To find the percent one number is of another, use the is/of method. The "is" number is the numerator, and the "of" number is the denominator.

Example:

18 is what percent of 24?

$$\frac{18}{24} = \frac{3}{4} \qquad \begin{array}{r} .75 \\ 4\overline{)3.00} = .75\% \\ \underline{28} \\ 20 \\ \underline{20} \\ 0 \end{array}$$

Example:

What percent of 500 is 125?

$$\frac{125}{500} = \frac{1}{4} \qquad 4\overline{)1.00} = .25\%$$

$$\begin{array}{r} .25 \\ 4\overline{)1.00} \\ \underline{8} \\ 20 \\ \underline{20} \\ 0 \end{array}$$

To find the percent of change, subtract to find the amount of change. Then find what percent is of the original amount using the is/of method.

Example:

A sweater is on sale for $42. The original price was $56. What is the percent of change?

$$\begin{array}{r} \$56 \\ -\ 42 \\ \hline \$14 \end{array} \qquad \frac{14}{56} = \frac{1}{4} = 4\overline{)1.00} = 25\%$$

$$\begin{array}{r} .25 \\ 4\overline{)1.00} \\ \underline{8} \\ 20 \\ \underline{20} \\ 0 \end{array}$$

Practice Exercise O

Change the following decimals to percents.

1. 0.225 = _____

2. 3.45 = _____

3. 0.7 = _____

4. 0.14 = _____

5. 4.5 = _____

6. 24 percent of 72 = _____

7. 5 percent of 12 = _____

8. 225 is what percent of 300? _____

9. What percent of 60 is 24? _____

10. What percent of 45 is 135? _____

ROMAN NUMERALS

Roman numerals are written using letters of the alphabet. The letters used to designate arabic numbers are:

Roman	Arabic Equivalent
I	1
V	5
X	10
L	50
C	100
D	500
M	1,000

Rules Governing the Use of Roman Numerals

Addition—placing one or more Roman numerals after the basic numeral adds to its value.

VII = 7

The same numeral cannot be repeated more than three times in succession. If this seems necessary, the rule for subtraction is used.

XXX = 30 XXXX—not allowed XL = 40.

Subtraction—placing one or more Roman numerals in front of the basic numeral removes value from it.

IV = 4

The symbols, V, D, and L are never used in subtraction.

Practice Exercise P

Write the proper Roman numerals:

1. 8 _____
2. 15 _____
3. 50 _____
4. 4 _____
5. 23 _____
6. 44 _____
7. 93 _____
8. 36 _____
9. 56 _____
10. 19 _____

11. 25 _____
12. 100 _____
13. 37 _____
14. 7 _____
15. 18 _____
16. 526 _____
17. 94 _____
18. 39 _____
19. 62 _____
20. 1980 _____

Write the proper Arabic numbers:

1. XXIV _____
2. XVII _____
3. L _____
4. XL _____
5. V _____
6. III _____
7. M _____
8. XIX _____
9. XXX _____
10. XXIX _____

11. VI _____
12. LXX _____
13. C _____
14. XCII _____
15. LXIX _____
16. XVII _____
17. XXII _____
18. XI _____
19. CCIV _____
20. MCXV _____

SOLUTIONS TO PRACTICE EXERCISES

PRACTICE EXERCISE A

1. $\dfrac{8}{16} = \dfrac{1}{2}$

2. $\dfrac{3}{12} = \dfrac{1}{4}$

3. $\dfrac{5}{10} = \dfrac{1}{2}$

4. $\dfrac{25}{100} = \dfrac{1}{4}$

5. $\dfrac{18}{72} = \dfrac{1}{4}$

6. $\dfrac{50}{60} = \dfrac{5}{6}$

7. $\dfrac{27}{54} = \dfrac{1}{2}$

8. $\dfrac{4}{64} = \dfrac{1}{16}$

9. $\dfrac{12}{144} = \dfrac{1}{12}$

10. $\dfrac{25}{150} = \dfrac{1}{6}$

PRACTICE EXERCISE B

1. $\dfrac{15}{4} = 3\dfrac{3}{4}$

2. $\dfrac{13}{6} = 2\dfrac{1}{6}$

3. $\dfrac{27}{5} = 5\dfrac{2}{5}$

4. $\dfrac{17}{3} = 5\dfrac{2}{3}$

5. $\dfrac{99}{10} = 9\dfrac{9}{10}$

6. $2\dfrac{1}{9} = \dfrac{19}{2}$

7. $6\dfrac{4}{5} = \dfrac{34}{5}$

8. $8\dfrac{3}{4} = \dfrac{35}{4}$

9. $3\dfrac{7}{8} = \dfrac{31}{8}$

10. $2\dfrac{1}{6} = \dfrac{13}{6}$

PRACTICE EXERCISE C

1.
$$\frac{1}{2} = \frac{3}{6}$$
$$\frac{1}{3} = \frac{2}{6}$$
$$\frac{1}{6} = \frac{1}{6}$$
$$\overline{}$$
$$\frac{6}{6} = 1$$

2.
$$\frac{3}{4} = \frac{9}{12}$$
$$\frac{1}{12} = \frac{1}{12}$$
$$\frac{2}{3} = \frac{8}{12}$$
$$\overline{}$$
$$\frac{18}{12} = 1\frac{6}{12} = 1\frac{1}{2}$$

3.
$$7\frac{2}{3} = 7\frac{16}{24}$$
$$3\frac{5}{24} = 3\frac{5}{24}$$
$$\frac{5}{12} = \frac{10}{24}$$
$$\overline{}$$
$$10\frac{31}{24} = 11\frac{7}{24}$$

4.
$$1\frac{1}{4} = 1\frac{12}{48}$$
$$5\frac{3}{16} = 5\frac{9}{48}$$
$$2\frac{5}{12} = 2\frac{20}{48}$$
$$\overline{}$$
$$8\frac{41}{48}$$

5.
$$26\frac{3}{5} = 26\frac{24}{40}$$
$$14\frac{1}{5} = 14\frac{8}{40}$$
$$5\frac{7}{8} = 5\frac{35}{40}$$
$$\overline{}$$
$$45\frac{67}{40} = = 46\frac{27}{40}$$

6.
$$7\frac{5}{8} = 7\frac{100}{160}$$
$$\frac{1}{32} = \frac{5}{160}$$
$$3\frac{1}{10} = 3\frac{16}{160}$$
$$\overline{}$$
$$10\frac{121}{160}$$

7.
$$4\frac{1}{2} = 4\frac{4}{8}$$
$$3\frac{1}{4} = 3\frac{2}{8}$$
$$9\frac{3}{8} = 9\frac{3}{8}$$
$$\overline{}$$
$$16\frac{9}{8} = 17\frac{1}{8}$$

8.
$$7\frac{11}{12} = 7\frac{33}{36}$$
$$16\frac{3}{4} = 16\frac{27}{36}$$
$$2\frac{4}{18} = 2\frac{8}{36}$$
$$\overline{}$$
$$25\frac{68}{36} = 26\frac{32}{36} = 26\frac{8}{9}$$

9.
$$1\frac{3}{24} = 1\frac{3}{24}$$
$$8\frac{1}{3} = 8\frac{8}{24}$$
$$3\frac{5}{6} = 3\frac{20}{24}$$
$$\overline{}$$
$$12\frac{31}{24} = 13\frac{7}{24}$$

10.
$$5\frac{5}{6} = 5\frac{100}{120}$$
$$7\frac{3}{8} = 7\frac{45}{120}$$
$$2\frac{3}{10} = 2\frac{36}{120}$$
$$\overline{}$$
$$14\frac{181}{120} = 15\frac{61}{120}$$

Practice Exercise D

1.
$$\frac{5}{8} = \frac{10}{16}$$
$$-\frac{3}{16} = \frac{3}{16}$$
$$\frac{7}{16}$$

2.
$$7\frac{5}{12} = 7\frac{5}{12}$$
$$-3\frac{1}{4} = 3\frac{3}{12}$$
$$4\frac{2}{12} = 4\frac{1}{6}$$

3.
$$\frac{1}{2} = \frac{4}{8}$$
$$-\frac{1}{8} = \frac{1}{8}$$
$$\frac{3}{8}$$

4.
$$3\frac{1}{8} = 3\frac{1}{8} = 2\frac{9}{8}$$
$$-1\frac{3}{4} = 1\frac{6}{8} = 1\frac{6}{8}$$
$$1\frac{3}{8}$$

5.
$$\frac{7}{9} = \frac{14}{18}$$
$$-\frac{1}{6} = \frac{3}{18}$$
$$\frac{11}{18}$$

6.
$$\frac{17}{20} = \frac{17}{20}$$
$$-\frac{3}{4} = \frac{15}{20}$$
$$\frac{2}{20} = \frac{1}{10}$$

7.
$$5\frac{3}{8} = 5\frac{6}{16} = 4\frac{22}{16}$$
$$-1\frac{7}{16} = 1\frac{7}{16} = 1\frac{7}{16}$$
$$3\frac{15}{16}$$

8.
$$\frac{2}{5} = \frac{18}{45}$$
$$-\frac{2}{9} = \frac{10}{45}$$
$$\frac{8}{45}$$

9.
$$4\frac{3}{4} = 4\frac{9}{12}$$
$$-2\frac{2}{3} = 2\frac{8}{12}$$
$$2\frac{1}{12}$$

10.
$$11\frac{7}{8} = 11\frac{7}{8}$$
$$-1\frac{3}{4} = 1\frac{6}{8}$$
$$10\frac{1}{8}$$

Practice Exercise E

1. $\dfrac{2}{3} \times \dfrac{1}{8} = \dfrac{1}{12}$

2. $\dfrac{2}{3} \times \dfrac{5}{12} = \dfrac{1}{6}$

3. $\dfrac{4}{21} \times \dfrac{7}{8} = \dfrac{1}{6}$

4. $\dfrac{15}{16} \times \dfrac{9}{10} = \dfrac{27}{32}$

5. $\dfrac{4}{6} \times \dfrac{2}{4} = \dfrac{1}{3}$

6. $3\dfrac{3}{8} \times \dfrac{27}{8} = \dfrac{27}{8} \times \dfrac{27}{8} = \dfrac{729}{64} = 11\dfrac{25}{64}$

7. $\dfrac{1}{2} \times 8 = \dfrac{1}{2} \times \dfrac{8}{1} = 4$

8. $6\dfrac{1}{2} \times 5\dfrac{4}{8} = \dfrac{13}{2} \times \dfrac{44}{8} = \dfrac{143}{4} = 35\dfrac{3}{4}$

9. $3\dfrac{2}{3} \times \dfrac{3}{4} = \dfrac{11}{3} \times \dfrac{3}{4} = \dfrac{11}{4} = 2\dfrac{3}{4}$

10. $9 \times 3\dfrac{1}{3} = \dfrac{9}{1} \times \dfrac{10}{3} = 30$

Practice Exercise F

1. $2\dfrac{1}{5} \div 11 = \dfrac{11}{5} \div \dfrac{11}{1} = \dfrac{11}{5} \times \dfrac{1}{11} = \dfrac{1}{5}$

2. $\dfrac{1}{50} \div \dfrac{1}{200} = \dfrac{1}{50} \times \dfrac{200}{1} = \dfrac{4}{1} = 4$

3. $6\dfrac{3}{5} \div 8\dfrac{3}{10} = \dfrac{33}{5} \div \dfrac{83}{10} = \dfrac{33}{5} \times \dfrac{10}{83} = \dfrac{66}{83}$

4. $\dfrac{3}{4} \div \dfrac{1}{8} = \dfrac{3}{4} \times \dfrac{8}{1} = \dfrac{6}{1} = 6$

5. $\dfrac{5}{12} \div \dfrac{5}{60} = \dfrac{5}{12} \times \dfrac{60}{5} = \dfrac{5}{1} = 5$

6. $10\dfrac{1}{2} \div \dfrac{1}{3} = \dfrac{21}{2} \times \dfrac{3}{1} = \dfrac{63}{2} = 31\dfrac{1}{2}$

7. $\dfrac{1}{60} \div \dfrac{1}{2} = \dfrac{1}{60} \times \dfrac{2}{1} = \dfrac{1}{30}$

8. $8 \div \dfrac{2}{3} = \dfrac{8}{1} \times \dfrac{3}{2} = \dfrac{12}{1} = 12$

9. $\dfrac{1}{6} \div \dfrac{1}{3} = \dfrac{1}{6} \times \dfrac{3}{1} = \dfrac{1}{2}$

10. $\dfrac{7}{8} \div \dfrac{3}{4} = \dfrac{7}{8} \times \dfrac{4}{3} = \dfrac{7}{6} = 1\dfrac{1}{6}$

Practice Exercise G

1. **The correct answer is 0.25.**

$$\frac{1}{4} = 4\overline{)1.00}^{.25}$$

2. **The correct answer is 0.875.**

$$\frac{7}{8} = 8\overline{)7.000}^{.875}$$
$$\underline{64}$$
$$60$$
$$\underline{56}$$
$$40$$
$$0$$

3. **The correct answer is 0.83.**

$$\frac{5}{6} = 6\overline{)5.00}^{.08\overline{3}}$$
$$\underline{48}$$
$$20$$
$$\underline{18}$$
$$2$$

4. **The correct answer is 0.04.**

$$\frac{5}{125} = 125\overline{)5.00}^{.04}$$
$$\underline{500}$$
$$00$$

5. **The correct answer is 0.3125.**

$$\frac{5}{16} = 16\overline{)5.000}^{.3125}$$
$$\underline{48}$$
$$20$$
$$\underline{16}$$
$$40$$
$$\underline{32}$$
$$80$$
$$\underline{80}$$

6. **The correct answer is 0.12.**

$$\frac{3}{25} = 25\overline{)3.00}^{.12}$$
$$\underline{25}$$
$$50$$
$$\underline{50}$$
$$0$$

7. **The correct answer is 0.45.**

$$\frac{9}{20} = 20\overline{)9.00}^{.45}$$
$$\underline{80}$$
$$100$$
$$\underline{100}$$
$$0$$

8. **The correct answer is 0.013.**

$$\frac{1}{75} = 75\overline{)1.000}^{.01\overline{3}}$$
$$\underline{75}$$
$$250$$
$$\underline{225}$$
$$25$$

9. **The correct answer is 0.375.**

$$\frac{3}{8} = 8\overline{)3.000}^{.375}$$
$$\underline{24}$$
$$60$$
$$\underline{56}$$
$$40$$
$$\underline{40}$$
$$0$$

10. **The correct answer is 0.3.**

$$\frac{3}{10} = 10\overline{)3.00}^{.30}$$
$$\underline{30}$$
$$00$$

PRACTICE EXERCISE H

1. $0.16 = \dfrac{16}{100} = \dfrac{4}{25}$

2. $0.04 = \dfrac{4}{100} = \dfrac{1}{25}$

3. $0.125 = \dfrac{125}{1000} = \dfrac{1}{8}$

4. $0.06 = \dfrac{6}{100} = \dfrac{3}{50}$

5. $0.257 = \dfrac{257}{1000}$

6. $0.75 = \dfrac{75}{100} = \dfrac{3}{4}$

7. $0.250 = \dfrac{250}{1000} = \dfrac{1}{4}$

8. $0.525 = \dfrac{525}{1000} = \dfrac{21}{40}$

9. $0.2 = \dfrac{2}{10} = \dfrac{1}{5}$

10. $4.75 = 4\dfrac{75}{100} = 4\dfrac{3}{4}$

PRACTICE EXERCISE I

1.
```
   7.2
   3.57
+ 10.8
─────
  21.57
```

2.
```
  48.3
  18.25
+  4.002
──────
  70.552
```

3.
```
   6.3
   0.005
+  2.67
─────
   8.975
```

4.
```
  25.4
  37.06
+ 41.0
─────
 103.46
```

5.
```
   8.50
  19.625
+  0.17
─────
  28.295
```

6.
```
  29.042
   2.6
+  3.12
─────
  34.762
```

7.
```
   5.4
   8.62
+  0.95
─────
  14.97
```

8.
```
   2.246
  16.8
+  4.26
─────
  23.306
```

9.
```
  16.1
   1.12
+  3.525
─────
  20.745
```

10.
```
  30.7
   4.05
+ 20.5
─────
  55.25
```

PRACTICE EXERCISE J

1. $\begin{array}{r} 5.67 \\ - 3.90 \\ \hline 1.77 \end{array}$

2. $\begin{array}{r} 37.20 \\ - 25.37 \\ \hline 11.83 \end{array}$

3. $\begin{array}{r} 17.400 \\ - 13.262 \\ \hline 4.138 \end{array}$

4. $\begin{array}{r} 58.940 \\ - 27.363 \\ \hline 31.577 \end{array}$

5. $\begin{array}{r} 2.425 \\ - 0.675 \\ \hline 1.750 \end{array}$

6. $\begin{array}{r} 15.00 \\ - 7.82 \\ \hline 7.18 \end{array}$

7. $\begin{array}{r} 205.60 \\ - 105.23 \\ \hline 100.37 \end{array}$

8. $\begin{array}{r} 246.520 \\ - 107.988 \\ \hline 138.532 \end{array}$

9. $\begin{array}{r} 35.25 \\ - 17.00 \\ \hline 18.25 \end{array}$

10. $\begin{array}{r} 1725.5000 \\ - 50.6325 \\ \hline 1674.8675 \end{array}$

PRACTICE EXERCISE K

1. $\begin{array}{r} 5.64 \\ \times 1.2 \\ \hline 1128 \\ 564 \\ \hline 6.768 \end{array}$

2. $\begin{array}{r} 4.25 \\ \times 12 \\ \hline 850 \\ 425 \\ \hline 51.00 \end{array}$

3. $\begin{array}{r} 35.6 \\ \times 2.5 \\ \hline 1780 \\ 712 \\ \hline 89.00 \end{array}$

4. $\begin{array}{r} 4.92 \\ \times 9.5 \\ \hline 2460 \\ 4428 \\ \hline 46.740 \end{array}$

5. $\begin{array}{r} 51 \\ \times 92 \\ \hline 102 \\ 459 \\ \hline 46.92 \end{array}$

6. $\begin{array}{r} 28.6 \\ \times 8.16 \\ \hline 1716 \\ 286 \\ 2288 \\ \hline 233.376 \end{array}$

7. $\begin{array}{r} 50.06 \\ \times 2.15 \\ \hline 25030 \\ 5006 \\ 10012 \\ \hline 107.6290 \end{array}$

8. $\begin{array}{r} 32.2 \\ \times 3.15 \\ \hline 1610 \\ 322 \\ 966 \\ \hline 101.430 \end{array}$

9.
```
      21.0
    × 41.6
    ──────
      1260
       210
       840
    ──────
    873.60
```

10.
```
       8.06
     × 3.654
     ───────
       3224
       4030
       4839
       2418
     ─────────
     29.45124
```

PRACTICE EXERCISE L

1. The correct answer is 40.

```
         40.
    2.5)100.0
```

2. The correct answer is 3.

```
       3.
    .3).9
```

3. The correct answer is 22.7.

```
        22.7
    1.7)38.6
        34
        ──
         46
         34
         ──
        120
        119
```

4. The correct answer is 76.66.

```
         76.66
    1.5)115.000
        105
        ───
         100
          90
          ──
         100
          90
          ──
          10
```

5. The correct answer is 2.2.

```
         2.2
    2.5)5.50
        50
        ──
         50
         50
         ──
```

6. The correct answer is 7.

```
        7.
    4.6)3.22
        322
        ───
          0
```

7. The correct answer is 3.1.

```
        3.1
    1.5)4.65
        4.5
        ───
         15
         15
         ──
```

8. The correct answer is 2.

```
        2.
    7.5)15.0
        150
        ───
          0
```

9. The correct answer is 0.14.

```
        .14
    .3).042
        3
        ──
        12
        12
        ──
```

10. The correct answer is 0.12.

```
         .12
    .05).0060
         5
         ──
         10
```

PRACTICE EXERCISE M

1. $\frac{4}{5} = 4 : 5$

2. $\frac{1}{3} = 1 : 3$

3. $\frac{3}{4} = 3 : 4$

4. $\frac{3}{8} = 3 : 8$

5. $\frac{1}{10} = 1 : 10$

6. $\frac{2}{3} = 2 : 3$

7. $\frac{1}{2} = 1 : 2$

8. $\frac{25}{50} = 25 : 50 = 1 : 2$

9. $\frac{3}{9} = 3 : 9 = 1 : 3$

10. $\frac{2}{5} = 2 : 5$

PRACTICE EXERCISE N

1. $8 : 10 = x : 30$
$10x = 240$
$x = 24$

2. $9 : 15 = x : 5$
$15x = 45$
$x = 3$

3. $x : 80 = 3 : 12$
$12x = 240$
$x = 20$

4. $8 : x = 8 : 24$
$8x = 72$
$x = 9$

5. $2 : 3 = x : 63$
$3x = 126$
$x = 42$

6. $5 : 15 = x : 60$
$15x = 300$
$x = 20$

7. $7 : x = 4 : 28$
$4x = 196$
$x = 49$

8. $0.2 : 8 = 25 : x$
$0.2x = 200$
$x = 1,000$

9. $5 : 7 = x : 28$
$7x = 140$
$x = 20$

10. $\frac{1}{10}x : 2000 = 1 : 100$
$10x = 2,000$
$x = 200$

Practice Exercise O

1. $0.225 = 22.5\%$

2. $3.45 = 345\%$

3. $0.7 = 70\%$

4. $0.14 = 14\%$

5. $4.5 = 450\%$

6. $\begin{array}{r} 72 \\ \times\ 24 \\ \hline 17.28 \end{array}$

7. $\begin{array}{r} 12 \\ \times\ .05 \\ \hline .60 \end{array}$

8. $\dfrac{\cancel{225}}{\cancel{300}} \genfrac{}{}{0pt}{}{3}{4} = \dfrac{3}{4} = 4\overline{)3.00} = 75\%$

$\begin{array}{r} .75 \\ \underline{20} \\ 20 \\ \underline{20} \\ 0 \end{array}$

9. $\dfrac{24}{60} = \dfrac{2}{4} = 5\overline{)2.0} = 40\%$

$\begin{array}{r} .4 \\ \underline{20} \\ 0 \end{array}$

10. $\dfrac{135}{45} = 3. = 300\%$

Practice Exercise P

Roman Numerals

1. The correct answer is VIII.

2. The correct answer is XV.

3. The correct answer is L.

4. The correct answer is IV.

5. The correct answer is XXIII.

6. The correct answer is XLIV.

7. The correct answer is XCIII.

8. The correct answer is XXXVI.

9. The correct answer is LVI.

10. The correct answer is XIX.

11. The correct answer is XXV.

12. The correct answer is C.

13. The correct answer is XXXVII.

14. The correct answer is VII.

15. The correct answer is XVIII.

16. The correct answer is DXXVI.

17. The correct answer is XCIV.

18. The correct answer is XXXIX.

19. The correct answer is LXII.

20. The correct answer is MCMLXXX.

Arabic Numbers

1. The correct answer is 24.

2. The correct answer is 17.

3. The correct answer is 50.

4. The correct answer is 40.

5. The correct answer is 5.

6. The correct answer is 3.

7. The correct answer is 1,000.

8. The correct answer is 19.

9. The correct answer is 30.

10. The correct answer is 29.

11. The correct answer is 6.

12. The correct answer is 70.

13. The correct answer is 100.

14. The correct answer is 92.

15. The correct answer is 69.

16. The correct answer is 17.

17. The correct answer is 22.

18. The correct answer is 11.

19. The correct answer is 204.

20. The correct answer is 1,115.

ANSWER SHEET

Test 2

1. Ⓐ Ⓑ Ⓒ Ⓓ   5. Ⓐ Ⓑ Ⓒ Ⓓ   9. Ⓐ Ⓑ Ⓒ Ⓓ   13. Ⓐ Ⓑ Ⓒ Ⓓ   17. Ⓐ Ⓑ Ⓒ Ⓓ

2. Ⓐ Ⓑ Ⓒ Ⓓ   6. Ⓐ Ⓑ Ⓒ Ⓓ   10. Ⓐ Ⓑ Ⓒ Ⓓ   14. Ⓐ Ⓑ Ⓒ Ⓓ   18. Ⓐ Ⓑ Ⓒ Ⓓ

3. Ⓐ Ⓑ Ⓒ Ⓓ   7. Ⓐ Ⓑ Ⓒ Ⓓ   11. Ⓐ Ⓑ Ⓒ Ⓓ   15. Ⓐ Ⓑ Ⓒ Ⓓ   19. Ⓐ Ⓑ Ⓒ Ⓓ

4. Ⓐ Ⓑ Ⓒ Ⓓ   8. Ⓐ Ⓑ Ⓒ Ⓓ   12. Ⓐ Ⓑ Ⓒ Ⓓ   16. Ⓐ Ⓑ Ⓒ Ⓓ   20. Ⓐ Ⓑ Ⓒ Ⓓ

Final Arithmetic and Mathematics Test

1. Ⓐ Ⓑ Ⓒ Ⓓ   5. Ⓐ Ⓑ Ⓒ Ⓓ   9. Ⓐ Ⓑ Ⓒ Ⓓ   13. Ⓐ Ⓑ Ⓒ Ⓓ   17. Ⓐ Ⓑ Ⓒ Ⓓ

2. Ⓐ Ⓑ Ⓒ Ⓓ   6. Ⓐ Ⓑ Ⓒ Ⓓ   10. Ⓐ Ⓑ Ⓒ Ⓓ   14. Ⓐ Ⓑ Ⓒ Ⓓ   18. Ⓐ Ⓑ Ⓒ Ⓓ

3. Ⓐ Ⓑ Ⓒ Ⓓ   7. Ⓐ Ⓑ Ⓒ Ⓓ   11. Ⓐ Ⓑ Ⓒ Ⓓ   15. Ⓐ Ⓑ Ⓒ Ⓓ   19. Ⓐ Ⓑ Ⓒ Ⓓ

4. Ⓐ Ⓑ Ⓒ Ⓓ   8. Ⓐ Ⓑ Ⓒ Ⓓ   12. Ⓐ Ⓑ Ⓒ Ⓓ   16. Ⓐ Ⓑ Ⓒ Ⓓ   20. Ⓐ Ⓑ Ⓒ Ⓓ

ARITHMETIC TESTS
TEST 1

30 QUESTIONS ▪▫ TIME—30 MINUTES

Directions: Work out each problem and fill in your answer in the space provided.

Reduce to lowest terms:

1. $\dfrac{3}{6} =$ _____

2. $\dfrac{10}{12} =$ _____

3. $\dfrac{40}{1,000} =$ _____

4. $\dfrac{15}{50} =$ _____

5. $\dfrac{75}{90} =$ _____

Change to improper fractions:

6. $2\dfrac{3}{5} =$ _____

7. $10\dfrac{3}{5} =$ _____

8. $6\dfrac{5}{6} =$ _____

9. $17\dfrac{1}{2} =$ _____

10. $9\dfrac{1}{3} =$ _____

Add:

11. $\begin{array}{r} \dfrac{2}{3} \\[4pt] \dfrac{1}{4} \\[4pt] +\dfrac{5}{6} \\ \hline \end{array}$

12. $\begin{array}{r} \dfrac{5}{9} \\[4pt] \dfrac{3}{8} \\[4pt] +\dfrac{1}{4} \\ \hline \end{array}$

13. $\begin{array}{r} \dfrac{4}{5} \\[4pt] \dfrac{3}{8} \\[4pt] +\dfrac{1}{20} \\ \hline \end{array}$

GO ON TO THE NEXT PAGE

14. $17\frac{2}{3}$

$\frac{8}{9}$

$+\ 2\frac{1}{12}$

_____

15. $1\frac{9}{10}$

$8\frac{4}{5}$

$+\ 9\frac{2}{3}$

_____

Subtract

16. $\frac{7}{8}$

$-\frac{1}{3}$

_____

17. $\frac{11}{18}$

$-\frac{2}{9}$

_____

18. $7\frac{1}{3}$

$-\ 2\frac{3}{4}$

_____

19. $2\frac{5}{6}$

$-\ \frac{8}{9}$

_____

20. $17\frac{1}{3}$

$-\ 8\frac{5}{15}$

_____

Multiply:

21. $\frac{1}{5} \times \frac{25}{50} =$ _____

22. $\frac{1}{3} \times \frac{3}{4} =$ _____

23. $\frac{7}{10} \times \frac{5}{6} =$ _____

24. $15 \times 2\frac{1}{3} =$ _____

25. $\frac{2}{3} \times \frac{9}{16} =$ _____

Divide:

26. $\frac{1}{2} \div \frac{1}{50} =$ _____

27. $\frac{1}{2} \div 6 =$ _____

28. $2\frac{1}{4} \div 3\frac{1}{2} =$ _____

29. $2\frac{4}{5} \div 7 =$ _____

30. $\frac{1}{2} \div \frac{3}{50} =$ _____

S T O P   If you finish before time is called, you may check your work on this section only. Do not turn to any other section in the test.

TEST 2

20 QUESTIONS ▪▫ TIME—20 MINUTES

Directions: Read each question carefully, then decide which choice is the best. Fill in the corresponding space on your answer sheet.

1. $23 + 4.67 + 19.2 + 0.365 =$
    - **(A)** 1047.0
    - **(B)** 47.235
    - **(C)** 1172.4
    - **(D)** 46.235

2. $2.37 \times 0.6 =$
    - **(A)** 14.22
    - **(B)** 1.282
    - **(C)** 1.422
    - **(D)** 12.82

3. The freshman nursing class consists of 40 students. $\frac{7}{8}$ of the class are women. How many women are in the class?
    - **(A)** 35
    - **(B)** 38
    - **(C)** 21
    - **(D)** 24

4. What percentage of 20 is 12?
    - **(A)** 12 percent
    - **(B)** 60 percent
    - **(C)** 14 percent
    - **(D)** 8 percent

5. What is the value of x in the proportion $1 : 5 = x : 1500$?
    - **(A)** 5
    - **(B)** $\frac{1}{3}$
    - **(C)** 750,000
    - **(D)** 300

6. Three percent of the 900 students in a school went on a trip. How many students remained in school?
    - **(A)** 27
    - **(B)** 30
    - **(C)** 873
    - **(D)** 773

7. The fraction $\frac{7}{16}$ expressed as a decimal is
    - **(A)** .1120
    - **(B)** .2286
    - **(C)** .4850
    - **(D)** .4375

8. If 30 is divided by .06, the result is
    - **(A)** 5
    - **(B)** 50
    - **(C)** 500
    - **(D)** 5,000

9. The sum of 637.894, 8352.16, 4.8673, and 301.5 is, most nearly
    - **(A)** 8989.5
    - **(B)** 9021.35
    - **(C)** 9294.9
    - **(D)** 9296.4

10. The sum of $82.79, $103.06, and $697.85 is
    - **(A)** $883.70
    - **(B)** $1,628
    - **(C)** $791
    - **(D)** $873

GO ON TO THE NEXT PAGE

11. One percent of $23,000 is
    (A) $23
    (B) $2.30
    (C) $230
    (D) $2300

12. If $1\frac{1}{2}$ pounds of candy are required to fill an Easter basket, how many baskets can be filled with $10\frac{1}{2}$ pounds of candy?
    (A) 7.5
    (B) 2.5
    (C) $5\frac{1}{2}$
    (D) 7

13. If 1 tee shirt costs $5.60, how many tee shirts can be bought for $61.60?
    (A) $8\frac{1}{2}$
    (B) 10
    (C) 9
    (D) 11

14. The decimal 410.07 less 38.49 equals
    (A) 372.58
    (B) 371.58
    (C) 381.58
    (D) 382.68

15. The fraction $\frac{3}{10}$ written as a decimal is
    (A) 0.3
    (B) 0.03
    (C) 0.003
    (D) 0.0003

16. The decimal 12.5 written as a fraction is
    (A) $\frac{1}{25}$
    (B) $12\frac{1}{2}$
    (C) $1\frac{1}{2}$
    (D) $\frac{125}{100}$

17. The product of 8.3×80 is
    (A) 6.64
    (B) 66.4
    (C) 664
    (D) 6,640

18. The fraction equal to 0.0625 is
    (A) $\frac{1}{16}$
    (B) $\frac{1}{15}$
    (C) $\frac{1}{14}$
    (D) $\frac{1}{13}$

19. The number 0.03125 equals
    (A) $\frac{3}{64}$
    (B) $\frac{1}{16}$
    (C) $\frac{1}{64}$
    (D) $\frac{1}{32}$

20. The quantity 21.70 divided by 1.75 equals
    (A) 124
    (B) 12.4
    (C) 1.24
    (D) .124

STOP   If you finish before time is called, you may check your work on this section only. Do not turn to any other section in the test.

FINAL ARITHMETIC AND MATHEMATICS TEST

20 QUESTIONS ▬▭ TIME—30 MINUTES

Directions: Work out each of the following problems. Fill in the corresponding space on your answer sheet.

1. Add $\frac{1}{4}$, $\frac{3}{8}$, and $\frac{7}{16}$.
    (A) $\frac{11}{16}$
    (B) $1\frac{1}{16}$
    (C) $\frac{11}{28}$
    (D) $\frac{18}{16}$

2. Multiply 25.5 by 0.326.
    (A) 83.13
    (B) 25.826
    (C) 0.2805
    (D) 8.313

3. Subtract 25.246 from 307.401.
    (A) 282.155
    (B) 54.941
    (C) 549.41
    (D) 28.2155

4. 14.75 + 15.1256 + 0.07 =
    (A) 299.46
    (B) 36.8756
    (C) 29.946
    (D) 268.756

5. Divide 36.36 by 0.0606.
    (A) .06
    (B) 0.6
    (C) 60
    (D) 600

6. Write the fraction $\frac{1}{8}$ as a ratio.
    (A) 8 : 1
    (B) 0.18
    (C) 1 : 8
    (D) 0.125

7. Solve for x in $2 : 8 = 11 : x$
    (A) 44
    (B) $2\frac{3}{4}$
    (C) $\frac{11}{16}$
    (D) 4.4

8. Change 85 percent to a fraction and reduce to lowest terms.
    (A) $\frac{85}{100}$
    (B) $\frac{17}{20}$
    (C) $\frac{100}{85}$
    (D) $\frac{20}{17}$

9. Change 0.12 to a percent.
    (A) 0.12 percent
    (B) 0.0012 percent
    (C) .12 percent
    (D) 12 percent

GO ON TO THE NEXT PAGE ▶

10. Subtract $\frac{1}{8}$ from $\frac{1}{6}$.

    (A) $\frac{2}{8}$

    (B) $\frac{3}{24}$

    (C) $\frac{1}{24}$

    (D) $\frac{1}{12}$

11. How many grains of codeine are there in $1\frac{1}{2}$ tablets of $\frac{1}{8}$ grain each?

    (A) $\frac{2}{8}$

    (B) $\frac{3}{16}$

    (C) $\frac{3}{8}$

    (D) $\frac{5}{8}$

12. Mary drank 8 ounces of milk from a quart containing 32 ounces of milk. What part of the quart had she consumed?

    (A) $\frac{1}{4}$

    (B) $\frac{1}{8}$

    (C) $\frac{1}{3}$

    (D) $\frac{1}{2}$

13. There are 75 nursing students in the freshman class, and 15 are men. What is the ratio of women to men?

    (A) $\frac{1}{4}$

    (B) $\frac{1}{5}$

    (C) $\frac{4}{1}$

    (D) $\frac{5}{1}$

14. If a recipe calls for 5 ounces of sugar for every 15 ounces of flour, what part of the mixture will be sugar?

    (A) $\frac{1}{2}$

    (B) $\frac{1}{5}$

    (C) $\frac{1}{3}$

    (D) $\frac{1}{4}$

15. If a suit is on sale for $120, and the original cost was $150, what percentage would you save by buying it on sale?

    (A) 40 percent
    (B) 30 percent
    (C) 10 percent
    (D) 20 percent

16. A seamstress bought $2\frac{2}{3}$ yards of wool material and $1\frac{3}{4}$ yards of crepe material. How many yards of material did she buy?

    (A) $4\frac{5}{12}$

    (B) $4\frac{2}{3}$

    (C) $5\frac{1}{4}$

    (D) $4\frac{1}{3}$

17. A sack contained 10 pounds of potatoes. Mrs. Brown used $1\frac{3}{4}$ pounds for french fries yesterday and $2\frac{1}{3}$ pounds for a casserole today. How many pounds of potatoes does she have left?

(A) $5\frac{1}{2}$

(B) $5\frac{11}{12}$

(C) $6\frac{2}{3}$

(D) $6\frac{11}{12}$

18. How many ounces is $\frac{3}{8}$ of a pound if a pound equals 16 ounces?

(A) 6 ounces

(B) 12 ounces

(C) 8 ounces

(D) 10 ounces

19. If John receives $\frac{2}{5}$ of $10, how much does he receive?

(A) $2

(B) $4

(C) $5

(D) $3

20. If there are 3,000 registered voters in Center City and $\frac{3}{5}$ of them are democrats, how many democrats are there in Center City?

(A) 500

(B) 600

(C) 1,800

(D) 1,500

STOP If you finish before time is called, you may check your work on this section only. Do not turn to any other section in the test.

ANSWER KEY

Test 1

1. $\frac{1}{2}$

2. $\frac{5}{6}$

3. $\frac{1}{25}$

4. $\frac{3}{10}$

5. $\frac{5}{6}$

6. $\frac{13}{5}$

7. $\frac{53}{5}$

8. $\frac{41}{6}$

9. $\frac{35}{2}$

10. $\frac{28}{3}$

11. $1\frac{3}{4}$

12. $1\frac{13}{72}$

13. $1\frac{9}{40}$

14. $20\frac{23}{36}$

15. $20\frac{11}{30}$

16. $\frac{13}{24}$

17. $\frac{7}{18}$

18. $4\frac{7}{12}$

19. $1\frac{17}{18}$

20. 9

21. $\frac{1}{10}$

22. $\frac{1}{4}$

23. $\frac{7}{12}$

24. 35

25. $\frac{3}{8}$

26. 25

27. $\frac{1}{12}$

28. $\frac{9}{14}$

29. $\frac{2}{5}$

30. $8\frac{1}{3}$

Test 2

1. B	5. D	9. D	13. D	17. C
2. C	6. C	10. A	14. B	18. A
3. A	7. D	11. C	15. A	19. D
4. B	8. C	12. D	16. B	20. B

Final Arithmetic and Mathematics Test

1. B	5. D	9. D	13. C	17. B
2. D	6. C	10. C	14. D	18. A
3. A	7. A	11. B	15. D	19. B
4. C	8. B	12. A	16. A	20. C

SOLUTIONS

TEST 1

1. $\dfrac{3}{6} = \dfrac{1}{2}$

2. $\dfrac{10}{12} = \dfrac{5}{6}$

3. $\dfrac{40}{1000} = \dfrac{1}{25}$

4. $\dfrac{15}{50} = \dfrac{3}{10}$

5. $\dfrac{75}{90} = \dfrac{5}{6}$

6. $2\dfrac{3}{5} = \dfrac{13}{5}$

7. $10\dfrac{3}{5} = \dfrac{53}{5}$

8. $6\dfrac{5}{6} = \dfrac{41}{6}$

9. $17\dfrac{1}{2} = \dfrac{35}{2}$

10. $9\dfrac{1}{3} = \dfrac{28}{3}$

11.
$$\dfrac{2}{3} = \dfrac{8}{12}$$
$$\dfrac{1}{4} = \dfrac{3}{12}$$
$$\dfrac{5}{6} = \dfrac{10}{12}$$
$$\rule{3cm}{0.4pt}$$
$$\dfrac{21}{12} = 1\dfrac{9}{12} = 1\dfrac{3}{4}$$

12.
$$\dfrac{5}{9} = \dfrac{40}{72}$$
$$\dfrac{3}{8} = \dfrac{27}{72}$$
$$+\;\dfrac{1}{4} = \dfrac{18}{72}$$
$$\rule{3cm}{0.4pt}$$
$$\dfrac{85}{72} = 1\dfrac{13}{72}$$

13.
$$\dfrac{4}{5} = \dfrac{32}{40}$$
$$\dfrac{3}{8} = \dfrac{15}{40}$$
$$\dfrac{1}{20} = \dfrac{2}{40}$$
$$\rule{3cm}{0.4pt}$$
$$\dfrac{49}{40} = 1\dfrac{9}{40}$$

14.
$$17\dfrac{2}{3} = 17\dfrac{24}{36}$$
$$\dfrac{8}{9} = \dfrac{32}{36}$$
$$2\dfrac{1}{12} = 2\dfrac{3}{36}$$
$$\rule{3cm}{0.4pt}$$
$$19\dfrac{59}{36} = 20\dfrac{23}{36}$$

15.
$$1\dfrac{9}{10} = 1\dfrac{27}{30}$$
$$8\dfrac{4}{5} = 8\dfrac{24}{30}$$
$$9\dfrac{2}{3} = 9\dfrac{20}{30}$$
$$\rule{3cm}{0.4pt}$$
$$18\dfrac{71}{30} = 20\dfrac{11}{30}$$

16.
$$\frac{7}{8} = \frac{21}{24}$$
$$-\frac{1}{3} = \frac{8}{24}$$
$$\frac{13}{24}$$

17.
$$\frac{11}{18} = \frac{11}{18}$$
$$-\frac{2}{9} = \frac{4}{18}$$
$$\frac{7}{18}$$

18.
$$7\frac{1}{3} = 7\frac{4}{12} = 6\frac{16}{12}$$
$$2\frac{3}{4} = 2\frac{9}{12} = 2\frac{9}{12}$$
$$4\frac{7}{12}$$

19.
$$2\frac{5}{6} = 2\frac{15}{18} = 1\frac{33}{18}$$
$$\frac{8}{9} = \frac{16}{18} = \frac{16}{18}$$
$$1\frac{17}{18}$$

20.
$$17\frac{1}{3} = 17\frac{5}{15}$$
$$8\frac{5}{15} = 8\frac{5}{15}$$
$$9$$

21. $\dfrac{1}{5} \times \dfrac{\overset{1}{\cancel{25}}}{\underset{2}{\cancel{50}}} = \dfrac{1}{10}$

22. $\dfrac{1}{\underset{1}{\cancel{3}}} \times \dfrac{\overset{1}{\cancel{3}}}{4} = \dfrac{1}{4}$

23. $\dfrac{7}{\underset{2}{\cancel{10}}} \times \dfrac{\overset{1}{\cancel{5}}}{6} = \dfrac{7}{12}$

24. $15 \times 2\frac{1}{3} = \overset{5}{\cancel{15}} \times \dfrac{7}{\underset{1}{\cancel{3}}} = \dfrac{35}{1}$

25. $\dfrac{\overset{1}{\cancel{2}}}{\underset{1}{\cancel{3}}} \times \dfrac{\overset{3}{\cancel{9}}}{\underset{8}{\cancel{16}}} = \dfrac{3}{8}$

26. $\dfrac{1}{2} \div \dfrac{1}{50} = \dfrac{1}{\underset{1}{\cancel{2}}} \times \dfrac{\overset{25}{\cancel{50}}}{1} = \dfrac{25}{1} = 25$

27. $\dfrac{1}{2} \div 6 = \dfrac{1}{2} \times \dfrac{1}{6} = \dfrac{1}{12}$

28. $2\frac{1}{4} \div 3\frac{1}{2} = \dfrac{9}{4} \div \dfrac{7}{2} = \dfrac{9}{\underset{2}{\cancel{4}}} \times \dfrac{\overset{1}{\cancel{2}}}{7} = \dfrac{9}{14}$

29. $2\frac{4}{5} \div 7 = \dfrac{14}{5} \div \dfrac{7}{1} = \dfrac{\overset{2}{\cancel{14}}}{5} \times \dfrac{1}{\underset{1}{\cancel{7}}} = \dfrac{2}{5}$

30. $\dfrac{1}{2} \div \dfrac{3}{50} = \dfrac{1}{\underset{1}{\cancel{2}}} \times \dfrac{\overset{25}{\cancel{50}}}{3} = \dfrac{25}{3} = 8\frac{1}{3}$

Test 2

1. **The correct answer is (B).**
$$\begin{array}{r} 23.0 \\ 4.67 \\ 19.2 \\ +\ 0.365 \\ \hline 47.235 \end{array}$$

2. **The correct answer is (C).**
$$\begin{array}{r} 2.37 \\ \times\ 0.6 \\ \hline 1.422 \end{array}$$

3. **The correct answer is (A).**
$$\dfrac{7}{\underset{1}{\cancel{8}}} \times \dfrac{\overset{5}{\cancel{40}}}{1} = 35$$

4. **The correct answer is (B).**

$$\frac{12}{20} = \frac{3}{5} = .6 = 60\%$$

$$x = 60\%$$

5. **The correct answer is (D).** $1 : 5 = x : 1{,}500$

$$5x = 1{,}500$$

$$x = 300$$

6. **The correct answer is (C).**

$$\begin{array}{r} 900 \\ \times\ .03 \\ \hline 27.00 \end{array} \qquad \begin{array}{r} 900 \\ -\ 27 \\ \hline 873 \end{array}$$

7. **The correct answer is (D).**

$$\frac{7}{16} = 16\overline{)7.0000}^{.4375}$$

$$\begin{array}{r} \underline{64} \\ 60 \\ \underline{48} \\ 120 \\ \underline{112} \\ 80 \\ \underline{80} \end{array}$$

8. **The correct answer is (C).**

$$.06\overline{)30.00}^{500.}$$

$$\begin{array}{r} \underline{30} \\ 00 \end{array}$$

9. **The correct answer is (D).**

$$\begin{array}{r} 637.8940 \\ 8352.1600 \\ 4.8673 \\ +\ 301.5000 \\ \hline 9296.4213 \end{array}$$

10. **The correct answer is (A).**

$$\begin{array}{r} \$\ 82.79 \\ 103.06 \\ +\ 697.85 \\ \hline \$883.70 \end{array}$$

11. **The correct answer is (C).**

$$\begin{array}{r} \$\ 230.000 \\ \times\ 0.01 \\ \hline \$230.00 \end{array}$$

12. **The correct answer is (D).**

$$\frac{1.5}{1} = \frac{10.5}{x}$$

$$1.5x = 10.5$$

$$x = 7$$

13. **The correct answer is (D).**

$$5.60\overline{)61.60}^{11.}$$

$$\begin{array}{r} \underline{560} \\ 560 \end{array}$$

14. **The correct answer is (B).**

$$\begin{array}{r} 410.07 \\ -\ 38.49 \\ \hline 371.58 \end{array}$$

15. **The correct answer is (A).**

$$\frac{3}{10} = 0.3$$

16. **The correct answer is (B).**

$$12.5 = 12\frac{5}{10} = 12\frac{1}{2}$$

17. **The correct answer is (C).**

$$\begin{array}{r} 8.3 \\ \times\ 80 \\ \hline 00 \\ 664 \\ \hline 664.0 \end{array}$$

18. **The correct answer is (A).**

$$.0625 = \frac{625}{10{,}000} = \frac{1}{16}$$

19. **The correct answer is (D).**

$$0.03125 = \frac{3125}{100{,}000} = \frac{1}{32}$$

20. **The correct answer is (B).**

$$1.75\overline{)21.700}^{12.4}$$

$$\begin{array}{r} \underline{17.5} \\ 4.20 \\ \underline{3.50} \\ 700 \\ \underline{700} \end{array}$$

Final Arithmetic and Mathematics Test

1. **The correct answer is (B).**

$$\frac{1}{4} = \frac{4}{16}$$

$$\frac{3}{8} = \frac{6}{16}$$

$$\frac{7}{16} = \frac{7}{16}$$

$$\frac{17}{16} = 1\frac{1}{16}$$

2. **The correct answer is (D).**

$$\begin{array}{r} 25.5 \\ \times\ .326 \\ \hline 1530 \\ 510 \\ 765 \\ \hline 8.3130 \end{array}$$

3. **The correct answer is (A).**

$$\begin{array}{r} 307.401 \\ -\ 25.246 \\ \hline 282.155 \end{array}$$

4. **The correct answer is (C).**

$$\begin{array}{r} 14.75 \\ 15.1256 \\ 0.07 \\ \hline 29.9456 = 29.946 \end{array}$$

5. **The correct answer is (D).**

$$0.0606\overline{)36.3600}\ \ \begin{array}{c}600.\\ \end{array}$$
$$\begin{array}{r}36.36\\\hline 00\end{array}$$

6. **The correct answer is (C).**

$$\frac{1}{8} = 1 : 8$$

7. **The correct answer is (A).**

$$2 : 8 = 11 : x$$
$$2x = 88$$
$$x = 44$$

8. **The correct answer is (B).**

$$85\% = 0.08 = \frac{85}{100} = \frac{17}{20}$$

9. **The correct answer is (D).**

$$0.12 = 12\%$$

10. **The correct answer is (C).**

$$\frac{1}{6} = \frac{4}{24}$$

$$-\frac{1}{8} = \frac{3}{24}$$

$$\frac{1}{24}$$

11. **The correct answer is (B).**

$$1\frac{1}{2} \times \frac{1}{8} = \frac{3}{2} \times \frac{1}{8} = \frac{3}{16}$$

12. **The correct answer is (A).**

$$\frac{8}{32} = \frac{1}{4}$$

13. **The correct answer is (C).**

$$\frac{60\ \text{women}}{15\ \text{men}} = \frac{4}{1}$$

14. **The correct answer is (D).**

$$\frac{5\ \text{oz. sugar}}{20\ \text{oz. total mixture}} = \frac{1}{4}$$

15. **The correct answer is (D).**

$$\frac{30}{150} = 150\overline{)30.00}\ \begin{array}{c}20\\\end{array} = 20\%$$
$$\begin{array}{r}300\\\hline 00\end{array}$$

16. **The correct answer is (A).**

$$2\frac{2}{3} = 2\frac{8}{12}$$

$$1\frac{3}{4} = 1\frac{9}{12}$$

$$3\frac{17}{12} = 4\frac{5}{12}$$

17. **The correct answer is (B).**

$$1\frac{3}{4} = 1\frac{9}{12}$$
$$+\ 2\frac{1}{3} = 2\frac{4}{12}$$
$$3\frac{13}{12} = 4\frac{1}{12}$$

$$10\text{ lbs}$$
$$-\ 4\frac{1}{12}\text{ lbs}$$
$$5\frac{11}{12}\text{ lbs}$$

18. **The correct answer is (A).**

$$\frac{3}{\cancel{8}}_{1} \times \frac{\cancel{16}^{2}}{1} = 6\text{ ounces}$$

19. **The correct answer is (B).**

$$\frac{2}{\cancel{5}}_{1} \times \frac{\cancel{10}^{2}}{1} = \$4.00$$

20. **The correct answer is (C).**

$$\frac{3}{\cancel{5}}_{1} \times \frac{\cancel{3000}^{600}}{1} = 1{,}800\text{ Democrats}$$

HEALTH AND SCIENCE

The Practical Nurse needs comprehensive knowledge of the basic concepts of the biological and physical sciences in order to understand body structure and functions and to recognize deviations from the norm. In order for the practical nurse to function as a competent health-care provider, basic principles of chemistry, physics, microbiology, and pathology must be included in the nursing curriculum. The questions in this section include facts and principles related to the following:

1. Knowledge of the body structure

2. Understanding of how the body functions

3. Knowledge of principles of nutrition

4. Knowledge of factors affecting health

HEALTH AND SCIENCE GLOSSARY

The purpose of this glossary is to acquaint the reader with some of the common terms that are used in body structure and functions.

A

abductor	A muscle that draws a part of the body away from the median line or normal position.
acetabulum	The socket of the hip bone.
adductor	A muscle that pulls a part of the body toward the median line.
adrenal glands	The two small glands that are on the upper part of the kidneys.
adrenalin	A hormone produced by the adrenal glands; a drug containing this hormone used to raise blood pressure.
alimentary canal	The passageway in the body extending from the mouth to the anus.
alveolus	An air cell of a lung; a tooth socket.
anatomy	The science of the structure of plants and animals.
aorta	The main artery of the body.
artery	A blood vessel carrying blood away from the heart to all parts of the body.
atrium	A chamber of the heart.
atrophy	A wasting away or failure of an organ to grow.
auditory	A term referring to the sense of hearing.
axilla	The armpit.

B

backbone	The column of bones (vertebrae) along the center of the back.
bile	A substance produced by the liver and stored in the gallbladder.
brachial	A term referring to the upper part of the forelimb of the vertebrae.
bronchus	Either of the two main branches or tubes extending from the trachea (windpipe).
bursa	A sac or cavity, especially between joints.

C

cardiac	Of or near the heart.
caudal	Near the tail.
cell	The basic unit of protoplasm.
cephalic	Of the head, skull, or cranium.
clavicle	The collarbone.
clonus	A series of muscle spasms.
colon	The part of the large intestine extending from the cecum to the rectum.
conjunctiva	The mucous membrane lining the inner surface of the eyelids and covering the front part of the eyeball.
cornea	The transparent outer coating of the eyeball.
cranium	The skull, especially that part containing the brain.
cutaneous	Of or on the skin; affecting the skin.

D

dactyl	A finger or toe.
dermis	The layer of skin just below the epidermis.
digit	A finger or toe.
duct	A tube through which secretions or excretions pass through the body.
duodenum	The first section of the small intestine below the stomach.

E

enamel	The hard, white coating of the crowns of teeth.
endothelium	A membrane that lines the heart, blood vessels, and lymphatic vessels.
epidermis	The outermost layer of the skin.
esophagus	The passage for food from the pharynx to the stomach; gullet.
eviscerate	To remove the entrails from; disembowel.

extensor A muscle that straightens some part of the body.

F

fascia A thin layer of connective tissue.

femur The thighbone.

fibrin A protein formed in the clotting of blood.

flexor A muscle that bends a part of the body.

foramen A small opening.

G

ganglion A mass of nerve cells serving as a center from which nerve impulses are transmitted.

gastric In or near the stomach.

genitals The sexual organs.

glottis The opening between the vocal cords in the larynx.

gullet The esophagus.

H

hemoglobin The red coloring matter of the red blood cells.

humerus The bone of the upper arm or forelimb, extending from the shoulder to the elbow.

hyoid A U-shaped bone at the base of the tongue.

hypophysis The pituitary gland.

I

ileum The lowest part of the small intestine.

ilium The uppermost part of the three sections of the hipbone.

insulin A secretion of the pancreas that helps the body use sugar.

intestines The lower part of the alimentary canal, extending from the stomach to the anus.

J

jejunum The middle part of the small intestine.

jugular Two large veins in the neck carrying blood from the head to the heart.

K

kidney Either of a pair of organs that separate water and products from the blood and excrete them as urine through the bladder.

L

lacrimal	Of, for, or producing tears.
larynx	A structure serving as an organ of the voice.
ligament	A band of tough tissue connecting bones or holding organs in place.
lumbar	Pertaining to the small of the back.
lymph	A clear, yellowish fluid found in the lymphatic system of the body.
lymphatic system	A system of vessels and nodes that leads from the tissue spaces to large veins entering the heart.

M

mastication	The act of chewing.
maxilla	The upper jawbone.
membrane	A thin, soft layer of tissue that covers or lines an organ or part.
meninges	The three membranes that enclose the brain and spinal cord.
meningitis	Inflammation of the meninges.
metacarpals	The bones in the hand between the wrist and the fingers.
metatarsals	The bones in the foot between the ankle and toes.
mucous	A membrane lining cavities leading to the outside of the body, such as to the mouth, membrane anus, etc.
mucus	The slimy secretion that moistens and protects the mucous membrane.

N

neural	Pertaining to the nerves or the nervous system.
nutrition	The series or processes by which an organism takes in and assimilates food for promoting growth and repairing tissues.

O

occiput	The back of the skull or head.
ocular	Pertaining to the eye.
olfactory	A term referring to the sense of smell.
ophthalmic	Of or connected with the eyes.
optic nerve	The nerve running from the brain to the eye.
orbit	The eye socket.
osteology	The study of bones.

P

pancreas   The gland that secretes insulin and other digestive juices.

parathyroid   Four small glands embedded in the thyroid gland; their secretions increase the calcium content in the blood.

pathogenic   Disease-producing.

pepsin   An enzyme secreted in the stomach, aiding in the digestion of proteins.

pharynx   The cavity extending from the mouth and nasal passages to the larynx and esophagus; throat.

placenta   The structure through which the fetus is nourished.

protoplasm   The essential living matter of animal and plant cells.

protozoa   A one-celled microscopic animal.

pubis   The bone that makes up the front part of the pelvis.

Q

quadrant   A term referring to four or part of four.

quadruped   A mammal or animal with four feet.

R

radius   The bone of the forearm on the same side as the thumb.

rectum   The lowest segment of the large intestine, ending at the anus.

retina   The innermost coating of the back part of the eyeball.

riboflavin   A factor of the vitamin B complex, found in milk, eggs, liver, fruits, leafy vegetables, etc.

S

scapula   The shoulder blade.

semen   The fluid secreted by the male reproductive organs containing sperm.

sphincter   A round muscle that can open or close a natural opening in the body by expanding and contracting.

sternum   The breastbone.

striated   Streaked with fine lines.

T

tarsals   The bones of the ankle.

tendons   The connective tissue that joins muscles to bones.

thrombin   A substance that aids in the clotting of blood.

thyroid gland   A large ductless gland near the trachea that produces thyroxine, which regulates metabolism.

tibia   The inner bone of the leg below the knee; shinbone.

trachea   The windpipe; the tube that conveys air from the larynx to the bronchi.

U

ulna   The bone of the forearm on the side opposite the thumb.

urea   A soluble, crystalline solid, found in urine.

urine   A yellowish fluid in mammals, containing urea and other waste products.

V

vagina   In female mammals, the canal leading from the vulva to the uterus.

vermiform   A small saclike appendage of the large intestine.

viscera   The internal organs of the body, such as the heart, lungs, stomach, etc.

vomer   A bone forming part of the nasal septum.

Z

zoology   The branch of biology dealing with the classification of animals and the study of animal life.

ANSWER SHEET

TEST 1

1. Ⓐ Ⓑ Ⓒ Ⓓ	9. Ⓐ Ⓑ Ⓒ Ⓓ	17. Ⓐ Ⓑ Ⓒ Ⓓ	25. Ⓐ Ⓑ Ⓒ Ⓓ	33. Ⓐ Ⓑ Ⓒ Ⓓ
2. Ⓐ Ⓑ Ⓒ Ⓓ	10. Ⓐ Ⓑ Ⓒ Ⓓ	18. Ⓐ Ⓑ Ⓒ Ⓓ	26. Ⓐ Ⓑ Ⓒ Ⓓ	34. Ⓐ Ⓑ Ⓒ Ⓓ
3. Ⓐ Ⓑ Ⓒ Ⓓ	11. Ⓐ Ⓑ Ⓒ Ⓓ	19. Ⓐ Ⓑ Ⓒ Ⓓ	27. Ⓐ Ⓑ Ⓒ Ⓓ	35. Ⓐ Ⓑ Ⓒ Ⓓ
4. Ⓐ Ⓑ Ⓒ Ⓓ	12. Ⓐ Ⓑ Ⓒ Ⓓ	20. Ⓐ Ⓑ Ⓒ Ⓓ	28. Ⓐ Ⓑ Ⓒ Ⓓ	36. Ⓐ Ⓑ Ⓒ Ⓓ
5. Ⓐ Ⓑ Ⓒ Ⓓ	13. Ⓐ Ⓑ Ⓒ Ⓓ	21. Ⓐ Ⓑ Ⓒ Ⓓ	29. Ⓐ Ⓑ Ⓒ Ⓓ	37. Ⓐ Ⓑ Ⓒ Ⓓ
6. Ⓐ Ⓑ Ⓒ Ⓓ	14. Ⓐ Ⓑ Ⓒ Ⓓ	22. Ⓐ Ⓑ Ⓒ Ⓓ	30. Ⓐ Ⓑ Ⓒ Ⓓ	38. Ⓐ Ⓑ Ⓒ Ⓓ
7. Ⓐ Ⓑ Ⓒ Ⓓ	15. Ⓐ Ⓑ Ⓒ Ⓓ	23. Ⓐ Ⓑ Ⓒ Ⓓ	31. Ⓐ Ⓑ Ⓒ Ⓓ	39. Ⓐ Ⓑ Ⓒ Ⓓ
8. Ⓐ Ⓑ Ⓒ Ⓓ	16. Ⓐ Ⓑ Ⓒ Ⓓ	24. Ⓐ Ⓑ Ⓒ Ⓓ	32. Ⓐ Ⓑ Ⓒ Ⓓ	40. Ⓐ Ⓑ Ⓒ Ⓓ

TEST 2

1. Ⓐ Ⓑ Ⓒ Ⓓ	7. Ⓐ Ⓑ Ⓒ Ⓓ	13. Ⓐ Ⓑ Ⓒ Ⓓ	19. Ⓐ Ⓑ Ⓒ Ⓓ	25. Ⓐ Ⓑ Ⓒ Ⓓ
2. Ⓐ Ⓑ Ⓒ Ⓓ	8. Ⓐ Ⓑ Ⓒ Ⓓ	14. Ⓐ Ⓑ Ⓒ Ⓓ	20. Ⓐ Ⓑ Ⓒ Ⓓ	26. Ⓐ Ⓑ Ⓒ Ⓓ
3. Ⓐ Ⓑ Ⓒ Ⓓ	9. Ⓐ Ⓑ Ⓒ Ⓓ	15. Ⓐ Ⓑ Ⓒ Ⓓ	21. Ⓐ Ⓑ Ⓒ Ⓓ	27. Ⓐ Ⓑ Ⓒ Ⓓ
4. Ⓐ Ⓑ Ⓒ Ⓓ	10. Ⓐ Ⓑ Ⓒ Ⓓ	16. Ⓐ Ⓑ Ⓒ Ⓓ	22. Ⓐ Ⓑ Ⓒ Ⓓ	28. Ⓐ Ⓑ Ⓒ Ⓓ
5. Ⓐ Ⓑ Ⓒ Ⓓ	11. Ⓐ Ⓑ Ⓒ Ⓓ	17. Ⓐ Ⓑ Ⓒ Ⓓ	23. Ⓐ Ⓑ Ⓒ Ⓓ	29. Ⓐ Ⓑ Ⓒ Ⓓ
6. Ⓐ Ⓑ Ⓒ Ⓓ	12. Ⓐ Ⓑ Ⓒ Ⓓ	18. Ⓐ Ⓑ Ⓒ Ⓓ	24. Ⓐ Ⓑ Ⓒ Ⓓ	30. Ⓐ Ⓑ Ⓒ Ⓓ

TEST 3

1. Ⓐ Ⓑ Ⓒ Ⓓ	7. Ⓐ Ⓑ Ⓒ Ⓓ	13. Ⓐ Ⓑ Ⓒ Ⓓ	19. Ⓐ Ⓑ Ⓒ Ⓓ	25. Ⓐ Ⓑ Ⓒ Ⓓ
2. Ⓐ Ⓑ Ⓒ Ⓓ	8. Ⓐ Ⓑ Ⓒ Ⓓ	14. Ⓐ Ⓑ Ⓒ Ⓓ	20. Ⓐ Ⓑ Ⓒ Ⓓ	26. Ⓐ Ⓑ Ⓒ Ⓓ
3. Ⓐ Ⓑ Ⓒ Ⓓ	9. Ⓐ Ⓑ Ⓒ Ⓓ	15. Ⓐ Ⓑ Ⓒ Ⓓ	21. Ⓐ Ⓑ Ⓒ Ⓓ	27. Ⓐ Ⓑ Ⓒ Ⓓ
4. Ⓐ Ⓑ Ⓒ Ⓓ	10. Ⓐ Ⓑ Ⓒ Ⓓ	16. Ⓐ Ⓑ Ⓒ Ⓓ	22. Ⓐ Ⓑ Ⓒ Ⓓ	28. Ⓐ Ⓑ Ⓒ Ⓓ
5. Ⓐ Ⓑ Ⓒ Ⓓ	11. Ⓐ Ⓑ Ⓒ Ⓓ	17. Ⓐ Ⓑ Ⓒ Ⓓ	23. Ⓐ Ⓑ Ⓒ Ⓓ	29. Ⓐ Ⓑ Ⓒ Ⓓ
6. Ⓐ Ⓑ Ⓒ Ⓓ	12. Ⓐ Ⓑ Ⓒ Ⓓ	18. Ⓐ Ⓑ Ⓒ Ⓓ	24. Ⓐ Ⓑ Ⓒ Ⓓ	30. Ⓐ Ⓑ Ⓒ Ⓓ

TEST 4

1. Ⓐ Ⓑ Ⓒ Ⓓ
2. Ⓐ Ⓑ Ⓒ Ⓓ
3. Ⓐ Ⓑ Ⓒ Ⓓ
4. Ⓐ Ⓑ Ⓒ Ⓓ
5. Ⓐ Ⓑ Ⓒ Ⓓ
6. Ⓐ Ⓑ Ⓒ Ⓓ
7. Ⓐ Ⓑ Ⓒ Ⓓ
8. Ⓐ Ⓑ Ⓒ Ⓓ
9. Ⓐ Ⓑ Ⓒ Ⓓ
10. Ⓐ Ⓑ Ⓒ Ⓓ
11. Ⓐ Ⓑ Ⓒ Ⓓ
12. Ⓐ Ⓑ Ⓒ Ⓓ
13. Ⓐ Ⓑ Ⓒ Ⓓ
14. Ⓐ Ⓑ Ⓒ Ⓓ

15. Ⓐ Ⓑ Ⓒ Ⓓ
16. Ⓐ Ⓑ Ⓒ Ⓓ
17. Ⓐ Ⓑ Ⓒ Ⓓ
18. Ⓐ Ⓑ Ⓒ Ⓓ
19. Ⓐ Ⓑ Ⓒ Ⓓ
20. Ⓐ Ⓑ Ⓒ Ⓓ
21. Ⓐ Ⓑ Ⓒ Ⓓ
22. Ⓐ Ⓑ Ⓒ Ⓓ
23. Ⓐ Ⓑ Ⓒ Ⓓ
24. Ⓐ Ⓑ Ⓒ Ⓓ
25. Ⓐ Ⓑ Ⓒ Ⓓ
26. Ⓐ Ⓑ Ⓒ Ⓓ
27. Ⓐ Ⓑ Ⓒ Ⓓ
28. Ⓐ Ⓑ Ⓒ Ⓓ

29. Ⓐ Ⓑ Ⓒ Ⓓ
30. Ⓐ Ⓑ Ⓒ Ⓓ
31. Ⓐ Ⓑ Ⓒ Ⓓ
32. Ⓐ Ⓑ Ⓒ Ⓓ
33. Ⓐ Ⓑ Ⓒ Ⓓ
34. Ⓐ Ⓑ Ⓒ Ⓓ
35. Ⓐ Ⓑ Ⓒ Ⓓ
36. Ⓐ Ⓑ Ⓒ Ⓓ
37. Ⓐ Ⓑ Ⓒ Ⓓ
38. Ⓐ Ⓑ Ⓒ Ⓓ
39. Ⓐ Ⓑ Ⓒ Ⓓ
40. Ⓐ Ⓑ Ⓒ Ⓓ
41. Ⓐ Ⓑ Ⓒ Ⓓ
42. Ⓐ Ⓑ Ⓒ Ⓓ

43. Ⓐ Ⓑ Ⓒ Ⓓ
44. Ⓐ Ⓑ Ⓒ Ⓓ
45. Ⓐ Ⓑ Ⓒ Ⓓ
46. Ⓐ Ⓑ Ⓒ Ⓓ
47. Ⓐ Ⓑ Ⓒ Ⓓ
48. Ⓐ Ⓑ Ⓒ Ⓓ
49. Ⓐ Ⓑ Ⓒ Ⓓ
50. Ⓐ Ⓑ Ⓒ Ⓓ
51. Ⓐ Ⓑ Ⓒ Ⓓ
52. Ⓐ Ⓑ Ⓒ Ⓓ
53. Ⓐ Ⓑ Ⓒ Ⓓ
54. Ⓐ Ⓑ Ⓒ Ⓓ
55. Ⓐ Ⓑ Ⓒ Ⓓ
56. Ⓐ Ⓑ Ⓒ Ⓓ

57. Ⓐ Ⓑ Ⓒ Ⓓ
58. Ⓐ Ⓑ Ⓒ Ⓓ
59. Ⓐ Ⓑ Ⓒ Ⓓ
60. Ⓐ Ⓑ Ⓒ Ⓓ
61. Ⓐ Ⓑ Ⓒ Ⓓ
62. Ⓐ Ⓑ Ⓒ Ⓓ
63. Ⓐ Ⓑ Ⓒ Ⓓ
64. Ⓐ Ⓑ Ⓒ Ⓓ
65. Ⓐ Ⓑ Ⓒ Ⓓ
66. Ⓐ Ⓑ Ⓒ Ⓓ
67. Ⓐ Ⓑ Ⓒ Ⓓ
68. Ⓐ Ⓑ Ⓒ Ⓓ
69. Ⓐ Ⓑ Ⓒ Ⓓ
70. Ⓐ Ⓑ Ⓒ Ⓓ

TEST 1

40 QUESTIONS ▪ TIME—35 MINUTES

Directions: Each question or incomplete statement below is followed by four suggested answers or completions. For each question, select the best choice and fill in the corresponding space on your answer sheet.

1. Muscles whose functions are to close off body openings are
   - (A) flexors.
   - (B) sphincters.
   - (C) extensors.
   - (D) adductors.

2. Bile aids in the digestion of
   - (A) amino acids.
   - (B) fats.
   - (C) starches.
   - (D) carbohydrates.

3. Urea is removed from the blood as it goes through the
   - (A) bladder.
   - (B) pancreas.
   - (C) spleen.
   - (D) kidney.

4. The blood group of a universal recipient is
   - (A) AB
   - (B) B
   - (C) O
   - (D) A

5. The stimulant in coffee is
   - (A) tannic acid.
   - (B) theobromine.
   - (C) theophylline.
   - (D) caffeine.

6. Which of the following foods is the most economical source of proteins?
   - (A) Dried milk
   - (B) Green leafy vegetables
   - (C) Meats
   - (D) Eggs

7. Connective tissue that attaches muscles to the bones is called
   - (A) tendons.
   - (B) ligaments.
   - (C) cartilage.
   - (D) osseous.

8. The hormone produced by the testes is
   - (A) progesterone.
   - (B) estrogen.
   - (C) testosterone.
   - (D) aldosterone.

9. The elbow joint is an example of
   - (A) ball-and-socket joint.
   - (B) hinge joint.
   - (C) pivot joint.
   - (D) saddle joint.

10. The movement that propels food down the digestive tract is called
    - (A) pyloraspasm.
    - (B) rugae.
    - (C) mastication.
    - (D) peristalsis.

11. In mumps, the gland affected is the
    - (A) parathyroid.
    - (B) pituitary.
    - (C) parotid.
    - (D) pineal.

12. The negative charged particle found within the atom is the
    - (A) proton.
    - (B) electron.
    - (C) nucleus.
    - (D) neutron.

GO ON TO THE NEXT PAGE

13. The exchange of nutrients and waste products occurs in the
    (A) venules.
    (B) capillaries.
    (C) arterioles.
    (D) arteries.

14. Hemoglobin is found in
    (A) basophils.
    (B) neutrophils.
    (C) monocytes.
    (D) erythrocytes.

15. Organic substances made up of several amino acids bound together are
    (A) carbohydrates.
    (B) fats.
    (C) proteins.
    (D) fatty acids.

16. The exchange of carbon dioxide and oxygen in the lungs occurs in the
    (A) venules.
    (B) alveoli.
    (C) bronchi.
    (D) bronchioles.

17. The pacemaker of the heart is the
    (A) Bundle of His.
    (B) AV node.
    (C) purkinje fibers.
    (D) SA node.

18. Mitral stenosis involves the
    (A) aortic valve.
    (B) pulmonary valve.
    (C) bicuspid valve.
    (D) tricuspid valve.

19. The smallest known microorganisms are
    (A) bacteria.
    (B) viruses.
    (C) fungi.
    (D) protozoa.

20. Which one of the following arteries carries deoxygenated blood?
    (A) Pulmonary
    (B) Coronary
    (C) Vena cava
    (D) Aorta

21. Electrolyte balance is maintained primarily by the action of the
    (A) testes.
    (B) kidney.
    (C) bladder.
    (D) liver.

22. The mineral that is necessary for the proper functioning of the thyroid gland is
    (A) sodium.
    (B) iodine.
    (C) calcium.
    (D) iron.

23. Vitamin C prevents
    (A) beriberi.
    (B) rickets.
    (C) pellagra.
    (D) scurvy.

24. The function of leukocytes is to
    (A) carry oxygen.
    (B) destroy bacteria.
    (C) carry food.
    (D) regulate metabolism.

25. Insulin is produced in the
    (A) pituitary gland.
    (B) thymus.
    (C) pancreas.
    (D) pineal gland.

26. The end product of protein metabolism is
    (A) amino acids.
    (B) glucose.
    (C) glycogen.
    (D) fatty acids.

27. Carbohydrates are absorbed into the blood as

   (A) glycogen.
   (B) amino acids.
   (C) glucose.
   (D) fatty acids.

28. When one muscle of a pair contracts, the opposing muscle must

   (A) also contract.
   (B) relax.
   (C) produce more energy.
   (D) remain in the same position.

29. The respiratory center is located in the part of the brain known as the

   (A) thalamus.
   (B) cerebrum.
   (C) pons.
   (D) medulla oblongata.

30. Rays pass through various parts of the eye in a process of bending called

   (A) refraction.
   (B) reflexion.
   (C) retraction.
   (D) retroversion.

31. The part of the eye commonly called the "window" is the

   (A) retina.
   (B) cornea.
   (C) lens.
   (D) pupil.

32. A calorie is a form of

   (A) light.
   (B) heat.
   (C) darkness.
   (D) sound.

33. The vitamin known as the "sunshine" vitamin is

   (A) vitamin E.
   (B) vitamin B.
   (C) vitamin K.
   (D) vitamin D.

34. The process by which the body changes food into substances that can be readily used by the body is

   (A) digestion.
   (B) deglutition.
   (C) micturition.
   (D) absorption.

35. The thyroid gland cannot function properly without

   (A) chloride.
   (B) iodine.
   (C) phosphorous.
   (D) iron.

36. The vitamin that is necessary for coagulation of the blood is

   (A) vitamin K.
   (B) vitamin C.
   (C) vitamin A.
   (D) vitamin E.

37. Another name for vitamin B_1 is

   (A) niacin.
   (B) thiamin.
   (C) riboflavin.
   (D) pyridoxine.

38. Food is moved through the alimentary canal by wave-like motions called

   (A) excretions.
   (B) mastication.
   (C) contractions.
   (D) peristalsis.

39. The femur is a bone located in the

   (A) forearm.
   (B) upper arm.
   (C) thigh.
   (D) lower leg.

40. The liquid portion of the blood is called

   (A) serum.
   (B) gamma globulin.
   (C) plasma.
   (D) lymph.

STOP   If you finish before time is called, you may check your work on this section only. Do not turn to any other section in the test.

TEST 2

30 QUESTIONS ▪▫ TIME—25 MINUTES

Directions: For each question, choose the answer that you consider correct or most nearly correct. Fill in the appropriate space on your answer sheet.

1. The force of the blood exerted against the wall of the blood vessel is called

   (A) pulse deficit.
   (B) apical pulse.
   (C) blood pressure.
   (D) pulse pressure.

2. The relative amount of moisture in the air is the

   (A) evaporation factor.
   (B) temperature.
   (C) dew.
   (D) humidity.

3. A laboratory sample is called a(n)

   (A) collection.
   (B) agar.
   (C) specimen.
   (D) symptom.

4. Defecation means

   (A) swallowing.
   (B) eliminating solid waste.
   (C) irrigating the colon.
   (D) relieving flatus.

5. An object completely free of all microorganisms is

   (A) sterile.
   (B) clean.
   (C) septic.
   (D) contaminated.

6. Carbon dioxide is a

   (A) respiratory depressant.
   (B) circulatory stimulant.
   (C) respiratory stimulant.
   (D) circulatory depressant.

7. The presence of protein in the urine is called

   (A) polyuria.
   (B) anuria.
   (C) albuminuria.
   (D) hematuria.

8. The substance basic to life is

   (A) carbohydrates.
   (B) proteins.
   (C) starches.
   (D) fats.

9. In diseases of the gallbladder, which of the following nutrients is limited?

   (A) Starches
   (B) Proteins
   (C) Fats
   (D) Carbohydrates

10. Water soluble vitamins include

    (A) vitamin A.
    (B) vitamin C.
    (C) vitamin D.
    (D) vitamin K.

11. Diets in the United States are most often deficient in

    (A) iron and calcium.
    (B) calcium and potassium.
    (C) iodine and sodium.
    (D) phosphorous and iron.

12. Tetany may be corrected by increasing the amount of

    (A) iron.
    (B) iodine.
    (C) calcium.
    (D) thiamine.

13. Which helps conserve body heat?

    (A) Increased sweat production
    (B) Increased respiratory activity
    (C) Dilation of the capillaries of the skin
    (D) Constriction of the capillaries of the skin

14. Milk is not a "perfect food" because it lacks

    (A) iron.
    (B) calcium.
    (C) phosphorous.
    (D) carbohydrates.

15. The body obtains most of its nitrogen from

    (A) carbohydrates.
    (B) proteins.
    (C) fats.
    (D) cellulose.

16. An ion is

    (A) one molecule of water.
    (B) one particle of hydrogen.
    (C) the same as a neutron.
    (D) an atom with an electric charge.

17. The basic unit of the living organism is

    (A) the brain.
    (B) the cell.
    (C) a tissue.
    (D) the nervous system.

18. The diffusion of water through a semiperme-able membrane is known as

    (A) anabolism.
    (B) synthesis.
    (C) mitosis.
    (D) osmosis.

19. A physician who specializes in diseases of the heart is known as a

    (A) dermatologist.
    (B) cardiologist.
    (C) pediatrician.
    (D) neurologist.

20. A fracture that occurs without breaking through the skin is called

    (A) complex.
    (B) compound.
    (C) greenstick.
    (D) comminuted.

21. Smoking and pollution, which have a deadly effect upon the lungs and pulmonary function, are classified as

    (A) environmental factors.
    (B) biological factors.
    (C) sociological factors.
    (D) physiological factors.

22. In the digestive process, almost all of the water is reabsorbed by the

    (A) sigmoid.
    (B) cecum.
    (C) colon.
    (D) rectum.

23. In what structure does fertilization normally occur?

    (A) Vagina
    (B) Cervix
    (C) Ovary
    (D) Fallopian tube

24. The process in which carbon dioxide and water is combined under the influence of light in green plants is called

    (A) respiration.
    (B) fermentation.
    (C) assimilation.
    (D) photosynthesis.

25. The most abundant gas in the atmosphere is

    (A) oxygen.
    (B) nitrogen.
    (C) carbon dioxide.
    (D) chlorine.

GO ON TO THE NEXT PAGE

26. A protein substance that initiates and accelerates a chemical reaction is called a(n)

    (A) gene.
    (B) enzyme.
    (C) hormone.
    (D) base.

27. Amino acids that cannot be manufactured by the body are called

    (A) essential amino acids.
    (B) synthetic amino acids.
    (C) basic amino acids.
    (D) dependent amino acids.

28. The instrument used to measure air pressure is called a

    (A) thermometer.
    (B) hydrometer.
    (C) barometer.
    (D) sphygmomanometer.

29. An elevation above normal body temperature is called

    (A) hypothermia.
    (B) pyrexia.
    (C) intermittent.
    (D) remittent.

30. The instrument used to examine the ears is called the

    (A) ophthalmoscope.
    (B) stethoscope.
    (C) cystoscope.
    (D) otoscope.

STOP If you finish before time is called, you may check your work on this section only. Do not turn to any other section in the test.

TEST 3

30 QUESTIONS ■□ TIME—25 MINUTES

Directions: For each question, choose the answer that you consider correct. Fill in the appropriate space on your answer sheet.

1. The body's continual response to changes in the external and internal environment is called

    (A) homeostasis.
    (B) diffusion.
    (C) osmosis.
    (D) filtration.

2. The ability of a cell to reproduce is called

    (A) osmosis.
    (B) crenation.
    (C) lysis.
    (D) mitosis.

3. The immunity that occurs when a person is given a substance containing antibodies or antitoxins is called

    (A) active.
    (B) autoimmune.
    (C) passive.
    (D) permanent.

4. The part of the cell necessary for reproduction is the

    (A) cytoplasm.
    (B) nucleus.
    (C) protoplasm.
    (D) cytoplasmic membrane.

5. The hormone that regulates the metabolic rate of the body cells is

    (A) oxytocin.
    (B) aldosterone.
    (C) thyroxin.
    (D) cortisone.

6. The sudoriferous glands secrete

    (A) sebum.
    (B) perspiration.
    (C) hormones.
    (D) synovial fluid.

7. Tanning of the skin is due to

    (A) keratin.
    (B) sebum.
    (C) sweat.
    (D) melanin.

8. The ovaries produce the hormones

    (A) estrogen and testosterone.
    (B) progesterone and testosterone.
    (C) estrogen and progesterone.
    (D) progesterone and prolactin.

9. The tissue that forms a protective covering for the body and lines the intestinal and respiratory tract is called the

    (A) periosteum.
    (B) pericardium.
    (C) epithelium.
    (D) connective tissue.

10. The hip joint is an example of a

    (A) ball and socket joint.
    (B) hinge joint.
    (C) pivot joint.
    (D) saddle joint.

11. The endocrine gland that prepares the body for the "fight or flight" response is the

    (A) adrenal cortex.
    (B) adrenal medulla.
    (C) pituitary.
    (D) thyroid.

GO ON TO THE NEXT PAGE

12. Tears drain into the nose through the
    (A) ciliary body.
    (B) lacrimal gland.
    (C) eustachian tube.
    (D) nasolacrimal duct.

13. Respiration and heart rate are controlled by the
    (A) cerebellum.
    (B) cerebrum.
    (C) medulla oblongota.
    (D) pons.

14. The main function of the large intestine is to
    (A) absorb digested food.
    (B) absorb water from waste materials.
    (C) produce digestive enzymes.
    (D) secrete digestive enzymes.

15. The hormone produced by the adrenal glands is
    (A) progesterone.
    (B) estrogen.
    (C) testosterone.
    (D) aldosterone.

16. The sloughing off of the endometrium is called
    (A) menarche.
    (B) menopause.
    (C) menstruation.
    (D) myometritis.

17. The dorsal cavity has two subdivisions, namely
    (A) thoracic and abdominopelvic.
    (B) cranial and spinal.
    (C) thoracic and spinal.
    (D) medial and lateral.

18. The chamber of the heart that receives venous blood from body tissue is the
    (A) right atrium.
    (B) left atrium.
    (C) right ventricle.
    (D) left ventricle.

19. The major work of the heart is completed by the
    (A) right ventricle.
    (B) left ventricle.
    (C) right atrium.
    (D) left atrium.

20. The shape of the eyeball is maintained by the
    (A) aqueous humor.
    (B) vitreous humor.
    (C) eye muscles.
    (D) eyelid.

21. The inner lining of the heart is the
    (A) endocardium.
    (B) myocardium.
    (C) pericardium.
    (D) pleura.

22. The muscular structure that forms the floor of the pelvis is the
    (A) peritoneum.
    (B) perineum.
    (C) mons pubis.
    (D) rectus abdominis.

23. The large, round portion at the upper and lateral portion of the femur most often involved in hip fractures is the
    (A) acetabulum.
    (B) acromiom.
    (C) greater trochanter.
    (D) tricuspid valve.

24. One of the large muscles that is used in climbing stairs and that forms most of the buttocks is the
    (A) gluteus maximus.
    (B) gluteus medius.
    (C) vastus lateralis.
    (D) vastus medialis.

25. The basic unit of function of the kidney is the
    (A) medulla.
    (B) hilus.
    (C) nephron.
    (D) cortex.

26. Which of the following is abnormal for urine?
    (A) Clear, amber liquid
    (B) Nitrogenous waste products
    (C) Slightly aromatic
    (D) High specific gravity

27. The hormone that regulates blood composition and blood volume by acting on the kidney is

    (A) antidiuretic (ADH).
    (B) aldosterone.
    (C) parathormone.
    (D) oxytocin.

28. Composition of urine normally includes

    (A) creatinine, urea, and water.
    (B) creatinine, ammonia, and sugar.
    (C) nitrogen wastes, sugar, and hormones.
    (D) nitrogen wastes, water, and pus cells.

29. An injury to the left motor area of the cerebrum would cause paralysis of

    (A) the right side of the body.
    (B) the left side of the body.
    (C) both arms and legs.
    (D) both arms.

30. Electrolyte balance is maintained chiefly by the action of the

    (A) bladder.
    (B) kidney.
    (C) islets of Langerhans.
    (D) gonads.

STOP If you finish before time is called, you may check your work on this section only. Do not turn to any other section in the test.

TEST 4

70 QUESTIONS ■□ TIME—70 MINUTES

Directions: Read each question carefully and consider all possible answers. When you have decided which choice is best, fill in the corresponding space on your answer sheet. There is only one best answer for each question.

1. Diabetes mellitus initially results from
   - (A) oversecretion of pancreatin.
   - (B) undersecretion of insulin.
   - (C) excessive intake of sugar.
   - (D) inadequate intake of fats.

2. The so-called "bag of water," which breaks during labor in the pregnant female, is the
   - (A) amniotic sac.
   - (B) yolk sac.
   - (C) placenta.
   - (D) chorionic membrane.

3. Sebaceous glands are most numerous in areas where
   - (A) there are small amounts of hair.
   - (B) there are large amounts of hair.
   - (C) the skin is thin.
   - (D) sweat glands are located.

4. Hereditary determiners are found in
   - (A) PKU.
   - (B) RNA.
   - (C) DNA.
   - (D) SMA.

5. Skin color varies with the amount of
   - (A) melanin.
   - (B) matrix.
   - (C) hair.
   - (D) keratin.

6. The deciduous teeth contain no
   - (A) cuspids.
   - (B) bicuspids.
   - (C) canines.
   - (D) incisors.

7. The material covering the surface of the tooth below the gum line is
   - (A) cementum.
   - (B) dentine.
   - (C) enamel.
   - (D) pulp.

8. Hemoglobin is a molecule composed principally of
   - (A) ferritin.
   - (B) amino acids.
   - (C) iron.
   - (D) myosin.

9. The sex of the new individual is determined by
   - (A) the female.
   - (B) the male.
   - (C) either the female or the male.
   - (D) neither the female nor the male.

10. The umbilical cord is cut immediately after a baby is born because
    - (A) of the need to stop circulation between the fetus and the placenta.
    - (B) the mother's blood will contaminate the baby's blood.
    - (C) the baby has less need for blood.
    - (D) the mother will hemorrhage.

11. The major difference between plasma and blood is
    - (A) cellular content.
    - (B) acid-base balance.
    - (C) anion-cation placement.
    - (D) solute-solvent concentrations.

12. The blood cells that cause blood clotting are called

    (A) leucocytes.
    (B) erythrocytes.
    (C) thrombocytes.
    (D) lymphocytes.

13. The longest, strongest, and heaviest bone in the body is the

    (A) tibia.
    (B) spinal column.
    (C) femur.
    (D) radius.

14. Iron is needed for

    (A) development of nervous tissue.
    (B) formation of red blood cells.
    (C) growth of hair and nails.
    (D) utilization of vitamins.

15. Which of the following is necessary for digestion?

    (A) Transamination
    (B) Glucogenolysis
    (C) Krebs cycle
    (D) Peristalsis

16. Which of the following organs is vital to life?

    (A) Adrenal glands
    (B) Thymus
    (C) Liver
    (D) Spleen

17. Gram-negative bacterial pathogens are generally more difficult to treat clinically than grampositive due to differences in

    (A) cell wall compositions.
    (B) ribosomes.
    (C) nucleon regions.
    (D) mesosomes.

18. Three-dimensional vision is related to which of the following structures?

    (A) Iris
    (B) Pupil
    (C) Optic chiasma
    (D) Retina

19. Urea formation is the human body's method of eliminating excess

    (A) carbon.
    (B) hydrogen.
    (C) nitrogen.
    (D) phosphorus.

20. Which of the following hormones is predominant in females?

    (A) Androgen
    (B) Testosterone
    (C) Gonadotrophin
    (D) Estrogen

21. Proteins are polymers of

    (A) hydrocarbons.
    (B) amino acids.
    (C) heterocyclics.
    (D) alcohols.

22. Which one of the following statements is true?

    (A) Bone marrow produces red blood cells in the adult.
    (B) The spleen synthesizes vitamins in the child.
    (C) The liver manufactures glucose and stores bile.
    (D) The lymphatic system refines fats and stores water.

23. The most widely distributed of all tissues is

    (A) epithelial.
    (B) muscle.
    (C) connective.
    (D) nervous.

24. The chemical reaction that supplies immediate energy for muscular contractions can be summarized as

    (A) ATP $\rightarrow$ ADP + P.
    (B) lactic acid $\rightarrow$ CO_2 + H_2O.
    (C) lactic acid $\rightarrow$ glycogen.
    (D) glycogen $\rightarrow$ ATP.

GO ON TO THE NEXT PAGE

25. The body's reaction to stress includes which of the following mechanisms?

    (A) Conversion of carbohydrates into glycogen
    (B) Decreased pumping action of the heart
    (C) Secretion of adrenalin
    (D) Pooling of blood in the veins

26. After rigorous exercise, the body is depleted of

    (A) Na and H_2O.
    (B) Glucose and H_2O.
    (C) H_2O and K.
    (D) H_2O and colloids.

27. Which of the following is related to the cause of heart disease?

    (A) Absence of serum transaminase
    (B) Accumulation of urea nitrogen
    (C) Decreased levels of bilirubin
    (D) Increased levels of blood cholesterol

28. The endocrine glands in the body have the function of

    (A) purifying the blood.
    (B) regulating bodily activities.
    (C) controlling the blood distribution.
    (D) preventing antigenic action.

29. Persons with overactive thyroids have which of the following changes in body functions?

    (A) Decrease in metabolic rate
    (B) Increase in metabolic rate
    (C) Loss of appetite
    (D) Gain in weight

30. The basic unit of the lung tissue is

    (A) lacuna.
    (B) nephron.
    (C) alveolus.
    (D) cyton.

31. Hemorrhoids, commonly called piles, affect which of the following structures?

    (A) Pyloric sphincter
    (B) Rectal sphincter
    (C) Urethral orifice
    (D) Mitral orifice

32. Before amino acids can be metabolized to release energy, which of the following must occur?

    (A) Fermentation
    (B) Hydrolysis
    (C) Deamination
    (D) Anabolism

33. A biochemical reaction, common to the digestion of carbohydrates, lipids, and proteins, is enzymatic

    (A) fermentation.
    (B) deamination.
    (C) glycogenolysis.
    (D) hydrolysis.

34. Fats yield more calories per gram and oxidize slower than carbohydrates, proteins, and nucleic acids due to excess atoms of

    (A) hydrogen.
    (B) oxygen.
    (C) nitrogen.
    (D) phosphorus.

35. In the circulatory system, oxygenated blood is pumped out of the heart from the

    (A) right ventricle.
    (B) left ventricle.
    (C) right atrium.
    (D) left atrium.

36. A person who escapes major infections and accidental death has an enhanced probability of living to age 100 if his or her apolipoprotein (E) allelic gene combination is

    (A) E-2/E-4
    (B) E-3/E-4
    (C) E-2/E-2
    (D) E-4/E-4

37. Smooth muscle tissue is found in the

    (A) heart.
    (B) kidneys.
    (C) intestines.
    (D) skeletal muscles.

38. The exchange of gases between the respiratory system and the circulatory system is by means of the pulmonary

    (A) arteries.
    (B) veins.
    (C) capillaries.
    (D) venules.

39. In the production of monoclonal antibodies, antigens, and lymphocytes from an experimental animal are fused with malignant cells to form an internseleate cell known as

    (A) hydroma.
    (B) polycloma.
    (C) hybridoma.
    (D) None of the above

40. In systemic circulation, venous blood is different from arterial blood in that the

    (A) CO_2 concentration is lower than the O_2 concentration.
    (B) CO_2 concentration is higher than the O_2 concentration.
    (C) overall concentration is high and the rate of flow is low.
    (D) overall concentration is low and the rate of flow is high.

41. Sperm and egg cells have the haploid number of chromosomes as a result of

    (A) meiosis.
    (B) cleavage.
    (C) mitosis.
    (D) fertilization.

42. Fraternal twins develop from

    (A) one fertilized egg.
    (B) two fertilized eggs.
    (C) one egg fertilized by two sperms.
    (D) two eggs fertilized by the same sperm.

43. The term *restriction fragment length polymorphism (RFLP)* refers to differences in length between

    (A) chromosome fragments.
    (B) fragments of DNA.
    (C) ribosomal fragments.
    (D) fragments of protein molecules.

44. The "pacemaker" of the heart is located in the

    (A) left atrium.
    (B) left ventricle.
    (C) right atrium.
    (D) right ventricle.

45. Which generalization concerning sex determination is true?

    (A) The female determines the sex of the offspring.
    (B) The XY chromosomes are found in the male.
    (C) The sex of the offspring is first determined during maturation.
    (D) There is a greater chance of getting female offspring than male offspring.

46. A decrease in the number of red corpuscles would result in a corresponding decrease in the blood's ability to

    (A) transport oxygen.
    (B) destroy disease germs.
    (C) form fibrinogen.
    (D) absorb glucose.

47. Heat shock proteins (HSPs) may enable structural and functional proteins, under conditions of elevated temperatures, to

    (A) expand their active sites.
    (B) re-establish their molecular geometry.
    (C) lower their optimal temperature.
    (D) crystallize.

48. In a normal person, the largest part of the central nervous system is the

    (A) cerebrum.
    (B) cerebellum.
    (C) medulla.
    (D) spinal cord.

49. Which one of the following terms is NOT directly associated with the same sense organ as the three others?

    (A) Stapes
    (B) Cochlea
    (C) Tympanic membrane
    (D) Cornea

GO ON TO THE NEXT PAGE

50. Human activity on the earth's biodiversity has caused

    (A) more species to occupy the total available space.
    (B) a decrease in biodiversity.
    (C) no change in overall space-species relationship.
    (D) an increase in biodiversity.

51. If the order of strength of the following bases is: $HCO_3 > C_2H_3O_2 > HSO_4 > Cl$, the weakest acid is

    (A) HCl ($H^+ + Cl^-$)
    (B) $HC_2H_3O_2$ ($H^+ + C_2H_3O_2^-$)
    (C) H_2SO_4 ($H^+ + HSO_4$)
    (D) H_2CO_3 ($H^+ + HCO_3^-$)

52. In a chemical reaction, [A] and [B] combine to form [C] and [D], as expressed by the reaction [A][B] = [C][D]. Select the statement that best describes the equilibrium condition.

    (A) Reaction is shifted to the right.
    (B) Concentrations of reactants and products are constant.
    (C) Reaction is shifted to the left.
    (D) Concentration of products is greater than the concentration reactants.

53. Down syndrome is a genetic disorder caused by

    (A) an extra copy of chromosome 21.
    (B) a defective gene on chromosome 21.
    (C) fragmentation of one copy of chromosome 23.
    (D) a missing copy of chromosome 23.

54. In cellular metabolism, glycolysis

    (A) requires O_2.
    (B) does not require O_2.
    (C) occurs only in animal cells.
    (D) produces $CO_2 + H_2O$.

55. If 5×10^5 lbs of NaCl were dumped into a 0.5 acre pond, what would happen to the water concentration inside the frog's body cells?

    (A) It would not change.
    (B) It would increase.
    (C) It would decrease.
    (D) It would approach boiling.

56. An astronaut, without a pressurized suit and with a blood pressure of 120/70, is accidentally sucked out of a spacecraft, halfway between the earth and the moon. He or she would

    (A) experience a collapse of blood vessels.
    (B) rapidly develop cancer.
    (C) experience an expansion of blood vessels.
    (D) experience no adverse medical effect.

57. Which of the following viruses have been associated with cancer in animals?

    (A) Adenovirus
    (B) Retrovirus
    (C) Papovavirus
    (D) All of the above

58. The major contributions of whole wheat or enriched bread or cereal to the diet are

    (A) carbohydrate and vitamin B complex.
    (B) protein and iron.
    (C) calcium and riboflavin.
    (D) protein and vitamin B complex.

59. A good label for canned goods always includes

    (A) picture of product to give idea of color, size, and appearance.
    (B) net contents, number of portions, and quality of product.
    (C) brief but specific instructions or directions for use.
    (D) brand name.

60. Caloric needs are highest during

    (A) infancy.
    (B) childhood.
    (C) adulthood.
    (D) middle age.

61. Isolated genes shown to initiate malignancies are known as

(A) carcinogens.

(B) oncogenes.

(C) prions.

(D) None of the above

62. One of the most contentious current problems relative to science ethics involves

(A) organ transplants.

(B) blood transfusion.

(C) human embryonic stem cell research.

(D) hospitalization time.

63. In the life cycle of the AIDS-causing virus (HIV), the pathogens bind to lymphocyte membrane receptors by their surface

(A) glycoproteins.

(B) capsids.

(C) reverse transcriptase molecules.

(D) prions.

64. After an AIDS virus enters a lymphocyte, it synthesizes viral DNA from a template composed of

(A) double-stranded DNA.

(B) double-stranded RNA.

(C) single-stranded DNA.

(D) single-stranded RNA.

65. In patients with cystic fibrosis, the accumulation of mucus around the membranes of cells in the lungs, liver, and pancreas has been shown to be caused by the blockage of ionic channels for

(A) CA^{++}

(B) Cl^-

(C) K^+

(D) Na^+

66. Choose the correct statement, relative to the distribution of sodium (Na^+) and potassium (K^+), on opposites of cell membranes.

(A) High Na^+ outside

(B) High K^+ outside

(C) Low Na^+ outside

(D) Low K^+ inside

67. Which of the following are requirements for cloning a gene?

(A) An enzyme to fragment DNA

(B) A vector (a bacterial plasmid or a virus)

(C) A host cell or organism

(D) All of the above

68. Small circular self-duplicating DNA molecule s found in bacterial cells are

(A) microbodies.

(B) oligaproteins.

(C) plasmids.

(D) None of the above

69. Enzymes necessary for fragmenting genes to be cloned are

(A) restriction enzymes.

(B) splicing enzymes.

(C) recombinases.

(D) polymerases.

70. In the formation of recombinant DNA, the DNA from two different sources is spliced by an enzyme

(A) polymerase.

(B) DNA ligase.

(C) recombinant dehydrogenase.

(D) None of the above

STOP   If you finish before time is called, you may check your work on this section only. Do not turn to any other section in the test.

ANSWER KEY

TEST 1

1. B	11. C	21. B	31. B
2. B	12. B	22. B	32. B
3. D	13. B	23. D	33. D
4. A	14. D	24. B	34. A
5. A	15. C	25. B	35. B
6. A	16. B	26. B	36. A
7. A	17. D	27. C	37. B
8. C	18. C	28. B	38. D
9. B	19. B	29. D	39. C
10. D	20. A	30. A	40. C

TEST 2

1. C	9. C	17. B	24. D
2. D	10. B	18. D	25. B
3. C	11. A	19. B	26. B
4. B	12. C	20. C	27. A
5. A	13. D	21. A	28. C
6. C	14. A	22. C	29. B
7. C	15. B	23. D	30. D
8. B	16. D		

TEST 3

1. A	9. C	17. B	24. A
2. D	10. A	18. A	25. C
3. C	11. B	19. B	26. D
4. B	12. D	20. B	27. B
5. C	13. C	21. A	28. A
6. B	14. B	22. B	29. A
7. D	15. D	23. C	30. B
8. C	16. C		

TEST 4

1. B	19. C	37. C	54. B
2. A	20. D	38. C	55. C
3. B	21. B	39. C	56. C
4. C	22. A	40. B	57. D
5. A	23. C	41. A	58. A
6. B	24. A	42. B	59. B
7. A	25. C	43. B	60. A
8. B	26. A	44. C	61. B
9. B	27. D	45. B	62. C
10. A	28. B	46. A	63. A
11. A	29. B	47. B	64. D
12. C	30. C	48. A	65. B
13. C	31. B	49. D	66. A
14. B	32. C	50. B	67. D
15. D	33. D	51. D	68. C
16. C	34. A	52. B	69. A
17. A	35. B	53. A	70. B
18. C	36. C		

EXPLANATORY ANSWERS

TEST 1

1. **The correct answer is (B).** Sphincters are circular muscles that contract when stimulated, closing and opening.

2. **The correct answer is (B).** Bile is released into the duodenum and breaks down the undigested fats into small droplets.

3. **The correct answer is (D).** Urea is filtered from the blood by the kidneys and excreted in urine.

4. **The correct answer is (A).** Group AB blood contains both group A and B antigens and neither A nor B antibodies; therefore, it cannot clump any donor red cells containing A and B antigens.

5. **The correct answer is (D).** Caffeine is a stimulant found in coffee.

6. **The correct answer is (A).** Dried milk is an inexpensive but valuable source of protein.

7. **The correct answer is (A).** Tendons, connective tissue made of dense fibers in the shape of a cord, have great strength.

8. **The correct answer is (C).** Testosterone is the hormone that regulates male sex characteristics.

9. **The correct answer is (B).** Hinge joints allow movement in only two directions.

10. **The correct answer is (D).** Peristalsis is the progressive, wavelike movement that occurs involuntarily to force food forward.

11. **The correct answer is (C).** The parotid gland is a large salivary gland that is affected by mumps.

12. **The correct answer is (B).** The electron is the unit of negative electricity.

13. **The correct answer is (B).** Capillaries connect arterioles with venules and function as exchange vessels.

14. **The correct answer is (D).** Erythrocytes (red blood cells) contain hemoglobin.

15. **The correct answer is (C).** Proteins are nutrients essential for growth and repair of tissue.

16. **The correct answer is (B).** The diffusion of gas occurs across the thin, squamous epithelium lining of the alveoli.

17. **The correct answer is (D).** The SA node, located in the right atrium, starts each heart beat.

18. **The correct answer is (C).** The mitral valve, located between the left atrium and left ventricle of the heart, is also called the bicuspid valve.

19. **The correct answer is (B).** Viruses are so small that they can be seen only through special electron microscopes.

20. **The correct answer is (A).** The pulmonary artery carries deoxygenated blood from the heart.

21. **The correct answer is (B).** When water intake is excessive, the kidneys excrete generous amounts of urine; if water intake is lost, they produce less urine. The process is regulated by hormones.

22. **The correct answer is (B).** Iodine makes up about 65 percent of thyroxine, a hormone secreted by the thyroid gland.

23. **The correct answer is (D).** Scurvy is a disease caused by a deficiency of vitamin C.

24. **The correct answer is (B).** Leukocytes (white blood cells) destroy bacteria when there is an infection in the body.

25. **The correct answer is (C).** The islets of Langerhans are located in the pancreas and produce insulin.

26. **The correct answer is (A).** Gastric and intestinal enzymes gradually break down the protein molecule into its separate amino acids.

27. **The correct answer is (C).** Glucose is the end product of carbohydrate digestion.

28. **The correct answer is (B).** When one muscle contracts, the opposing muscle must relax; in this way, movements are coordinated and normal functions are carried out.

29. **The correct answer is (D).** The medulla oblongata is located between the pons and the spinal cord, and the vital centers are located in it.

30. **The correct answer is (A).** Rays pass through a series of transparent, colorless eye parts. On the way, they undergo a process of bending called refraction, which makes it possible for light from a large area to focus on the retina.

31. **The correct answer is (B).** The cornea is referred to frequently as the "window" of the eye.

32. **The correct answer is (B).** A calorie is the unit of measure of heat—the amount of heat required to raise the temperature of 1 kilogram of water by 1°C.

33. **The correct answer is (D).** Vitamin D is referred to as the "sunshine" vitamin because it is formed in the body by the action of the sunshine on the cholesterol products in the skin.

34. **The correct answer is (A).** Digestion is the process whereby the enzymes in the body change food into simple substances that can be readily used by the body.

35. **The correct answer is (B).** The thyroid gland needs iodine for the formation of thyroxine.

36. **The correct answer is (A).** Vitamin K helps the liver to produce substances necessary for the clotting of blood.

37. **The correct answer is (B).** Thiamine is another name for vitamin B_1.

38. **The correct answer is (D).** Peristalsis is a wave-like progression of muscular contractions that moves food through the alimentary canal.

39. **The correct answer is (C).** The thigh bone is the femur. It is the longest and strongest bone in the body.

40. **The correct answer is (C).** Plasma is the liquid portion of the blood in which corpuscles are suspended.

TEST 2

1. **The correct answer is (C).** Blood pressure is the force of the blood exerted against the wall of the blood vessel.

2. **The correct answer is (D).** Relative humidity refers to the amount of moisture in the air in relation to the temperature.

3. **The correct answer is (C).** Specimen is a laboratory sample used to help the physician make a diagnosis.

4. **The correct answer is (B).** Defecation means the act of having a bowel movement or removing solid waste materials from the body.

5. **The correct answer is (A).** Sterile means that an object is completely free of all microorganisms. Steam under pressure (autoclave) will give complete sterilization.

6. **The correct answer is (C).** Carbon dioxide stimulates the respiratory center in the brain (medulla oblongata).

7. **The correct answer is (C).** Protein substance in the urine is called albuminuria. It results from the failure of the kidneys to filter.

8. **The correct answer is (B).** Protein, the body's vital building material, makes up the basic structure of all cells.

9. **The correct answer is (C).** The gallbladder stores and concentrates bile, which is used to break down fats into droplets and aids in the absorption of fatty acids and glyceral. Therefore, fats are restricted when there are diseases of the gallbladder.

10. **The correct answer is (B).** Water-soluble vitamins include vitamin C and vitamin B complex.

11. **The correct answer is (A).** Iron and calcium are the minerals most often deficient in the American diet.

12. **The correct answer is (C).** Tetany, which is due to lack of calcium, may be corrected by increasing milk or milk products, which are rich in calcium salts. Drugs containing high amounts of calcium may be given intravenously in emergencies.

13. **The correct answer is (D).** Constriction of the blood vessels prevents loss of heat from the blood through the skin.

14. **The correct answer is (A).** Milk contains only about 0.1 milligram of iron per cup. The recommended daily amount is 15–18 milligrams.

15. **The correct answer is (B).** Food proteins supply our bodies with nitrogen to replace that lost in urine, feces, and perspiration.

16. **The correct answer is (D).** The electrical charge results when a neutral atom or group of atoms loses or gains one or more electrons during chemical reactions.

17. **The correct answer is (B).** The cell is the unit of structure and function of all living things. The simplest organisms consist of only one cell.

18. **The correct answer is (D).** Osmosis is the diffusion of water through a semipermeable membrane from a region of greater concentration to a region of lesser concentration.

19. **The correct answer is (B).** *Cardiologist* comes from the word *cardiology*, meaning the study of the heart's physiology and pathology.

20. **The correct answer is (C).** Greenstick fractures are incomplete fractures with a longitudinal split of the shaft. They usually occur in long bones of children.

21. **The correct answer is (A).** Environmental factors are the relationships of living things to their surroundings.

22. **The correct answer is (C).** The fluid-like residue of digestion found in the colon contains valuable water, which is absorbed into the blood stream.

23. **The correct answer is (D).** After ovulation, the egg travels into the fallopian tube. If sperms are present, the union of the sperm and the egg (fertilization) takes place in the fallopian tube.

24. **The correct answer is (D).** Photosynthesis is the process by which certain living plant cells combine carbon dioxide and water, in the presence of chlorophyll and light energy, to form carbohydrates and release oxygen as a waste product.

25. **The correct answer is (B).** The atmosphere is composed of about 78 percent nitrogen.

26. **The correct answer is (B).** Enzymes are protein substances that act as biochemical catalysts. They affect the rate at which a specific reaction occurs.

27. **The correct answer is (A).** Essential amino acids are those that cannot be manufactured by the body and, therefore, must be included in the daily diet.

28. **The correct answer is (C).** The barometer is an instrument used to measure air pressure and to forecast weather.

29. **The correct answer is (B).** An elevation of body temperature above normal is referred to as fever or pyrexia.

30. **The correct answer is (D).** The otoscope is a lighted instrument used to examine the ear canal, eustachian tube, eardrum, and the middle ear.

TEST 3

1. **The correct answer is (A).** The body is constantly stabilizing and equalizing its environment to prevent any sudden or severe changes.

2. **The correct answer is (D).** The DNA molecules in the nucleus of a cell duplicate themselves and the cell divides, forming two cells.

3. **The correct answer is (C).** In acquiring passive immunity, the body of the recipient plays an active part in response to an antigen.

4. **The correct answer is (B).** The functional unit is suspended near the center of the cell and has the property of division.

5. **The correct answer is (C).** Produced by the thyroid gland, thyroxin controls the rate at which glucose is burned and converts it to heat and energy.

6. **The correct answer is (B).** Sweat glands are distributed in the skin and produce perspiration, primarily water.

7. **The correct answer is (D).** Melanin, a brown pigment, increases when exposed to sun.

8. **The correct answer is (C).** Estrogen and progesterone promote development of female sex characteristics and regulate menstruation.

9. **The correct answer is (C).** Epithelial tissue has many forms—flat and irregular, square, long and narrow—that are arranged in single or multiple layers to form a protective covering and lining.

10. **The correct answer is (A).** The ball-shaped head of the femur fits into the concave socket of the hipbone and allows for a wide range of motion.

11. **The correct answer is (B).** Adrenaline is released from the adrenal medulla to prepare the body for emergency situations.

12. **The correct answer is (D).** A small opening into the nose at the inner corner of the eye allows the fluid to drain through.

13. **The correct answer is (C).** Many gray-matter areas that form the cranial nerves are located in the medulla oblongota and are involved in the control of vital activities.

14. **The correct answer is (B).** As peristalsis moves content along, water is absorbed through the walls into the circulation, and the remaining cellulose passes on to the rectum.

15. **The correct answer is (D).** Aldosterone is the hormone released from the adrenal cortex that helps regulate sodium and potassium balance.

16. **The correct answer is (C).** The shedding of the lining of the uterus occurs if the egg has not been fertilized by the sperm.

17. **The correct answer is (B).** Dorsal pertains to the back; the cranial and spinal cavities contain the brain and the spinal cord.

18. **The correct answer is (A).** Deoxygenated blood returns from the body tissues via the superior and inferior vena cava into the right atrium.

19. **The correct answer is (B).** The left ventricle has the major responsibility for pumping blood into the aorta to be dispersed throughout the body.

20. **The correct answer is (B).** The jellylike substance prevents the eyeball from collapsing inward.

21. **The correct answer is (A).** The endocardium is a smooth lining, which helps blood flow smoothly through the heart.

22. **The correct answer is (B).** The perineum, which forms the pelvic floor, is the external region between the vulva and anus in the female or between the scrotum and anus in the male.

23. **The correct answer is (C).** The greater trochanter is the ball-like head that articulates with the hipbone.

24. **The correct answer is (A).** The gluteus maximus is part of the hips and buttocks.

25. **The correct answer is (C).** Nephrons are responsible for the processes of filtration, absorption, and secretion.

26. **The correct answer is (D).** Normal urine has a low specific gravity.

27. **The correct answer is (B).** Aldosterone is released by the adrenal cortex in response to decreased blood volume, decreased blood sodium ions, or increased potassium ions.

28. **The correct answer is (A).** Water plus creatinine and urea, which are nitrogenous wastes, are normal substances in urine.

29. **The correct answer is (A).** The left motor control center in the brain controls the right side of the body because of the crossing of the nerve tracts within the brain.

30. **The correct answer is (B).** When the water intake is excessive, the kidneys excrete generous amounts of urine; if the water intake is lost, they produce less urine. The process is regulated by hormones.

TEST 4

1. **The correct answer is (B).** Insulin increases the permeability of the cell membrane to glucose, thus enhancing the uptake of glucose from the blood by the cells. If insulin is deficient, glucose is not removed from the blood and utilized by the cells, resulting in an excess of glucose in the blood and leading to other symptoms of diabetes.

2. **The correct answer is (A).** The amnion is one of the extraembryonic structures formed during embryonic development. It surrounds the embryo and becomes filled with fluid in which the embryo floats. The amniotic fluid probably provides protection from mechanical shock for the embryo.

3. **The correct answer is (B).** Sebaceous glands are associated with hair follicles: the cells lining the glands form the secretion, and the entire cellular lining, plus the fatty secretion, form sebum, which is expelled into the hair follicle. Sebum serves to keep the hair and skin pliable.

4. **The correct answer is (C).** DNA (deoxyribonucleic acid) is found in the nucleus of each cell and "stores" genetic information, or the genetic code. DNA replicates itself before mitosis or meiosis begins, and genetic information is distributed equally to the daughter nuclei. RNA (ribonucleic acid), transcribed on DNA, translates the genetic or hereditary information.

5. **The correct answer is (A).** Melanin is a dark pigment found in the cells of the basal layers of the skin. Skin color varies with the size and density of the melanin particles: the more melanin present, the darker the skin.

6. **The correct answer is (B).** Each person has a set of 20 deciduous teeth, as contrasted to 32 permanent or nondeciduous teeth. The set of deciduous teeth contains no bicuspids, and only two molars per quadrant rather than three. A set per quadrant of deciduous teeth includes two incisors, one canine, and two molars; a set per quadrant of nondeciduous teeth includes two incisors, one canine, two premolars (bicuspids), and three molars.

7. **The correct answer is (A).** Cementum covers the surface of roots of teeth; enamel covers the surface of the crowns of teeth.

8. **The correct answer is (B).** The bulk of a hemoglobin molecule consists of 4 subunits, each one of which is a chain of amino acids. Iron is also present in hemoglobin but does not comprise as large a part of the entire molecule as the 4 chains of amino acids. Ferritin is an iron-containing molecule stored in the liver. Myosin is a major component of muscle cells.

9. **The correct answer is (B).** The XY chromosomes are found in the male, while the female carries XX. As a result of meiosis, a sperm will carry either an X or Y chromosome; all eggs will carry one X. Fertilization of an X-bearing egg by a Y-bearing sperm produces an XY zygote, which develops into a male. Fertilization of an X-bearing egg by an X-bearing sperm produces an XX zygote, which develops into a female.

10. **The correct answer is (A).** The fetus and the mother have independent circulatory systems. Fetal blood passing to and from the placenta by way of the umbilical blood vessels is separated from the mother's blood in the placenta by thin tissues; food, gases, and metabolic wastes can diffuse through these tissues between the two bloodstreams. After birth, the placenta's function has ended, and as the baby's systems become "active," there is no longer an exchange of materials between the two bloodstreams.

11. **The correct answer is (A).** *Plasma* is the liquid portion of the blood. *Whole blood* consists of plasma with its dissolved materials and the blood cells.

12. **The correct answer is (C).** Thrombocytes disintegrate when blood flows from a blood vessel, releasing a phospholipid, thrombokinase, that acts to convert prothrombin in the plasma to thrombin. Thrombin acts enzymatically on fibrinogen in the plasma, converting it to fibrin, which is insoluble and forms a mesh, trapping blood cells. This mesh is the blood clot.

13. **The correct answer is (C).** The femur is the thigh bone of the leg. It is the longest, strongest, and heaviest bone of the body.

14. **The correct answer is (B).** Iron is a part of the hemoglobin molecule, the red, oxygen-carrying pigment of red blood cells. If iron is deficient, hemoglobin cannot be produced, and the formation of red blood cells is inhibited..

15. **The correct answer is (D).** *Peristalsis* is the wave of muscular contractions that pushes food through the esophagus into the stomach and through the intestine. Food must reach the digestive sites, the stomach and small intestine, for digestion to occur. The other possible answer choices are involved in metabolic processes, not in digestion.

16. **The correct answer is (C).** The liver is the largest glandular organ of vertebrates and has the important function of regulating organic materials such as wastes, glucose, and proteins in the blood. It can also perform other essential functions, such as fat digestion and storage functions, immune responses, protein metabolism, and detoxifying blood by converting toxic substances into harmless wastes. It is essential for life.

17. **The correct answer is (A).** The cell walls of gram-negative bacteria are more complex than gram-positives—with less peptidoglycan and more lipopolysaccharides—which renders them more difficult for drugs to cross.

18. **The correct answer is (C).** Nerve fibers from the retina of the eye form the optic nerve of the eye; at the crossover point (*optic chiasma*), fibers from the nasal halves (inner halves) of each retina cross to the opposite side of the brain, while fibers of the temporal halves (outer halves) of each retina remain uncrossed. Thus, each optic nerve, after the chiasma, contains fibers from both retinas. This means that objects in one field of vision (either left or right) produce effects in two eyes that are transmitted to one side of the brain. In other words, the two halves of the retina of each eye are represented on opposite sides of the brain, producing a stereoscopic effect and permitting perception of depth.

19. **The correct answer is (C).** Many aquatic animals excrete ammonia as their nitrogenous waste, egg-laying animals excrete uric acid, and intra-uterine animals excrete urea.

20. **The correct answer is (D).** *Estrogen* is a complex of female sex hormones responsible for the appearance of secondary sex characteristics, such as widening of the pelvis, breasts, etc. Estrogen also functions in the menstrual cycle, preparing the uterus for implantation of the embryo.

21. **The correct answer is (B).** A *polymer* is a large, chain-like organic molecule formed by bonding together many smaller organic molecules of the same kind. A protein is a chain of many amino acid molecules joined to one another by peptide bonds. The amino acid molecules present, and the sequence in which they are joined, are considered the *primary structure* of the protein and determine its physical or chemical properties.

22. **The correct answer is (A).** Red blood cells are produced in the bone marrow in the adult. The other statements are incorrect as follows: vitamins typically are consumed with food (two possible exceptions); glucose is a product of digestion, and bile is stored in the gallbladder; water is a part of almost all tissues; and fats are refined by the bile from the liver.

23. **The correct answer is (C).** *Connective tissues* are those whose cells are not contiguous but scattered throughout a noncellular matrix. Connective tissues can bind and support other tissues; therefore, they are widely distributed. Some examples of connective tissues are blood, bone, cartilage, adipose, and tissues composing tendons or ligaments.

24. **The correct answer is (A).** The limited amount of ATP stored in muscle tissue supplies immediate energy for contraction when the ATP is converted to ADP. When the ATP is used up, it is recreated by energy from a reserve, creatine phosphate. When the creatine phosphate is consumed, oxidation of glucose to CO_2 and water provides energy for muscle contraction and for the resynthesis of creatine phosphate. Lactic acid can form anaerobically during severe muscle exertion, and its accumulation is partly responsible for the feeling of fatigue. Lactic acid diffuses out of the muscle tissue into the bloodstream and thus to the liver, where some of it is oxidized to produce further energy, and some can be converted to glycogen for carbohydrate storage.

25. **The correct answer is (C).** Adrenalin, or epinephrine, secreted by the adrenal medulla, is normally released in small quantities and helps to regulate blood circulation and carbohydrate metabolism. Under stressful conditions, the adrenal medulla is stimulated to release larger amounts of adrenalin, which increases blood pressure, heart rate, carbohydrate metabolism, and conversion of glycogen to sugar, thus raising the blood sugar level, etc. This prepares the body to cope with the stressful situation—hence, the "flight or fight" response.

26. **The correct answer is (A).** Exercise will cause perspiration, which evaporates from the skin. *Perspiration* is a liquid composed of water, salt, and a small amount of urea and is drawn from the bloodstream (from capillaries in the sweat glands) and released to the body surface through pores. Thus, rigorous exercise will cause the body to lose sodium (salt) and water.

27. **The correct answer is (D).** Cholesterol is a lipid that is insoluble in fluids such as blood; therefore, it is bound to proteinaceous carriers for transport. Evidence indicates that cholesterol is involved in the fatty deposits in arteries, even infiltrating cells and the intercellular spaces of arterial walls, if carried by certain carriers. This can lead to plaque and clot formation, blocking off the arteries and interfering with blood circulation. This same plaque and clot formation can occur in the coronary artery supplying heart muscle, causing a heart attack.

28. **The correct answer is (B).** The endocrine glands secrete hormones directly into the bloodstream. The hormones are transported throughout the body, but only specific "target" cells or tissues can pick up a specific hormone. Thus, the hormone may regulate cellular activities in tissues some distance from the cells that secreted it. By regulating cellular activities of tissues, hormones regulate bodily activities.

29. **The correct answer is (B).** The thyroid hormone controls the rate of cellular metabolism for the release of energy. An overactive gland secretes an excess of hormone, which will increase the metabolic rate. A deficiency of thyroid hormone causes the rate of metabolism to be lowered.

30. **The correct answer is (C).** The *alveolus* is a small, thin-walled sac of the lung; it is the blind end of the smallest bronchioles. Each alveolus (approximately 300 million are present in human lungs) is surrounded by, or adjacent to, small capillaries. It is here that gaseous exchange between the blood and lungs occur. Carbon dioxide passes into the alveolus from the blood, and oxygen passes from the alveolus into the bloodstream through the capillary walls.

31. **The correct answer is (B).** A *hemorrhoid* is a dilation of veins in the anal region. This can lead to a enlargement of tissue, especially the rectal sphincter, which is a ring-shaped muscle controlling the anal opening.

32. **The correct answer is (C).** The amino nitrogen must be removed from amino acids in order to give them the basic hydrocarbon skeleton similar to carbohydrates. After the amino group is removed, the resulting compounds may enter the same metabolic pathways used by carbohydrates.

33. **The correct answer is (D).** The chemistry of life is closely dependent upon the chemistry of water. Water, in the presence of the proper enzymes, must be added to the bonds that bind monosaccharides in carbohydrates, amino acids in proteins, and fatty acids and glycerol in fats to degrade these polymers to their subunits.

34. **The correct answer is (A).** Energy production, in the degradation of foods, is associated with the release of hydrogen (oxidation). The ratio of hydrogen to oxygen is significantly greater in fats than in carbohydrates and proteins.

35. **The correct answer is (B).** Oxygenated blood passes from the lungs to the left atrium of the heart by way of the pulmonary veins. From the left atrium, blood moves to the left ventricle, from which it is pumped through the aorta to the arterial system of the body, and thus throughout the body, where oxygen is diffused into the cells and carbon dioxide is picked up by the blood. The carbon dioxide–laden blood is returned to the heart, entering the right atrium, and passing to the right ventricle. From the right ventricle, it is pumped to the lungs through the pulmonary arteries, where it becomes oxygenated again.

36. **The correct answer is (C).** Studies conducted by Dr. Allan Roses and D. Warren Stuttmatter at the Duke University Medical Center and reported in the Wall Street Journal (October 19, 1995) indicated that the apoliprotein (E) gene occurs as E-2, E-3, and E-4 subtypes. The potential of gene E for promoting cell maintenance and protection against Alzheimer's, heart disease, and diabetes is in order of potency of E-2 > E-3 > E-4. Therefore, E-2 is the good gene and E-4 is the bad form.

37. **The correct answer is (C).** The three basic kinds of muscle tissue are *smooth*, *skeletal*, and *cardiac*. Smooth muscle is characteristic of the digestive tract and arteries, organs not under voluntary control. Cardiac muscle is found in the heart. Skeletal muscle (striated) makes up the muscles associated with voluntary movement. The kidney is nonmuscular.

38. **The correct answer is (C).** Gaseous exchange between the respiratory system and the circulatory system occurs by means of the capillaries present in the lungs surrounding alveoli. These are referred to as the *pulmonary capillaries*.

39. **The correct answer is (C).** Thy hybridoma, formed by fusing lymphocytes with cancer cells, produces a single type of antibody. The hybridoma can be injected into a mouse or cultured, in vitro, to increase production of the single antibody type.

40. **The correct answer is (B).** Blood in systemic veins is returning to the right atrium of the heart from the cells of the body. Therefore, it is high in concentrations of carbon dioxide and metabolic wastes that were received from the cells as a result of cellular metabolism. Venous blood of the pulmonary system is returning to the left atrium of the heart from the lungs, where it gave up carbon dioxide to be expelled from the body and acquired oxygen. Therefore, it has a higher concentration of oxygen.

41. **The correct answer is (A).** The first division of *meiosis* results in a reduction of the number of chromosomes, because the members of each pair of chromosomes are separated from one another. Each daughter nucleus resulting from meiosis receives only one chromosome of each pair present in the parent nucleus, or one half the number of chromosomes of the parent nucleus. Nuclei resulting from meiosis are *haploid*, as contrasted to the *diploid* condition of the parent nucleus.

42. **The correct answer is (B).** *Fraternal*, or nonidentical, twins result from two fertilized eggs, or *zygotes*. If two eggs are released during ovulation and both are fertilized (one sperm per egg), fraternal twins result. These twins are like ordinary siblings, whereas identical twins resulting from a single *zygote* are genetically identical.

43. **The correct answer is (B).** *Restriction fragment length polymorphisms* are differences in the lengths of fragments of DNA produced by exposing DNA from genetically different individuals to a bacterial restriction enzyme that cuts DNA at specific points.

44. **The correct answer is (C).** Specialized muscle cells, known as the "pacemaker" of the heart, make up a region of the right atrium. When these cells are excited, the atria are stimulated to contract, emptying the blood into the ventricles. Certain muscle fibers then carry the excitation stimulus, by way of the atrio-ventricular node, to muscles of the ventricles, stimulating them to contract and force blood from the heart.

45. **The correct answer is (B).** The XY chromosomes are found in the male, while the female carries XX. As a result of meiosis, a sperm will carry either an X or a Y chromosome; all eggs will carry an X. Fertilization of an X-bearing egg by a Y-bearing sperm produces an XY zygote, which develops into a male. Fertilization of an X-bearing egg by an X-bearing sperm produces an XX zygote, which develops into a female.

46. **The correct answer is (A).** Red blood cells contain the pigment hemoglobin, which has as its function the transport of oxygen. If the number of red blood cells is decreased, the ability of the blood to transport oxygen is decreased.

47. **The correct answer is (B).** Temperatures greater than 40°C will denature (destroy) the molecular geometry of most proteins. In many plant and animal cells, special proteins (heat shock proteins) are synthesized to prevent denaturation at these temperatures.

48. **The correct answer is (A).** The cerebrum is the largest division of the central nervous system of humans. It originates thinking and controls learning, memory, thought, some voluntary movements, and the senses. In the animal kingdom, observations indicate that intelligence increases with cerebrum size. Humans have the largest cerebrum, in proportion to body size, in the animal kingdom.

49. **The correct answer is (D).** The stapes, cochlea, and tympanic membrane are all parts of the ear: The *stapes* is one of the vibrating bones of the middle ear, the *cochlea* is the receptor portion of the inner ear from which electrical impulses ("messages") are transmitted to the brain through the auditory nerve, and the *tympanic membrane* is the eardrum. The *cornea*, on the other hand, is the transparent covering over the front of the lens of the eye.

50. **The correct answer is (B).** Human activities (e.g., agricultural and industrial) generally destroy food and alter physical conditions required to complete the life cycle in some species. The overall effect is a reduction in the total number of species that occupy a habitat.

51. **The correct answer is (D).** Acidity is determined by the concentration of hydrogen ion H^+s per unit of volume. Strong bases allow fewer H^+s to escape in aqueous solution than weak bases, producing weaker acids (e.g., Cl^- is a weak base, making HCl and strong acid, whereas HCO_3 is a strong base, making H_2CO_3 a weak acid).

52. **The correct answer is (B).** The arrows directed to the right in chemical equations represent products generated from the forward reaction, and those directed to the left represent reactants produced by the reverse reaction. The arrow length symbolizes the concentration of the substances on both sides of the equation.

53. **The correct answer is (A).** In humans and other animals, it is normal for an individual to have two copies of each type of chromosome in the nucleus of any body cell, except an egg or a sperm. There are 23 different types of chromosomes in humans; therefore, the normal complement of chromosomes in human cells is 46. Individuals with Down's syndrome receive an extra copy of chromosome 21 from one of their parents. They have three copies of chromosome 21 and a total of 47 chromosomes in the nuclei of their cells.

54. **The correct answer is (B).** In cellular metabolism, glycolysis is an anaerobic process (requires no O_2), produces reduced nicotinamide adeninedinucleotide ($NADH_2$) and small amounts of ATP, and occurs in all types of cells.

55. **The correct answer is (C).** Osmosis is the movement of water across cell membranes from solutions of low solute concentration to solutions with higher concentrations of solute. The salt gives the water a higher solute concentration than the frog's intracellular fluids. Therefore, the water concentration inside the cells would decrease as water flowed to the outside.

56. **The correct answer is (C).** The air (atmosphere) around the earth exerts a normal pressure of 760 mmHg (1.0 atmosphere). The pressure in interplanetary space is zero (a vacuum). Since the pressure inside the astronaut's blood vessels is greater than zero, the vessels would push outward.

57. **The correct answer is (D).** All of these viruses have been associated with cancer: adenoviruses (respiratory tract tumors), retroviruses (leukemia and AIDS), and papovaviruses (cervical cancer).

58. **The correct answer is (A).** Cereals (grains) are rich in certain members of the vitamin B complex; because of the starchy endosperm in seeds, cereals also are high in carbohydrates.

59. **The correct answer is (B).** Labels on canned goods may include a variety of information about the product, but the net contents by weight or volume and the quality should always be included. The number of portions may vary per net contents, according to the nature of the product, so knowledge of the number of servings is useful information. Other information may also be included on the label.

60. **The correct answer is (A).** Caloric needs vary with age as well as with physiological state, activity, and the size of the individual. Both physical and mental growth and development are more rapid during infancy and early childhood than at any other time in one's life. Therefore, more food is needed in proportion to size to provide the needed calories of energy and to provide the materials for growth. A proper diet is essential for normal development.

61. **The correct answer is (B).** Genes shown to cause cancerous growths are called oncogenes.

62. **The correct answer is (C).** Many individuals believe that the use of tissues from aborted fetuses is ethically unacceptable.

63. **The correct answer is (A).** The AIDS virus uses its surface glycoproteins to bind to membrane receptors of host cells, initiating the infection by infusing viral RNA into the host cell.

64. **The correct answer is (D).** The AIDS virus uses an enzyme—reverse transcriptase—as the normal pattern of synthesis (using DNA as a template to produce RNA) to a reverse method (using RNA as a template to form DNA).

65. **The correct answer is (B).** The inability to pass Cl^- to the outside of cells in cystic fibrosis patients causes water to enter the cells by osmosis, making the intercellular mucus thicker than normal.

66. **The correct answer is (A).** Cell membranes maintain their high external Na^+ and high internal K^+ concentrations by using ATP to energize membrane carrier proteins that form the sodium-potassium pump. This is an active transport mechanism, which moves both ions against concentration gradients.

67. **The correct answer is (D).** The general procedure for cloning includes: isolating DNA plasmid from a bacterium, isolating the DNA comprising the gene of interest from a different cell type, mixing the gene of interest with the plasmid to form a hybrid type of DNA called recombinant DNA, infecting a vector (bacteria or virus) with the recombinant DNA, and culturing the vector (containing the recombinant DNA) to produce many identical copies of itself (clones).

68. **The correct answer is (C).** Plasmids—small, circular self-duplicating DNA molecules isolated from bacteria—are major requirements for recombinant DNA technology.

69. **The correct answer is (A).** The restriction enzymes recognize and fragment the DNA (at the proper location) of the genes to be cloned.

70. **The correct answer is (B).** The splicing of DNA from two different sources is accomplished by the enzyme, DNA ligase, which catalyzes bonding by the complementarity of base pairing.

READING COMPREHENSION

ANSWER SHEET

TEST 1

1. Ⓐ Ⓑ Ⓒ Ⓓ
2. Ⓐ Ⓑ Ⓒ Ⓓ
3. Ⓐ Ⓑ Ⓒ Ⓓ
4. Ⓐ Ⓑ Ⓒ Ⓓ
5. Ⓐ Ⓑ Ⓒ Ⓓ

TEST 2

1. Ⓐ Ⓑ Ⓒ Ⓓ
2. Ⓐ Ⓑ Ⓒ Ⓓ
3. Ⓐ Ⓑ Ⓒ Ⓓ
4. Ⓐ Ⓑ Ⓒ Ⓓ
5. Ⓐ Ⓑ Ⓒ Ⓓ
6. Ⓐ Ⓑ Ⓒ Ⓓ

TEST 3

1. Ⓐ Ⓑ Ⓒ Ⓓ
2. Ⓐ Ⓑ Ⓒ Ⓓ
3. Ⓐ Ⓑ Ⓒ Ⓓ
4. Ⓐ Ⓑ Ⓒ Ⓓ
5. Ⓐ Ⓑ Ⓒ Ⓓ
6. Ⓐ Ⓑ Ⓒ Ⓓ

TEST 4

1. Ⓐ Ⓑ Ⓒ Ⓓ
2. Ⓐ Ⓑ Ⓒ Ⓓ
3. Ⓐ Ⓑ Ⓒ Ⓓ
4. Ⓐ Ⓑ Ⓒ Ⓓ
5. Ⓐ Ⓑ Ⓒ Ⓓ

TEST 5

1. Ⓐ Ⓑ Ⓒ Ⓓ
2. Ⓐ Ⓑ Ⓒ Ⓓ
3. Ⓐ Ⓑ Ⓒ Ⓓ
4. Ⓐ Ⓑ Ⓒ Ⓓ
5. Ⓐ Ⓑ Ⓒ Ⓓ

TEST 1

5 QUESTIONS ▬ TIME—8 MINUTES

Please review Unit 4, Reading Comprehension, before completing this section.

Directions: Following the passage below, you will find a number of incomplete statements about the passage. Select the word or expression that most satisfactorily completes each statement. Fill in the corresponding space on your answer sheet.

How can we know that the birds we see in the South in the winter are the same ones that come north in the spring? John J. Audubon, a bird lover, wondered about this. Every year he watched a pair of little phoebes nesting in the same place. He wondered if they were the same birds and so decided to put tiny silver bands on their legs. The next spring, back came the birds with the bands to build their nests on the walls of farm buildings in the neighborhood. The phoebe, it was learned, wintered wherever it was warm enough to find flies. In summer, phoebes could be seen from Georgia to Canada; in winter, anywhere from Georgia to Florida and Mexico. The phoebe was the first kind of bird to be banded, and Mr. Audubon was the first birdbander. Today there are thousands of birdbanders all over America, people who band all kinds of birds.

The government of the United States has a special birdbanding department that makes all the birdbands. The bands do not hurt the birds because they are made of aluminum and are very light. They come in different sizes for different-sized birds. Each band has a special number and the words, "Notify Fish and Wildlife Service, Washington, DC." Anyone who finds a dead bird with a band on one of its legs is asked to send the band to Washington with a note telling where and when the bird was found. In this way naturalists add to their knowledge of the habits and needs of birds.

1. The title below that best expresses the main theme or subject of this selection is
   - **(A)** "The Migration of Birds."
   - **(B)** "The Work of John Audubon."
   - **(C)** "The Habits and Needs of Birds."
   - **(D)** "Studying Bird Life Through Birdbanding."

2. According to the selection, Audubon proved his theory that
   - **(A)** birds prefer a diet of flies.
   - **(B)** birds return to the same nesting place each spring.
   - **(C)** silver is the best material for birdbands.
   - **(D)** phoebes are the most interesting birds to study.

3. Audubon's purpose in banding the phoebes was to
   - **(A)** satisfy his curiosity.
   - **(B)** notify the government.
   - **(C)** start a birdbanding department.
   - **(D)** gain fame as the first birdbander.

4. The migration habits of phoebes depend upon
   (A) nesting places.
   (B) the help of bird lovers.
   (C) the available food supply.
   (D) the number of young birds.

5. Which statement is true according to the selection?
   (A) Residents of Georgia may expect to see phoebes all year long.
   (B) The weight of a band causes a bird considerable discomfort.
   (C) The government offers a reward for information about dead birds.
   (D) Phoebes are more plentiful in the East than any other kind of bird.

STOP If you finish before time is called, you may check your work on this section only. Do not turn to any other section in the test.

TEST 2

6 QUESTIONS ■□ TIME—10 MINUTES

Directions: Following the passage below, you will find a number of incomplete statements about the passage. Select the word or expression that most satisfactorily completes each statement. Fill in the corresponding space on your answer sheet.

It is important to understand just what we mean when we talk about stress, and theoretical definitions of stress abound. Probably the best definition was offered by the renowned stress researcher Hans Selye, who summarized stress as ". . . any bodily change produced as a response to a perceived demand being placed upon the individual." This definition highlights the notion that there are two important facets to stress: the psychological (or menial) and the physiological (or physical).

Stress can be typically negative events, called "distress," as well as the more positive happenings in life that nonetheless demand change and adjustment. After a demand is perceived, bodily or physical changes occur as a reaction. These biological responses typically include increased heart rate, respiration rate, blood pressure, and muscular tension, shallow (rather than deep) breathing, and the increased release of certain so-called stress hormones such as adrenaline and cortisol.

Such bodily changes occur for what is commonly known as the "fight-or-flight" response. The fight-or-flight response served a purpose ages ago, when acute, sudden stressors such as animal predators immediately threatened a person's existence. Successfully fighting off or fleeing from the threat greatly increased one's chance of survival. And, as with other creatures, our fight-or-flight stress reaction became "wired in" as a protective mechanism.

Stress continues to serve us today, as mild to moderate levels of stress can sharpen our alertness and motivate positive growth, spur the need to accept challenges, and promote change in our lives. Stress becomes a problem only when you consider the nature of some of our stressors. Unlike the saber-tooth tigers of long age, today's stressors tend to be more chronic in nature. Most people struggle with the demands of health problems, interpersonal difficulties, financial worries, and negative or critical self-imaging, to name just a few.

These concerns have a propensity to stick around. When you begin to experience any one of them, your body reacts with predictable changes. However, because these stressors usually stay around and dominate parts of our existence for long stretches of time, the bodily changes that get "turned on," stay "turned on," which can cause or influence numerous undesirable consequences.

Chronic stress can contribute to such physical problems as migraine headaches, lower back pain, ulcers, digestive disorders, TMJ (temporomandibular joint) syndrome, suppressed immunity, and, of particular concern to people with diabetes, difficulty controlling blood sugar. There is even some evidence that cardiovascular disease, high blood pressure, and certain types of cancer can be adversely affected by stress. Chronic stress also appears to contribute to many psychological and behavioral disorders such as depression anxiety disorders, and low self-esteem.

Everyone attempts to cope with the stress in their lives, whether they do so consciously and deliberately or not. Unfortunately, many of the strategies people use to deal with stress actually produce additional sources of stress. Overeating, excessive alcohol consumption, cigarette smoking, and drug use are examples of stress management attempts gone awry.

Any effective strategy of stress management needs to do more than just distract you from that which is causing the stress. It needs to address both the physical and the psychological aspects of stress. To efficiently deal with stress, you must first get to know yourself and observe how stress tends to affect you, both physically and psychologically.

—*"Women and Diabetes:*
Strategies for Handling Stress"
Reprinted with permission from
Diabetes Self-Management
Copyright © 1997 R.A. Rapaport Publishing, Inc.

1. According to Hans Selye, stress is stimulated by a(n)

   (A) environmental change.
   (B) bodily change.
   (C) perceived demand.
   (D) physiological and psychological conflict.

2. The physiological symptoms of stress are a result of

   (A) secretion of adrenalin and cortisol.
   (B) suppression of adrenaline.
   (C) accumulation of cortisol.
   (D) absence of adrenaline and cortisol.

3. The main problem presented by stress in diabetics is that the

   (A) blood sugar rises.
   (B) blood pressure drops.
   (C) immune system is suppressed.
   (D) stomach develops ulcers.

4. The theoretical basis for the effects of stress is based on the

   (A) interaction of the physiological and psychological self.
   (B) interaction of the self with the environment.
   (C) relationship between change and coping.
   (D) relationship between change and growth.

5. An effective method of coping with stress would be

   (A) focusing on the pleasure of eating.
   (B) inducing relaxation by drinking alcoholic beverages.
   (C) delaying stopping smoking.
   (D) adapting to change.

6. According to this passage,

   (A) stress causes cancer.
   (B) stress can be controlled.
   (C) all stress is harmful.
   (D) all stress is continuous.

STOP   If you finish before time is called, you may check your work on this section only. Do not turn to any other section in the test.

TEST 3

6 QUESTIONS ▪▭ TIME—10 MINUTES

Directions: Following the passage below, you will find a number of incomplete statements about the passage. Select the word or expression that most satisfactorily completes each statement. Fill in the corresponding space on your answer sheet.

Since 1910, more American women have died of heart disease than of any other cause. But for most of this century, physicians and researchers treated heart disease almost exclusively as a man's problem. When the American Heart Association held its first public conference for women in 1964, it focused on how women could help protect their *husbands'* hearts.

How could doctors and scientists overlook such a clear threat to women's health for so long?

For many years, heart-disease researchers concerned themselves primarily with *premature* heart attacks—heart attacks that strike down the young or middle-aged rather than the elderly. When women get heart disease, however, they tend to develop it 10 to 15 years later than men; thus, they are more likely to have heart attacks when they are past middle age.

For much of their lives, the sex hormone estrogen offers women substantial protection from heart disease. Only around age 55 does the rate of heart disease in women start to climb, both because estrogen levels drop after menopause and because other risk factors for heart disease become more common at the same age.

The age difference makes heart disease appear a more dramatic problem in men than in women; it's somehow more shocking when a heart attack hits a 50-year-old than when a 65-year-old is the victim. Indeed, the fact that men develop heart disease earlier than women means the disease may have a greater impact on their lives, and offers some justification for putting a greater emphasis on studying heart disease in men than in women. But until recently, researchers have done much more than that: They have systematically and almost completely excluded women from studies of all aspects of coronary heart disease.

One major heart-disease study did include women in virtually equal numbers with men, but the data were misinterpreted in a way that actually added to the confusion over women's risks. The Framingham Heart Study has been following more than 5,000 men and women since 1948 to chart the causes and course of heart disease. Among other factors, the researchers identified people with chest pain, and assumed that they were suffering from angina, a symptom indicating that narrowed coronary arteries are supplying inadequate amounts of oxygen to the heart muscle.

Angina often precedes a heart attack. But in the mid-1950s, the Framingham researchers found that men with chest pain were much more likely than women with chest pain to have a heart attack within five years. They concluded that heart disease was simply not much of a threat to women.

There are two problem with that conclusion. First, many women with chest pain turn out not to have angina at all. A major study published in 1982 revealed that fully half of all women with chest pain who underwent coronary angiography—an X-ray procedure for visualizing the arteries of the heart—did not have blockages. (The same was true of only 17 percent of the men.) And second, in the 1950s most of Framingham's women were still too young to be at high risk for heart attack. A later analysis of the Framingham data showed that heart disease in women develops more gradually than in men. Women are more likely to experience angina for an extended period of time before suffering a heart attack.

Clinical trials—studies that test the effects of different treatments on a disease, rather than simply trying to understand the factors that lead to illness—have also tended to exclude women. Investigators have traditionally steered clear of testing any new treatments on women of childbearing age to avoid the confounding effects their hormonal cycles might have on test results, and to avoid unwittingly exposing a fetus by giving a drug to a woman who doesn't yet know she is pregnant. Many researchers have also excluded people over age 65, the age when women have the greatest heart-disease risk, out of concern that other illnesses in these older people would muddy the data. In clinical trials conducted over the past 30 years to evaluate treatments for heart attack, fewer than 20 percent of the total 151,000 subjects were women, according to a recent analysis in the *Journal of the American Medical Association*.

As a result, physicians have proceeded on the assumption that a treatment tested in men will work about equally well in women. Not necessarily. It is now clear, for instance, that the drug propranolol (*Inderal*), a beta-blocker commonly prescribed for high blood pressure and angina, is broken down far more slowly in women's bodies—an important consideration for dosage. Moreover, the potential of estrogen treatment to prevent heart disease in postmenopausal women is only now being tested in large clinical trials.

In 1985, the U.S. Public Health Service Task Force on Women's Health Issues ordered the National Institutes of Health to include more women in research, particularly research on heart disease. After several years of foot-dragging, the NIH established an office to ensure that women are appropriately represented in NIH-funded studies. Several large-scale clinical trials including women are now in the planning stage or underway. The clinical trial portion of the Women's Health Initiative—a $600 million, 14-year effort—will study the effects of a low-fat diet and hormonal therapy in preventing cardiovascular disease (as well as cancer and osteoporosis). It may be many years, however, before the decades of neglect are overcome.

—*"Heart Disease: Women at Risk"*
Copyright © 1993 by Consumers Union of U.S., Inc.,
Yonkers, NY 10703-1057
Reprinted by permission from
Consumer Reports, May 1993

1. The theory that estrogen protects women heart disease is supported by the fact that
   (A) the rate of heart disease in women drops after age 55.
   (B) the rate of heart disease in women increases after age 55.
   (C) the incidence of heart disease in women is far less than in men.
   (D) only post-menopausal women have heart disease.

2. Physicians and researchers have placed emphasis on heart disease in men more than in women because
   (A) men develop heart disease earlier than women.
   (B) more men die from heart disease than women.
   (C) men are more prone to heart disease than women.
   (D) men respond to treatment more readily than women.

3. When comparing the occurrence of angina in men and women,
   (A) angina often proceeds a heart attack in men.
   (B) angina usually proceeds a heart attack in both men and women.
   (C) the occurrence is more frequent in females.
   (D) the occurrence is less frequent in males.

4. The age when women are at greatest risk for heart disease is
   (A) 45–50
   (B) 50–55
   (C) 65–70
   (D) 70–75

GO ON TO THE NEXT PAGE

5. It is important to conduct clinical research on both men and women because

   (A) preventative techniques are the same for both men and women.

   (B) age differences in occurrence of heart disease indicate differences in causes.

   (C) physiological differences lead to differences in responses to treatment.

   (D) the impact of heart disease on an individual's life is the same for men and women.

6. The focus of the NIH clinical trials for Women's Health Initiative is to study the

   (A) relationship between the aging process and the occurrence of heart disease.

   (B) factors that lead to high risk for heart disease.

   (C) female responses to drugs used to treat heart disease.

   (D) effects of diet and hormonal therapy on prevention of heart disease.

STOP   If you finish before time is called, you may check your work on this section only. Do not turn to any other section in the test.

TEST 4

5 QUESTIONS ▬ TIME—8 MINUTES

Directions: Following the passage below, you will find a number of incomplete statements about the passage. Select the word or expression that most satisfactorily completes each statement. Fill in the corresponding space on your answer sheet.

Can creativity evolve with aging—maybe even flower with aging? If you belong to the "can't teach an old dog new tricks" school of thought, you may think that unless you have been an artist or writer or musician your whole life you are unlikely to be one in midlife—that increased creativity isn't compatible with growing old.

But research into fields as varied as neurology, behavioral science and art history says otherwise. So do the thousands of people who are finding that different types of creativity can accompany aging.

There is the artistic creativity of people like Bill Traylor, a folk art painter who did not pick up a paintbrush until he was 85 years old.

There is the exhilaration of the 81-year-old whose late-life burst of creativity led to her discovery of literature, a discovery she felt changed her life.

Then there is social creativity, a deftness with interpersonal relationships, that older people, the keepers of the culture, have traditionally offered.

The point is not that every older person can or should be a Picasso, but that aging precludes neither productivity nor creative energy. Moreover, creative capacity after age 65 is considerably more common than most people realize.

Creativity at older ages is not just a matter of anecdote; science has shown that the potential for intellectual growth with aging has biological underpinnings. Studies of the brain show that, in response to a more stimulating or challenging environment, brain cells sprout new extensions, improving their communication with other brain cells.

The same studies, along with behavioral research, indicate that brain cells respond to mental exercise just as muscle cells respond to physical exercise. Science, in short, supports the maxim "use it or lose it" when it comes to the aging brain.

There are several ways of categorizing the creative impulses of older persons:

- creativity that continues with aging;
- creativity that commences with aging;
- creativity that changes with aging;
- creativity in response to late-life loss.

There are famous examples of older people exuding creativity throughout their lives—Picasso experimenting with new styles of painting in his 90s, Verdi composing new operas in his 80s, George Bernard Shaw writing new plays in his 90s.

—*"Contemplating Creativity"*
by Dr. Gene Cohen
Reprinted with permission from
AARP Bulletin, April 1997
Copyright © 1997 by AARP

1. According to this passage, the relationship between aging and creativity can be
   (A) direct.
   (B) indirect.
   (C) mutually exclusive.
   (D) unpredictable.

2. Bill Traylor is an example of which one of the following types of creativity?
   (A) Composing music
   (B) Social creativity
   (C) Literature discovery
   (D) Folk art painting

GO ON TO THE NEXT PAGE

3. A theoretical basis for creativity at older ages is that
   (A) intercommunication among brain cells expands in response to physical exercise.
   (B) intercommunication among brain cells expands in response to stimulating environments.
   (C) intellectual growth increases in the aging brain.
   (D) intellectual growth decreases in the aging brain.

4. According to this passage, one would expect to see more creativity in the aged when the person
   (A) is a bus driver.
   (B) works with embroidery.
   (C) is a teacher.
   (D) is a bird-watcher.

5. Which one of the following statements is true?
   (A) All aged people are creative.
   (B) Only people who have been creative in younger life can be creative in older life.
   (C) The first sign of creativity may occur in older life.
   (D) Only one type of creativity is seen in aged people.

STOP If you finish before time is called, you may check your work on this section only. Do not turn to any other section in the test.

TEST 5

5 QUESTIONS ▪▫ TIME—9 MINUTES

Directions: Following the passage below, you will find a number of incomplete statements about the passage. Select the word or expression that most satisfactorily completes each statement. Fill in the corresponding space on your answer sheet.

A nearby flow of water is a very convenient place to dispose of waste materials, and people have been doing this for many years. If the right chemicals are dumped into the water, it can be beneficial. Lakes tend to follow a course from being deep, clear, nutrient-poor lakes to becoming shallow and more productive nutrient-rich lakes. This is the natural course of most lakes, and the addition of chemicals such as phosphates and nitrates can actually accelerate this process. To a certain extent, this is beneficial, and it has been done intentionally in some cases: but when carried to extremes, it can lead to a man-made natural disaster. The water produces so much algae that most other forms of life cannot exist, and the lake chokes to death. In most cases, factories and sewage drains have carried this addition of chemicals too far.

Another consequence of dumping waste material into waterways, especially lakes, occurs when the waste contains metals, such as copper. Some metals literally cover the lake bottom and kill off all the bottom-dwelling organisms. Since many of these organisms are responsible for the decomposition of organic material on the bottom, the removal of these animals results in a great deal of the organic material remaining undecomposed, decreasing the nutrient content of the environment.

The dumping of waste materials from combustion into the air is quite obvious every time you look at the skyline of any major industrial area: Dumping poisonous materials into the environment has resulted in the destruction of many of our oxygen-producing plants and has driven many animals from our immediate environment. Another result that strikes perhaps closer to home is the increase in lung disease attributed to air pollution. Moreover, the propellants from aerosol cans cause problems by deteriorating the ozone layer of the atmosphere. This depletion allows greater amounts of ultraviolet radiation to reach the surface of the earth. This higher level of radiation reputedly causes an increase in skin cancer.

Both air and water pollution are a retaliation by nature to human abuse. We assume that the dumping of wastes into the environment is a one-way process, and we do not count on any repercussions. But the cost of dumping garbage into the environment is slowly coming back to haunt us. Whether it be by the return of mercury and DDT to us in our food, or the destruction of shields in the atmosphere that protect us from being burned by the sun's radiation, we will pay for our assaults on the environment.

1. The title that best expresses the main idea of this section is

   (A) "Save Our Lakes."
   (B) "Man's Responsibility Toward Nature."
   (C) "Air Pollution."
   (D) "How Pollution Causes Cancer."

2. According to this passage, one of the negative results of dumping waste chemicals into lakes is the

   (A) increased growth of algae, which kills other organisms.
   (B) discoloration of water.
   (C) limitation of recreational activities.
   (D) increased temperature in the water.

3. Two causes of air pollution are
   (A) smoke and copper.
   (B) aerosol cans and recycling of waste materials.
   (C) decomposition of organisms and deoxygenation of plants.
   (D) dumping of waste materials and use of aerosol cans.

4. The author's attitude toward environmental protection is
   (A) complacency.
   (B) pro-conservation.
   (C) indifference.
   (D) apathetic.

5. The author's reference to the driving of animals from our immediate environment implies
   (A) migration.
   (B) extinction.
   (C) destruction.
   (D) poaching.

STOP   If you finish before time is called, you may check your work on this section only. Do not turn to any other section in the test.

ANSWER KEY

TEST 1

1. D	2. B	3. A	4. C	5. A

TEST 2

1. C	2. A	3. A	4. A	5. D	6. B

TEST 3

1. B	2. A	3. A	4. C	5. C	6. D

TEST 4

1. A	2. D	3. B	4. C	5. C

TEST 5

1. B	2. A	3. D	4. B	5. A

NOTES

NOTES

NOTES

NOTES

NOTES

NOTES

NOTES

NOTES

NOTES

NOTES

NOTES

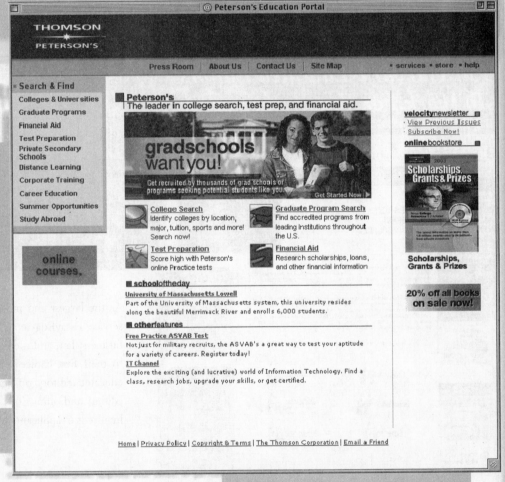